Atlas of single-port, la~
and robo*i~ ~~   ~ ~

Atlas of Single-Port, Laparoscopic, and Robotic Surgery

Pedro F. Escobar • Tommaso Falcone
Editors

Atlas of Single-Port, Laparoscopic, and Robotic Surgery

A Practical Approach in Gynecology

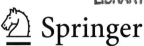 Springer

Editors
Pedro F. Escobar, MD
Director of Gynecologic Oncology
Instituto Gyneco-Oncológico
Hospital HIMA-Oncologico
Caguas, PR
USA

Clinical Associate Professor of Surgery
Cleveland Clinic Lerner
College of Medicine
Cleveland, OH
USA

Tommaso Falcone, MD, FRCSC
FACOG
Department of Obstetrics
and Gynecology
Women's Health Institute
Cleveland Clinic
Cleveland, OH
USA

ISBN 978-1-4614-6839-4   ISBN 978-1-4614-6840-0   (eBook)
DOI 10.1007/978-1-4614-6840-0
Springer New York Heidelberg Dordrecht London

Library of Congress Control Number: 2014940544

Printed on acid-free paper

Springer is part of Springer Science+Business Media (www.springer.com)

Preface

Over the years, minimally invasive surgery, namely operative laparoscopy, has emerged as the standard treatment for many gynecologic conditions. Innovations in minimally invasive surgical technology—such as multichannel ports, articulating instruments, and flexible high-definition endoscopes—have allowed laparoscopic surgeons to perform increasingly complex surgeries through smaller incisions utilizing robotic and single-site technology. The collaborative efforts that we, the editors, have had together from novel surgical instrumentation development and working together on multiple national and international events have resulted in this surgical atlas.

We are honored to have a group of world experts in conventional laparoscopic, robotic, and single-site gynecologic surgery contribute to our surgical atlas. This atlas is unique in that it includes illustrative pictures, drawings, and images that cover all contemporary minimally invasive techniques in gynecology.

Caguas, PR, USA   Pedro F. Escobar, MD
Cleveland, OH, USA   Tommaso Falcone, MD, FRCSC, FACOG

Acknowledgment

Allison Siegel, for her immense contribution to the editing of the book.

Contents

Contributors

Mauricio S. Abrao, MD Department of Obstetrics and Gynecology, University of São Paulo, São Paulo, SP, Brazil

Arnold P. Advincula, MD, FACOG, FACS Department of Obstetrics and Gynecology, Columbia Presbyterian Hospital, New York, NY, USA

Mohamed A. Bedaiwy, MD, PhD Department of Obstetrics and Gynaecology, The University of British Columbia, Vancouver, BC, Canada

Fariba Behnia-Willison Department of Obstetrics, Gynecology, and Reproductive Medicine, Flinders Medical Centre, Flinders University, Adelaide, SA, Australia

Elizabeth Buescher, MD, MEd Department of OBGYN, Center for Special Minimally Invasive and Robotic Surgery, Stanford University Medical Center, Palo Alto, CA, USA

Luiz Fernando Pina Carvalho Department of Obstetrics and Gynecology, University of São Paulo, São Paulo, SP, Brazil

Leticia Cox, MD Department of Obstetrics and Gynecology, University Hospitals Case Medical Center, Case Western Reserve University, Cleveland, OH, USA

Teresa P. Díaz-Montes, MD, MPH The Gynecology Oncology Center, Mercy Medical Center, Baltimore, MD, USA

Pedro F. Escobar, MD Director of Gynecologic Oncology, Instituto Gyneco-Oncológico, Hospital HIMA-Oncologico, Caguas, PR, USA

Clinical Associate Professor of Surgery, Cleveland Clinic Lerner College of Medicine, Cleveland, OH, USA

Anna Fagotti, MD Division of Minimally Invasive Gynecologic Surgery, St. Maria Hospital, University of Perugia, Terni, Italy

Tommaso Falcone, MD, FRCSC, FACOG Department of Obstetrics and Gynecology, Women's Health Institute, Cleveland Clinic, Cleveland, OH, USA

Francesco Fanfani Department of Obstetrics and Gynecology, Catholic University of the Sacred Heart, Rome, Italy

Rebecca Flyckt, MD Department of Obstetrics and Gynecology, Cleveland Clinic, Cleveland, OH, USA

Michael Frumovitz, MD, MPH Department of Gynecologic Oncology, Unit 1362, M. D. Anderson Cancer Center, Houston, TX, USA

Anirudha Garg, MD Department of Obstetrics, Gynecology, and Reproductive Medicine, Flinders Medical Centre, Flinders University, Adelaide, Australia

M. Brigid Holloran-Schwartz, MD Department of Obstetrics, Gynecology, and Women's Health, St. Louis University, St. Louis, MO, USA

Jason A. Knight, MD Women's Health Institute, Section of Gynecologic Oncology, Cleveland Clinic, Cleveland, OH, USA

Javier F. Magrina, MD Department of Gynecology, Division of Gynecologic Oncology, Mayo Clinic in Arizona, Phoenix, AZ, USA

Jillian Main, MD Department of OBGYN, Center for Special Minimally Invasive and Robotic Surgery, Stanford University Medical Center, Palo Alto, CA, USA

Chad M. Michener, MD Department of Obstetrics and Gynecology, Women's Health Institute, Cleveland Clinic, Cleveland, OH, USA

Magdy Milad, MD, MS Department of Obstetrics and Gynecology, Northwestern University Feinberg School of Medicine, Chicago, IL, USA

Anjana R. Nair, MD Department of Obstetrics and Gynecology, Carolinas HealthCare System, Charlotte, NC, USA

Camran Nezhat, MD Department of OBGYN, Center for Special Minimally Invasive and Robotic Surgery, Stanford University Medical Center, Palo Alto, CA, USA

Amanda Nickles Fader, MD Department of Gynecology and Obstetrics, Johns Hopkins Hospital, Baltimore, MD, USA

Mona Orady Department of Obstetrics, Gynecology, Women's Health Institute, Cleveland Clinic, Cleveland, OH, USA

Marie Fidela Paraiso, MD Department of Obstetrics and Gynecology, Women's Health Institute, Cleveland Clinic, Cleveland, OH, USA

Elizabeth W. Patton, MD, MPhil Department of Obstetrics and Gynecology, University of Michigan, Ann Arbor, MI, USA

Michael C. Pitter, MD, FACOG Department of Minimally Invasive & Gynecologic Robotic Surgery, Newark Beth Israel Medical Center, Newark, NJ, USA

Beri Ridgeway, MD Department of Obstetrics, Gynecology, Women's Health Institute, Cleveland Clinic, Cleveland, OH, USA

Rebecca Rossener Department of Obstetrics and Gynecology, University of São Paulo, São Paulo, SP, Brazil

Cristiano Rossitto Department of Obstetrics and Gynecology, Catholic University of the Sacred Heart, Rome, Italy

Juan Luis Salgado, MD Department of Obstetrics and Gynecology, Universidad Central Caribe School of Medicine, Bayamon, PR, USA

Jesus Manuel Salgueiro Bravo Attending Physician, HIMA San Pablo Oncologico, Caguas, PR, USA

Giovanni Scambia Department of Obstetrics and Gynecology, Catholic University of the Sacred Heart, Rome, Italy

Stacey A. Scheib, MD Department of Gynecology and Obstetrics, Johns Hopkins Hospital, Baltimore, MD, USA

Rose Soliemannjad Department of OBGYN, Center for Special Minimally Invasive and Robotic Surgery, Stanford University Medical Center, Palo Alto, CA, USA

Kevin J.E. Stepp, MD Department of Obstetrics and Gynecology, Carolinas HealthCare System, Charlotte, NC, USA

Amanda Stevens, MD Department of OBGYN, Center for Special Minimally Invasive and Robotic Surgery, Stanford University Medical Center, Palo Alto, CA, USA

Edward J. Tanner, MD Department of Gynecology and Obstetrics, The Kelly Gynecologic Oncology Service, Johns Hopkins Hospital, Baltimore, MD, USA

Megan E. Tarr, MD, MS Department of Obstetrics and Gynecology, Women's Health Institute, Cleveland Clinic, Cleveland, OH, USA

Jill H. Tseng, MD Department of Gynecology and Obstetrics, Johns Hopkins Hospital, Baltimore, MD, USA

Cecile A. Unger, MD, MPH Division of Female Pelvic Medicine and Reconstructive Surgery, Department of Obstetrics and Gynecology, Cleveland Clinic, Cleveland, OH, USA

Mary Jean Uy-Kroh, MD Department of Obstetrics and Gynecology, Cleveland Clinic, Cleveland, OH, USA

Jessica R. Woessner, MD Women's Health Institute, Cleveland Clinic, Cleveland, OH, USA

Patrick P. Yeung Jr, MD Department of Obstetrics, Gynecology, and Women's Health, St. Louis University, St. Louis, MO, USA

Stephen E. Zimberg, MD, MSHA Department of Gynecology, Women's Health Institute, Cleveland Clinic Florida, Fort Lauderdale, FL, USA

Part I

Conventional Laparoscopy

Basic Principles and Anatomy for the Laparoscopic Surgeon

M. Jean Uy-Kroh and Tommaso Falcone

As we push open the barriers of minimally invasive surgery and incorporate new platforms, the gynecologic surgeon must utilize steadfast surgical and anatomic principles to optimize outcomes and reduce complications. In this chapter, we review laparoscopic principles and practical anatomy that allow one to safely operate in even the most challenging surgical landscapes. There is an emphasis on clearly labeled anatomy and illustration of critical anatomic relationships. We include a thorough discussion and demonstration of the anterior abdominal wall, vasculature, and innervations of the abdomen and pelvis, peritoneal landmarks, pelvic viscera, and the pelvic diaphragm.

The common objective of single-port, laparoscopic, and robotic gynecologic surgery is to treat conditions using techniques that safely maximize operative exposure and minimize patient recovery time and pain. No matter what approach is used, the surgeon requires an intimate knowledge of abdominal and pelvic anatomy to achieve optimal outcomes and reduce complications. This chapter reviews basic principles and practical surgical anatomy encountered by the laparoscopic, gynecologic surgeon.

M.J. Uy-Kroh, MD, FACOG (✉)
T. Falcone, MD, FRCSC, FACOG
Department of Obstetrics and Gynecology,
Women's Health Institute, Cleveland Clinic,
9500 Euclid Avenue, A81,
Cleveland, OH 44195, USA
e-mail: falcont@ccf.org; uykrohm@ccf.org

P.F. Escobar, T. Falcone (eds.), *Atlas of Single-Port, Laparoscopic, and Robotic Surgery*,
DOI 10.1007/978-1-4614-6840-0_1, © Springer Science+Business Media New York 2014

1.1   Surface Landmarks

Surface anatomy and osseous structures are important markers for surgeons. Once identified, they can be used to avoid underlying vasculature and plan safe surgical points of entry. A surgeon should always begin with a brief survey of the supine patient. The osseous landmarks of the anterior abdominal wall are fixed (Table 1.1) and frame the clinical decisions that are made prior to surgery, such as port placement. The osseous landmarks include the xyphoid process, the inferior margins of the tenth costal cartilages, the anterior superior iliac spines (ASIS), and the pubic symphysis (Fig. 1.1).

The nonosseous landmarks are in variable relationship to each other and the bony landmarks. Their anatomic positions are influenced by patient habitus, skin laxity, and patient positioning (i.e., supine versus Trendelenburg).

The umbilicus is an important nonosseous landmark that is a common point of surgical entry. It has a variable position and is influenced by patient habitus. Owing to its relationship to the adjacent vasculature, the angle of trocar entry must be planned. The umbilicus lies in close proximity to the aorta and its bifurcation into the right and left common iliac arteries [1, 2]. While the patient is supine, the aortic bifurcation is located cephalad to the umbilicus in almost 90 % of patients. In contrast, when the patient is in the Trendelenburg position, the aortic bifurcation is located cephalad to the umbilicus in only 70 % of patients. When the bifurcation lies caudal to the

Table 1.1 Anterior landmarks and corresponding vertebral levels

Landmark	Vertebral level
Xyphoid process	T9
Tenth costal cartilage inferior margin	L2/L3
Umbilicus	Variable
Ideal body weight	Intervertebral disc between L3/L4
Anterior superior iliac spine (ASIS)	Sacral promontory
Inguinal ligament	
Pubic symphysis	

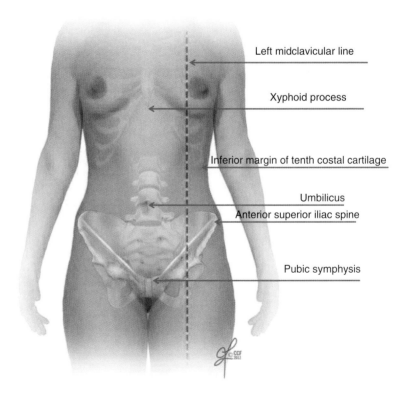

Fig. 1.1 Supine abdomen with osseus and nonosseus landmarks

Left midclavicular line

Xyphoid process

Inferior margin of tenth costal cartilage

Umbilicus

Anterior superior iliac spine

Pubic symphysis

umbilicus, the iliac vessels, in particular the left common iliac vein, are more susceptible to trocar injury. Patients are therefore usually placed in the supine position in order to minimize vessel injury during initial surgical entry at the umbilicus.

Furthermore, several studies have confirmed the effect of obesity on the position of the umbilicus, trocar angle, and distance to the retroperitoneal structures during initial umbilical entry. For patients of ideal body weight (body mass index [BMI] <25 kg/m^2), the umbilicus is often at the level of the intervertebral disc between the L3 and L4 vertebrae. For these patients, the trocar or Veress needle should be introduced at a 45-degree angle to protect the retroperitoneal vessels, since these vessels can be as close as 4 cm from the skin. In contrast, for obese patients a more vertical, almost 90-degree trocar entry is necessary to traverse the increased width of the abdominal wall (Fig. 1.2) [3].

The inguinal ligament, formed by the aponeurosis of the external oblique, marks the anatomic boundary between the abdomen and the thigh. The abdominal wall midline is the area between the xyphoid and the pubic symphysis. The left midclavicular line refers to a line drawn from the middle of the left clavicle to the middle of the left inguinal ligament.

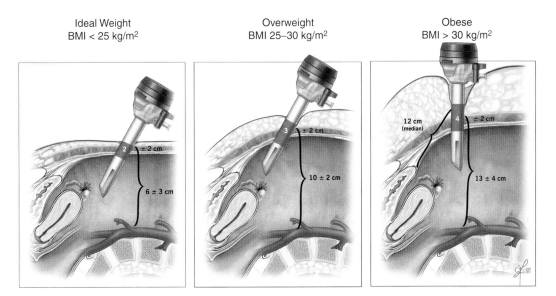

Fig. 1.2 The effect of increasing weight on anterior abdominal wall anatomy. These sagittal views illustrate that as a patient's body mass index increases, the distance from the base of the umbilicus to the peritoneum and the distance from the base of the umbilicus to retroperitoneal structures increase. To accommodate for these increased distances, the trocar angle must move from a 45-degree angle in an ideal weight patient to almost a 90-degree angle in an obese patient in order to traverse the abdominal wall. The purple trocar area denotes the distance from the base of the umbilicus to the peritoneum at a 45-degree angle in ideal and overweight patients. In the obese patient, this distance is measured at a 90-degree angle, to mimic the recommended trocar trajectory. Furthermore, if one were to utilize a standard 45-degree trocar for insertion in the obese patient, the median distance from the base of the umbilicus to the peritoneum is 12 cm (Adapted from Hurd et al. [3])

1.2 Anterior Abdominal Wall

The abdominal wall from superficial to deep includes skin, subcutaneous tissue/superficial fascia, rectus sheath and muscles, transversalis fascia, extraperitoneal fascia, and parietal peritoneum. Several important nerves and blood vessels course through these layers.

1.2.1 Subcutaneous Tissue

Camper's fascia is the superficial fatty layer and Scarpa's fascia is the deeper, thin fibrous layer; collectively they represent the "superficial fascia" or subcutaneous tissue. Superficial abdominal wall vessels course through the fascia. This tissue layer tends to be deceptively prominent in obese patients.

1.2.2 Muscles and Fascia

The abdominal wall is composed of five pairs of interconnected muscles. There are two midline muscles (the rectus abdominis and pyramidalis) and three sets of lateral muscles (the external and internal obliques and the transversus abdominis). In the midline, the rectus abdominis originates from the xiphoid process and costal cartilages of the fifth to seventh ribs and extends to the pubic symphysis. This broad strap muscle is encased within the anterior and posterior rectus sheath. The aponeuroses of the rectus muscles fuse in the midline as the linea alba and fuse laterally as the linea semilunares.

The pyramidalis muscle is a small triangular muscle that lies in the rectus sheath, anterior to the inferior aspect of the rectus abdominis. Occasionally this muscle is absent on one or both sides. When it is present, it arises from the pubis and inserts into the lower linea alba.

The three lateral muscles, found bilaterally, are also referred to as flat muscles. The most superficial of these is the external oblique. It arises from the lower eighth rib, where its fibers interdigitate with the serratus anterior muscle

and extend inferiorly to the linea alba and pubic tubercle, creating a broad fibrous swath known as an aponeurosis.

Aponeuroses are tendon-like membranes that bind muscles to each other or to bones. Posterior to the external oblique lies the internal oblique muscle, whose fibers arise from the lumbar fascia, the iliac crest, and the lateral two-thirds of the inguinal ligament. The internal oblique fibers are at right angles to the external oblique fibers. The anterior and posterior layers of the internal oblique separate into the anterior and posterior rectus sheath and are responsible for creating the arcuate line landmark. The deepest lateral muscle is the transversus abdominis. Its muscle fibers run in a transverse fashion across the abdomen. The fibers arise from the costal cartilages of the sixth to eighth ribs, interlocking with the diaphragm, the lumbodorsal fascia, the lateral third of the inguinal ligament, and from the anterior three-fourths of the iliac crest and terminate anteriorly as an aponeurosis. The transversalis fascia lies deep to the transversus abdominis and is a continuous layer that lines the abdominal and pelvic cavity (Fig. 1.3).

The arcuate line is a transverse line located midway between the umbilicus and the pubic symphysis. Above the arcuate line, the rectus abdominis muscles possess both anterior and posterior sheaths formed by the aponeuroses of the midline and lateral muscles. Below the arcuate line, all layers of the sheaths course anterior to the rectus abdominis muscles.

The extraperitoneal fascia is the layer of connective tissue that separates the transversalis fascia from the parietal peritoneum. It contains a varying amount of adipose tissue and lines the abdominal and pelvic cavities. Viscera in the extraperitoneal fascia are referred to as retroperitoneal. Last, the parietal peritoneum lines the abdominal cavity. Remarkably, it is only one cell layer thick. Inward reflections of this peritoneum form a double cell layer known as mesentery.

The inguinal ligament is formed by the aponeuroses of the external oblique. It arises from the ASIS and inserts into the pubic tubercle. The inguinal canal runs parallel to the inguinal ligament. The inguinal canal is classically described by its four walls. Its anterior wall is formed by the aponeurosis of the external

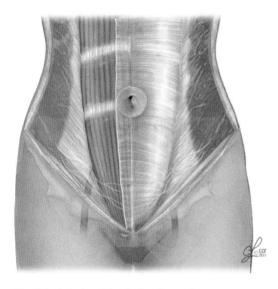

Fig. 1.3 Anterior abdominal wall muscles

oblique, the inferior wall (floor) is formed by the inguinal ligament, the superior wall (roof) is formed by arching fibers of the internal oblique and transversus abdominis muscles, and the posterior wall is formed by the transversalis fascia.

The deep internal inguinal ring is the tubular evagination of the transversalis fascia, located halfway between the ASIS and the pubic symphysis. The inferior epigastric vessels lie medial to the deep internal inguinal ring. The round ligament dives through this deep internal ring, enters the inguinal canal, exits through the superficial external inguinal ring, and terminates at the labia majora. In addition, the terminal aspect of the ilioinguinal nerve and the genital branch of the genitofemoral nerve exit the inguinal canal via the superficial external inguinal ring. The superficial external inguinal ring is created by the opening of the external oblique aponeurosis and is located superior and lateral to the pubic tubercle (Fig. 1.4).

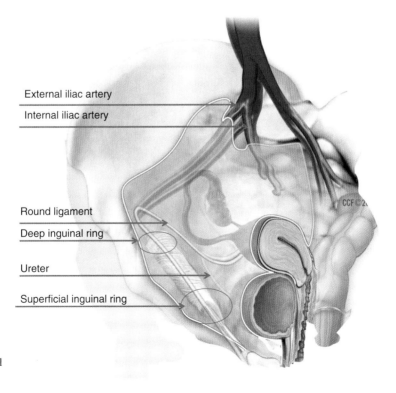

External iliac artery

Internal iliac artery

Round ligament

Deep inguinal ring

Ureter

Superficial inguinal ring

Fig. 1.4 The peritoneum drapes over the ureters, vital blood vessels, and large organs within the pelvis. The round ligament is seen entering the deep inguinal ring and exiting the superficial inguinal ring

1.2.3 Nerves

The clinically relevant upper and lower anterior abdominal wall nerves contain both motor and sensory fibers. The thoracoabdominal and subcostal nerves originate from T7 to T11 and T12, respectively. Their distributions are summarized in Table 1.2.

The iliohypogastric nerve and ilioinguinal nerve originate from L1 and accompany the thoracoabdominal and subcostal nerves as they course between the internal oblique and transversus abdominis muscles. At the ASIS, they traverse the internal oblique and run between the internal and external oblique muscles. The iliohypogastric nerves innervate the lateral abdominal wall, inferior to the umbilicus. The ilioinguinal nerve runs within the inguinal canal and emerges from the superficial, or external, inguinal ring to provide sensory innervation to the labia majora, inner thigh, and groin.

During laparoscopic and robotic surgery, the iliohypogastric and ilioinguinal nerves are particularly susceptible to injury because of their close proximity to traditional, lower quadrant trocar sites. Nerve damage may result from trocar placement or nerve entrapment secondary to lateral closure of transverse incisions or scar tissue (Table 1.3). The nerve injury usually results in chronic neuropathic pain (Fig. 1.5) [4].

Postoperative nerve damage should be suspected if the patient reports a burning or searing pain in the lower abdominal, pelvic, or medial thigh areas. The pain may be worsened by the Valsalva maneuver and is often relieved by hip and trunk flexion. A diagnostic and therapeutic injection of local anesthetic at the origin of the affected nerves, 3 cm medial to the ASIS, may provide relief.

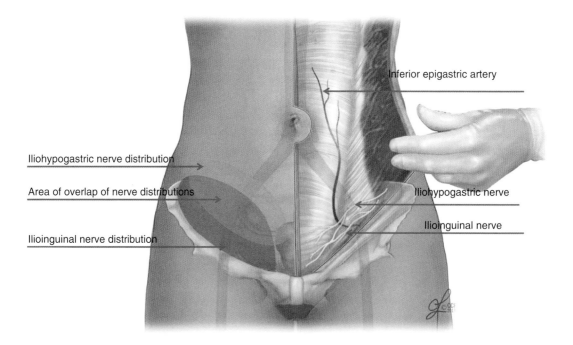

Fig. 1.5 Laparoscopic port placement two fingerbreadths superior and medial to the anterior superior iliac spine usually avoids ilioinguinal and iliohypogastric nerves and the inferior epigastric vessels

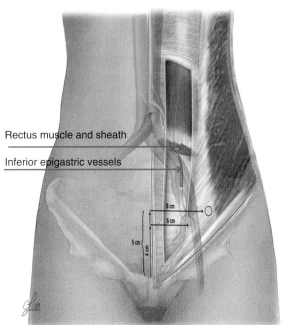

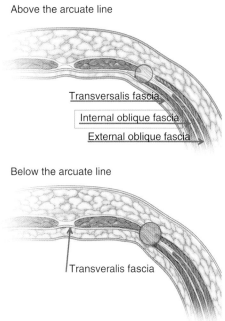

Above the arcuate line

Transversalis fascia

Internal oblique fascia

External oblique fascia

Below the arcuate line

Transveralis fascia

Rectus muscle and sheath

Inferior epigastric vessels

8 cm

6 cm

5 cm

4 cm

Fig. 1.6 Lower abdominal trocars should be placed lateral to the inferior epigastric vessels. These vessels travel medially from their origin off the external iliac artery and course toward the umbilicus. The vessels penetrate the transversus abdominis fascia and muscle approximately 4 cm superior and 6–7 cm lateral from the pubic symphy-sis. They then continue to run obliquely for an additional 7 cm and enter the posterior rectus sheath. Given these landmarks, a safe area for trocar entry is 5 cm superior and 8 cm lateral to the pubic symphysis (Modified from Park and Barber [7])

Table 1.2 Anterior abdominal wall innervations

Thoracoabdominal n.
   T7–T9 superior to the umbilicus
   T10 – at level of umbilicus
   T11 – inferior to umbilicus
Subcostal n. (anterior and lateral branches)
   T12 – inferior to the umbilicus
Iliohypogastric n.
   L1 lateral and inferior to the umbilicus
Ilioinguinal n.
   L1 labia majora, inner thigh, and groin

Table 1.3 Basic principle: decrease the risk of neuropathy

Basic principle: Reduce the risk of iliohypogastric and ilioinguinal nerve damage by utilizing transverse skin incisions and small trocars.

If possible, place laparoscopic trocars at or above the level of the ASIS [5].

If necessary, place lower abdominal trocars 2 cm medial and superior to the ASIS

1.2.4   Blood Vessels

The most notable anterior abdominal wall arteries are the epigastric vessels and the circumflex iliac vessels. Both pairs of vessels can be further classified into superficial and deep vessels. The deep epigastric vessels include the superior and inferior epigastric arteries and veins. The superior epigastric artery originates from the internal mammary artery and descends through the thorax into the rectus muscle, where it anastomoses with the inferior epigastric artery. The superior epigastric artery is accompanied by two superior epigastric veins. The deep inferior epigastric artery arises from the external iliac artery, just above the inguinal ligament. The inferior epigastric artery and vein travel in a medial and oblique fashion along the peritoneum to pierce the transversalis fascia and the rectus muscle. Owing to the absence of the posterior rectus sheath below the arcuate line, the inferior epigastric vessels can be seen within the lateral umbilical fold (Table 1.4) [6]. Accidental laceration of these deep vessels may result in life-threatening hemorrhage that must be swiftly occluded using electrosurgery or sutures (Fig. 1.6) [7].

In contrast, the superficial epigastric artery originates from the femoral artery and courses through the superficial fascia toward the umbilicus. Prior to placing secondary laparoscopic trocars, the superficial epigastric vessels are often identified by intra-abdominal transillumination in order to avoid vessel injuries (Table 1.5) [8].

Vascular trauma to the superficial epigastric vessels may result in a hematoma or abscess and, on rare cases, may even expand to the labia majora [9].

The circumflex iliac arteries consist of the deep and superficial circumflex iliac arteries. They arise from the femoral and external iliac arteries, respectively.

Table 1.4 Basic principle: decrease the risk of vascular injury

Always identify the deep, inferior epigastric vessels as they course along the parietal peritoneum. The deep vessels are located lateral to the medial umbilical folds but medial to the deep inguinal ring. Identify the deep inguinal ring by locating where the round ligament enters the inguinal canal and continues into the deep inguinal ring.

If the deep epigastric vessels are obscured by excess tissue and cannot be easily identified, one of two strategies may be employed:

1. Place the trocars approximately 8 cm lateral to the midline and 5 cm above the pubic symphysis [6]. These right and left anterior abdominal areas approximate "McBurney's point" and "Hurd's point," respectively.

Or,

2. Place the trocar medial to the medial umbilical fold, as the inferior epigastrics are consistently lateral to these. One problem with positioning the trocar this medially, however, is poor access to the adnexa.

Table 1.5 Basic principle: identify the vasculature

To avoid vessel injury, transilluminate the superficial epigastric and circumflex vessels, and identify their course prior to placing secondary trocars.

1.2.5 Peritoneal Landmarks

Distorted anatomy and severe surgical scarring challenge even experienced laparoscopic surgeons. When difficult situations are encountered, it is imperative to identify key structures that will facilitate safe surgical dissection and avoid injury to retroperitoneal vessels and viscera (Table 1.6). In the midline, there are two peritoneal folds. In the upper abdomen, the falciform ligament extends from the umbilicus to the liver and includes the obliterated umbilical vein. It is a remnant of the ventral mesentery. In the pelvis, the median umbilical fold extends from the umbilicus to the apex of the bladder and encases the urachus. Occasionally, the urachus fails to close after birth and continues to communicate with the bladder. Therefore, one should avoid this fibrous fold during laparoscopic trocar placement. In addition, a pair of bilateral, medial, and lateral umbilical folds encase the obliterated umbilical arteries and inferior epigastric vessels (Figs. 1.7 and 1.8).

There are two naturally occurring peritoneal pouches within the pelvis. Located anteriorly, the vesicouterine pouch is found between the uterus and the bladder. In a pristine pelvis, the ventral aspect of the bladder may be seen behind the anterior abdominal wall peritoneum. However, after cesarean sections, myomectomies, and previous abdominal surgery this area may be scarred and the ventral bladder margin may be more cephalad than expected. Similarly, the dorsal bladder margin usually lies on the anterior surface of the uterus. It is an important landmark for avascular dissection, but after pelvic surgery it may be adherent and require meticulous dissection (Table 1.7).

Located posteriorly, the rectouterine pouch, or the pouch of Douglas, lies posterior to the vagina, cervix, uterus, and anterior to the rectum. This pocket can be completely obliterated in cases of advanced endometriosis. The scarring may extend inferiorly to the posterior wall of the vagina and the anterior wall of the rectum. This area is an extraperitoneal fascial plane known as the rectovaginal septum. On pelvic examination, endometriosis can be appreciated as palpable nodularity along this fascial plane that runs from the rectouterine pouch to the perineal body (Fig. 1.9).

Fig. 1.7 Peritoneal folds of the anterior abdominal wall. The nonmidline folds aid in identifying critical vasculature. The medial umbilical folds lie on each side of the median fold and extend from the umbilicus to the anterior division of the internal iliac artery. The medial folds contain the obliterated umbilical arteries and form the boundaries of the bladder dome. Lateral to the medial folds are the lateral umbilical folds that extend from the arcuate line to the inguinal ring. The lateral umbilical folds are vital landmarks that contain the large, inferior epigastric vessels

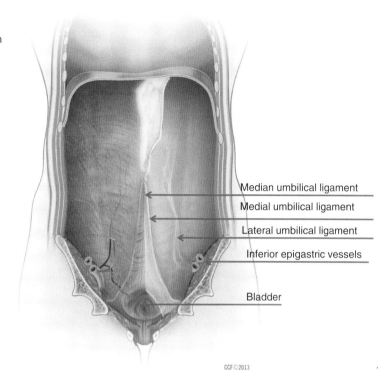

Median umbilical ligament
Medial umbilical ligament
Lateral umbilical ligament
Inferior epigastric vessels
Bladder

CCF©2013

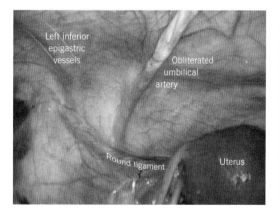
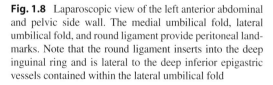

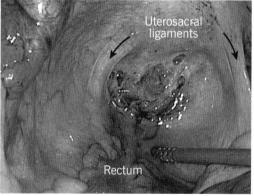

Fig. 1.8 Laparoscopic view of the left anterior abdominal and pelvic side wall. The medial umbilical fold, lateral umbilical fold, and round ligament provide peritoneal landmarks. Note that the round ligament inserts into the deep inguinal ring and is lateral to the deep inferior epigastric vessels contained within the lateral umbilical fold

Fig. 1.9 The rectouterine pouch is shown after resection for endometriosis. Bilateral uterosacral ligaments (*black arrows*) as well as the rectum are visible

Table 1.6 Peritoneal landmarks: their location and clinical significance

Peritoneal landmark	Anatomic location	Clinical significance
Median umbilical fold	Midline	Contains the fibrous and potentially patent urachus
	From umbilicus to bladder apex	
Medial umbilical fold	Bilateral	Forms the boundaries of the bladder dome
	From umbilicus to the anterior division of the internal iliac artery	Contains the fetal/obliterated umbilical artery
Lateral umbilical fold	Bilateral	Lie lateral to the medial folds but medial to the deep inguinal ring
	From arcuate line to inguinal ring	Contains the deep inferior epigastric vessels

Table 1.7 Basic principle: avoid vesical injury

To decrease bladder injury, incise the peritoneum laterally, and work medially. Keep in mind, that the bladder apex is most cephalad at the midline and is triangular in shape. The medial umbilical ligaments mark the bladder dome boundaries and are contiguous with the parietal peritoneum.

1.3 Upper Abdomen

Historically, laparoscopists only utilized the left upper quadrant as the initial entry point in patients with previous surgeries, suspected umbilical adhesions, or a large pelvic mass. However, today the left upper quadrant and other upper abdominal sites are routinely used in laparoscopic and robotic surgery. To perform a left upper quadrant entry, a Veress needle or trocar is introduced at Palmer's point, located in the midclavicular line just below the left subcostal margin. Anatomic structures at the greatest risk of injury are the stomach, left lobe of the liver, and the splenic flexure of the colon [10, 11]. Hence, prior to attempting this entry, the patient should be placed in the supine position and the stomach decompressed. Although the upper abdomen has become a more familiar landscape in recent years, caution should be exercised when using this entry in patients with relative contraindications such as hepatosplenomegaly, portal hypertension, and gastric or pancreatic masses (Fig. 1.10).

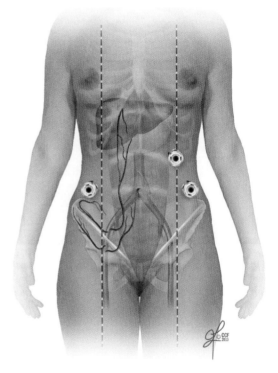

Fig. 1.10 The relationship of standard lower and upper abdominal trocar sites to important vascular landmarks and organs

1.4 Posterior Abdominal Wall and Pelvic Side Walls

Thorough knowledge of the posterior abdominal wall and the pelvic side wall structures is necessary for safe retroperitoneal dissection and effective management of surgical complications.

1.4.1 Muscles

There are six clinically relevant muscles of the posterior abdominal wall and pelvic side wall. Beginning superiorly, the diaphragm is a dome-shaped muscle that separates the thorax from the abdomen. The psoas major muscle originates from the transverse processes of the lumbar vertebrae and runs longitudinally to insert onto the lesser trochanter of the femur. The psoas major muscle constitutes a substantial portion of the posterior and medial walls. The psoas minor muscle lies anterior to the psoas major and its tendon is seen during dissection near the external iliac vessels. The quadratus lumborum muscle is located lateral and posterior to the psoas major. It spans the transverse process of lumbar vertebrae and ribs to the iliac crest. The iliacus muscle is a flat, triangular muscle that fills the iliac fossa and joins the psoas major to form the iliopsoas muscle. Ending inferiorly, the piriformis muscle lies immediately posterior to the internal iliac vessels. It originates from the anterior sacrum, passes through the greater sciatic foramen, and inserts into the greater trochanter of the femur.

1.4.2 Nerves

There are many nerves that innervate and course along the pelvic side wall. Deep nerves, such as the superior and inferior gluteal nerves, supply the pelvic muscles but are not visible during reproductive surgery. The obturator nerve, however, can easily be identified during pelvic side wall dissections. It provides sensory innervation to the medial thigh and is responsible for thigh adduction (Fig. 1.11).

The genitofemoral nerve (from spinal cord levels L1 and L2) lies on the anterior surface of the psoas major muscle and as its name implies, it divides into two branches: the femoral and the genital nerves (Fig. 1.12). The genitofemoral nerve provides sensory innervation over the anterior surface of the thigh.

The femoral nerve (spinal cord levels L2–L4) is usually not seen during pelvic surgery, but it may be injured during laparotomy. The femoral nerve is a branch of the lumbar plexus. It dives into the psoas major muscle and then emerges at its lower lateral border. The nerve courses between the psoas and iliacus muscles and then passes posterior to the inguinal ligament to supply the motor and sensory nerves of the anterior thigh. Prolonged pressure on the psoas major muscle may cause temporary or permanent damage to the femoral nerve. Therefore, it is imperative to ensure that the lateral blades of a self-retaining retractor do not exert excessive pressure on the pelvic side walls.

The sacral and coccygeal nerve plexuses are located beneath the branches of the internal iliac artery and are found anterior to the piriformis muscle. The sciatic and pudendal nerves are the most important nerves in this area. The sciatic nerve (from spinal cord levels L4–S3) lies anterior to the piriformis muscle and exits the pelvis through the greater sciatic foramen. The pudendal nerve (from spinal cord levels S2–S4) also lies anterior to the piriformis muscle and exits the pelvis through the greater sciatic foramen. It then courses around the sacrospinous ligament and ischial spine, through the lesser sciatic foramen, and continues into the perineum. At this level, endometriosis may involve the sciatic nerve and cause pain related to the course of the nerve.

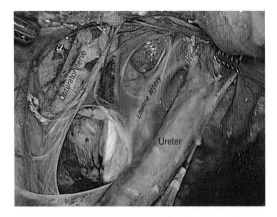

Fig. 1.11 The obturator nerve originates at spinal cord levels L2–L4 and descends through the psoas major muscle and emerges medially to course over the obturator internus muscle. The obturator nerve remains lateral to the anterior division of the internal iliac artery and ureter and then enters the thigh through the obturator canal

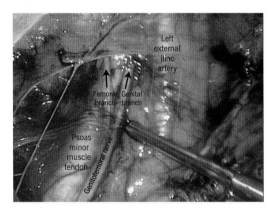

Fig. 1.12 The genitofemoral nerve lies lateral to the external iliac artery. The femoral branch enters the thigh under the inguinal ligament, and the genital branch enters the inguinal canal. The genitofemoral nerve is at risk when the peritoneal fold between the sigmoid colon and the psoas major muscle is incised

1.4.3   Blood Vessels

The aorta descends from the thorax into the abdominal cavity slightly left of the midline. It bifurcates at the level of L4 to L5, into the left and right common iliac arteries and also gives rise to the much smaller, middle sacral artery (Fig. 1.13). The inferior vena cava (IVC) lies to the right of the aorta. In the abdomen, the IVC is anterior to the aorta at the level of the renal veins. It then runs posterior to the aorta by the level of the aortic bifurcation and divides into the left and right common iliac veins (Table 1.8).

The common iliac artery courses anterior and lateral to the common iliac vein before dividing into the external and internal iliac arteries (Fig. 1.14). The external iliac artery is medial to the psoas muscle and gives rise to two vessels: the inferior epigastric artery and the deep circumflex iliac artery. Once the external iliac artery passes under the inguinal ligament, it becomes the femoral artery. Of note, its venous counterpart, the external iliac vein, is a much larger vessel, and it is situated posterior and medial to the artery, over the obturator fossa.

The internal iliac artery is the predominant artery within the pelvis. In addition to supplying the pelvic viscera, its smaller branches veer in and out of the greater and lesser sciatic foramina to perfuse the gluteal muscles and the perineum.

The internal iliac arteries split into anterior and posterior divisions that are readily seen with a retroperitoneal dissection. The anterior division of the internal iliac artery has several branches of clinical relevance. The obturator artery branches anterolaterally and dives into the obturator canal, posterior to the obturator nerve. The obliterated umbilical artery and uterine artery emerge from a common trunk and then diverge along their distinct paths. The distal portion of the obliterated umbilical artery is contained within the medial umbilical fold and serves as a peritoneal landmark. The superior vesical artery arises from the same internal iliac trunk and courses inferiorly and medially to supply the superior portion of the bladder and the distal ureter. Knowledge of these anatomic relationships is particularly useful when dealing with distorted anatomy (Table 1.9).

The uterine artery supplies the uterus and the adnexa and is of great clinical importance. In the retroperitoneum, the proximal uterine artery travels lateral and parallel to the ureter. As the uterine artery descends into the pelvis, it crosses over the ureter in a medial and anterior fashion at the level of the cervix (Fig. 1.15). The most distal aspect of the uterine artery is usually identified within the cardinal ligament, at the level of the internal os, as it propagates into smaller spiral arteries that form a network toward the uterine corpus and cervix.

The vaginal artery usually originates from the uterine artery, but it may arise directly from the internal iliac artery.

Other important branches of the anterior trunk of the internal iliac artery are the middle rectal, internal pudendal, and inferior gluteal arteries. The inferior gluteal artery is the largest branch of the anterior trunk.

The posterior division travels toward the ischial spine and gives rise to the iliolumbar, lateral sacral, and superior gluteal arteries. The superior gluteal artery is the largest branch of the internal iliac artery as it supplies the skin and muscles of the gluteal region. During uterine fibroid embolization, accidental occlusion of the superior gluteal artery can result in necrosis of the gluteal region.

The uterus and the adnexa are perfused by the uterine, vaginal, and ovarian arteries and their anastomoses with each other.

The ovarian arteries originate directly from the abdominal aorta. They descend over the pelvic brim, lateral to the ureters, and then course within the infundibular pelvic ligaments. The right ovarian vein drains directly into the IVC, while the left ovarian vein drains to the left renal vein.

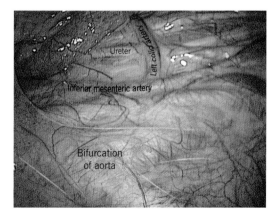

Fig. 1.13 Vessels of the abdomen and pelvis. The aorta is seen bifurcating into the iliac vessels. The left colic artery and inferior mesenteric artery are visible lateral to this bifurcation

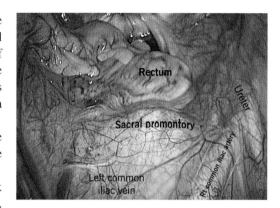

Fig. 1.14 A laparoscopic view of vessels posterior to the umbilicus. The left and right iliac vessels are seen in relationship to the sacral promontory, rectum, and ureter. Appreciation of this proximity and control of the trocar speed, angle, and depth are necessary to avoid serious complications

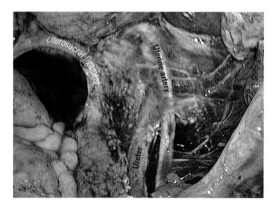

Fig. 1.15 Uterine artery crossing over the ureter

Table 1.8 Basic principle: considerations prior to inserting an umbilical trocar

When placing the initial umbilical trocar, remember that the left common iliac vein lies in the midline, just caudad to the aortic bifurcation and the umbilicus (see Fig. 1.14). Also see previous section on the impact of increasing weight on anterior abdominal wall anatomy.

Table 1.9 Basic principle: utilize peritoneal landmarks for orientation

Identification of the ureters and major vessels is critical before any ligation or cauterization is performed. When distorted anatomy poses a challenge, first identify a medial umbilical fold as a fibrous band on the anterior abdominal wall. Then apply gentle traction on this fold (and the encased obliterated umbilical artery) and follow it to its origin, the internal iliac artery. In this vicinity, the superior vesical artery and uterine artery can be identified and followed toward their terminal organs.

1.4.4 Ureters

The ureters measure approximately 25–30 cm from the renal pelvis to the bladder. They are located in the retroperitoneum and are occasionally duplicated on one or both sides. In the abdomen, the ureters descend on the medial aspect of the psoas major muscle and cross the common iliac vessels at their bifurcation into the internal and external iliac arteries at the pelvic brim (Fig. 1.16).

In the pelvis, the ureters lie in close proximity to the ovarian vessels. The ureter is located medial to the internal iliac and its anterior division (Fig. 1.17). The ureter is usually found medial to the infundibulopelvic ligament. Broad ligament dissection may be necessary to identify the ureter and to ensure the safe ligation of the ovarian vessels during a salpingo-oophorectomy (Fig. 1.18).

The ureter then dives deep into the parametrium and travels under the uterine artery. This anatomic relationship is classically referred to as "water under the bridge." It traverses the cardinal ligament, then crosses over the vaginal fornix, and finally inserts into the bladder trigone.

The average distance between the ureter and cervix is more than 2 cm. However, this distance can be less than 0.5 cm in about 10 % of women [12]. This variable distance partially explains the relatively common occurrence of ureteral injury during hysterectomy.

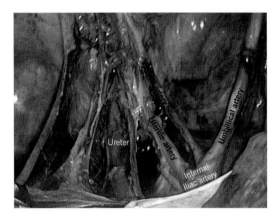

Fig. 1.17 A more caudad view of the internal iliac artery and its anterior division. Here the uterine, vaginal, and umbilical arteries are seen in relationship to the ureter. Note how the ureter moves from a lateral (in Fig. 1.16) to a medial position in relationship to the internal iliac artery as it courses from the pelvic brim to deep within the pelvis

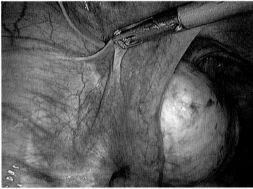

Fig. 1.18 Incising the left broad ligament to facilitate ureter identification. Retroperitoneal dissection may begin at the pelvic brim and is carried caudad to follow the course of the ureter. Alternatively, in the event of a salpingo-oophorectomy, the broad ligament may be grasped and incised between the round ligament and the infundibular pelvic ligament to access the retroperitoneum and aid in ureter identification prior to securing the vascular ovarian pedicle. The ureter is located on the medial leaf of the broad ligament

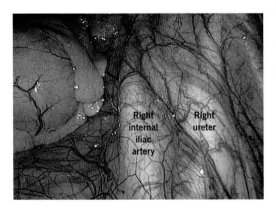

Fig. 1.16 A view of the ureter and internal iliac vessels from the pelvic brim

1.5 Muscles of the Pelvic Floor

The pelvic floor contains a series of muscles and endopelvic fascia that provide pelvic support to the uterus, vagina, bladder, and rectum. Disruption of these varying levels of pelvic support, described as Levels 1, 2, and 3, result in pelvic organ prolapse, paravaginal defects, and voiding and defecatory dysfunction. Pelvic floor relaxation occurs with increasing age but may be hastened by stressors such as the physiologic rigors of pregnancy, increasing parity, obesity, and birth trauma [13].

1.5.1 Pelvic Diaphragm

The pelvic diaphragm refers to the levator ani muscle complex and the coccygeus muscle. The levator ani consists of the puborectalis, pubococcygeus, and the iliococcygeus muscles (Fig. 1.19).

The thick anterior and posterior condensations of white fascia that surround the vagina are known as the arcus tendineus fascia pelvis (ATFP) and the arcus tendineous rectovaginalis (ATRV). These fasciae, together with the levator ani muscles, attach the midvagina to the pelvic side walls and support the bladder and rectum. Note the almost perpendicular axis of the puborectalis and pubococcygeus muscles to the vagina and rectum in a standing woman. Defects of Level 2 support result in cystoceles and rectoceles (Fig. 1.20) [14].

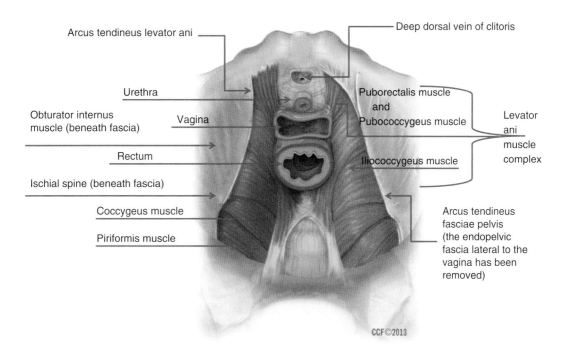

Fig. 1.19 Components of the pelvic diaphragm. The puborectalis muscle encircles the rectum and is attached to the pubic symphysis. The pubococcygeus muscle stretches in an anteroposterior fashion, from the pubis to the coccyx, and is attached to the obturator internus muscle by a dense band of connective tissue known as the arcus tendineus fascia pelvis (ATFP). The ATFP runs from the ischial spine and inserts on the pubic symphysis, and its posterior support is mirrored by the arcus tendineus rectovaginalis. The lateral iliococcygeus muscle extends from the arcus tendineus fascia pelvis and ischial spine to the coccyx. The coccygeus muscle is the most posteriolateral component and spans from the ischial spine to the coccyx and sacrum

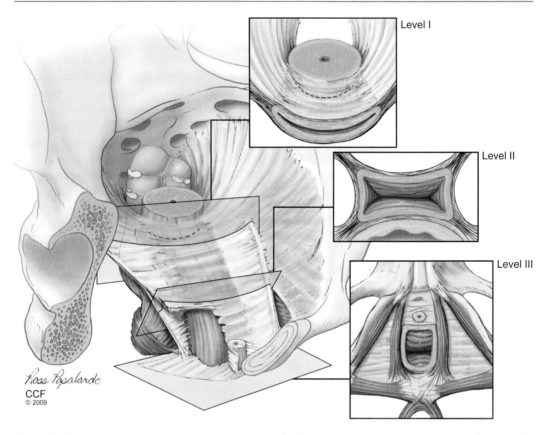

Level I

Level II

Level III

Ross Papalardo
CCF
© 2009

Fig. 1.20 Three integrated levels of uterine and vaginal support in a standing woman. *Level 1* support relies on the uterosacral and cardinal ligament complex to suspend the uterus, cervix, and upper vagina vertically and posteriorly toward the sacrum. *Level 2* utilizes the arcus tendineus fascia pelvis and arcus tendineus rectovaginalis to provide lateral support to the midportion of the vagina. *Level 3* support is provided by the network of connective tissue surrounding the vagina. These connective tissues bind the vagina to the urethra, perineum, and levator ani muscles

1.5.2 Deep and Superficial Perineal Pouches and the Perineal Membrane

The deep perineal pouch is somewhat of a misnomer as there is no true pouch. It refers to the area superior to the perineal membrane located between the inferior pubic rami and the perineal body. The connective tissues in this region provide the most distal level of pelvic organ support. Anteriorly, the ATFP unifies the vagina to the contiguous striated muscles of the urethra. Posteriorly, the ATRV merges the vagina to the deep transverse perineal muscles, perineal membrane, and the perineal body. And laterally, the connective fibers attach the vagina to the levator ani muscles. Defects of this Level 3 support result in perineal body descent and can cause urethral hypermobility, stress incontinence, and defecatory dysfunction [14].

The perineal membrane is a fascial layer that separates the deep and superficial perineal pouches but still allows passage of the vagina and urethra to the pelvic outlet.

The superficial perineal pouch includes the greater vestibular glands (Bartholin glands), and the ischiocavernosus, bulbospongiosus, and superficial transverse perineal muscles.

1.6   Presacral Space

Appreciation of the innervations and vascular anatomy of the presacral space is required prior to presacral dissection. Surgeries performed within this region include presacral neurectomy, sacral colpopexy, and rectal resection. In this space lies the superior hypogastric plexus that contains prelumbar sympathetic and parasympathetic nerve fibers. The superior hypogastric plexus divides into two branches at the level of the bifurcation of the aorta. These nerves carry visceral afferent fibers from the uterus in addition to parasympathetic fibers that stimulate bladder contraction and modulate activity of the distal colon. Therefore, patients undergoing presacral neurectomy must be counseled that surgery can result in both bladder and bowel dysfunction.

Vascular injury in this confined, deep space is problematic at the very minimum and at times can be life-threatening. The left common iliac vein marks the left superior margin of the presacral space. The median sacral vessels that originate from the aorta and descend in the midline into the presacral area are at risk during dissection. Laceration and bleeding from any of these vessels and the presacral venous plexus may result in hemorrhage.

1.7   Pelvic Viscera

The pelvic viscera include the rectum, urinary organs, the vagina, uterus, uterine tubes, and ovaries.

1.7.1   The Rectum

The rectum of the adult is approximately 12–15 cm in length. It begins at the rectosigmoid junction at the level of S3 and ends at the level of the coccyx. It is distinguished from the colon by its lack of taenia coli, haustra, and omental appendices.

The upper third of the rectum projects into the peritoneal cavity. At its midpoint, the rectouterine pouch is formed by the extension of the rectum's anterior peritoneum onto the vaginal fornix. The distal one-third of the rectum is located in the retroperitoneum.

The blood supply to the rectum includes the superior rectal artery, a branch from the inferior mesenteric artery, the middle rectal artery, a branch from the internal iliac artery and the inferior rectal artery, and a branch from the internal pudendal artery. Sympathetic fibers from the inferior hypogastric plexus, parasympathetic fibers from S2 to S4, and sensory fibers from the rectum all join the inferior hypogastric plexus to innervate the rectum.

1.7.2   Vagina

The vagina is a muscular membranous cylinder that extends anteroinferiorly from the uterine cervix to the vestibule and is approximately 7–9 cm in length. The vagina is separated from the bladder and rectum by the vesicouterine and rectouterine pouch. The vagina receives its blood supply from the uterine, vaginal, and middle rectal arteries. The inferior hypogastric plexus and pelvic splanchnic nerves innervate the vagina.

1.7.3   Uterus

The uterus is a dynamic, fibromuscular organ that varies in size and weight according to life stage and parity. The uterus is composed of a body (corpus) and a cervix. The fundus is the portion of the uterine body above the fallopian tubes. The uterine cavity is triangular in shape. The length of the uterine cavity changes according to life stage owing to the profound effect of hormones on uterine size. In premenarchal females the uterine length from the external os to the fundus is 1–3 cm. During the reproductive years, this increases to 6–7 cm, and in postmenopausal women the uterus decreases to 3–5 cm in length. Similarly, the inner lining of the uterus is hormonally active and varies throughout a woman's life cycle. The endometrium varies from 5 to 15 mm during a single menstrual cycle during the reproductive years but should measure less than 5 mm in thickness during the postmenopausal period.

The myometrium is thickest in the midportion of the corpus and thinnest in the cornua. The outer and innermost layers are composed mostly of longitudinal fibers in contrast to the middle layer, which consists of circular and oblique fibers that enwrap blood vessels and loose connective tissue.

The majority of the uterine blood supply is from the uterine artery, a branch of the internal iliac artery. Uterine arteries run along the lateral borders of the uterus and form anastomoses with the ovarian and vaginal arteries. The anterior and posterior arcuate arteries branch off the uterine arteries and run circumferentially around the uterine corpus and anastomose in the midline. Interestingly, no large blood vessels are found in the uterine midline. Radial arteries develop from the arcuate arteries and deeply penetrate the myometrium to reach the endometrium. The spiral arteries, which arise from the radial arteries, supply the endometrium and are the terminal blood vessels of the uterus.

1.7.4   Uterine Tubes

The uterine tubes are enshrouded within the uppermost aspect of the broad ligament and measure about 10–12 cm. Each tube is divided into four anatomic segments: intramural (or interstitial), isthmic, ampullary, and infundibulum.

The intramural portion is usually 1.5 cm long and less than 1 mm in diameter and may be tortuous. The isthmic portion is often the segment excised or ligated during tubal ligation and therefore is also the site of tubal anastomosis. The lumen is approximately 0.5 mm. Subsequent pregnancy rates are highest for procedures done in this area.

The ampulla comprises two-thirds of the length of the tube and is characterized by 4–5 longitudinal ridges. It is the site of fertilization. Not surprisingly, it is also the most common site of ectopic pregnancy. Tubal ligations are often performed at this more distal site. Pregnancy rates after anastomosis are lower in this segment despite the larger lumen.

The infundibulum is the most distal section of the tube. It is open to the peritoneal cavity and is readily identified by its fimbriae. The lumen diameter may reach 10 mm.

The tubal wall is made up of three layers: mucosa, muscularis, and serosa. The muscular layer possesses an external longitudinal layer and an inner circular layer of smooth muscle. Branches of the uterine and ovarian arteries course though the mesosalpinx and provide the blood supply for the fallopian tube.

1.7.5   Ovaries

The ovaries are hormonally dynamic ovoid structures suspended from the posterior aspect of the broad ligament by the mesovarium. This fold of peritoneum contains a complex of blood vessels. The ovarian ligament enters the ovary along its inferior pole and the suspensory ligament of the ovary, or infundibulopelvic ligament, enters the ovary along its superior pole. The infundibulopelvic ligament carries the ovarian vessels, lymphatics, and nerves from the pelvic side wall and lies in close proximity to the ureter at the pelvic brim. The ovary is attached to the broad ligament by the well-vascularized mesovarium. The highly coiled, cascading anastamoses of uterine and ovarian vessels are prominent in the gravid uterus or a uterus laden with leiomyomata.

1.8   Pelvic Fasciae and Ligaments

The pelvic viscera are attached to the pelvic side walls by (1) peritoneal folds, (2) condensations of pelvic fascia, and (3) remnants of embryonic structures. Historically, these structures were called ligaments because it was believed that they supported the uterus and prevented genital prolapse. However, it has become clear that they do not provide significant support for the pelvic viscera in the presence of pelvic floor defects.

1.8.1   Peritoneal Folds

The broad ligament is a double-layered transverse fold of peritoneum that drapes the uterus, fallopian tubes, lateral pelvic side walls, and pelvic floor. On the lateral aspects of the uterus, the mesometrium encloses the uterine vessels and the ureters. Posteriorly, the mesovarium attaches the ovary to the broad ligament, while the mesosalpinx connects the fallopian tube near the base of the mesovarium.

The suspensory ligament of the ovary, or the infundibulopelvic ligament, is a lateral continuation of the broad ligament beyond the fallopian tube that connects the ovary to the pelvic brim and contains the ovarian vessels. The ureter crosses beneath these vessels near the ligament's insertion into the pelvic side wall (Fig. 1.21).

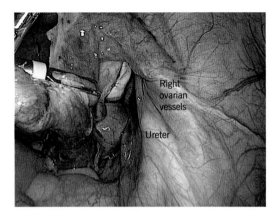

Fig. 1.21 Proximity of the ureter to the ovarian vessel. In order to minimize ureteral injury a surgeon may perform ureterolysis or create a clear window between the ovarian vessels and the ureter prior to ligation and incision of the blood vessels. Damage to the ureter most commonly occurs at the following locations: at the pelvic brim while securing the ovarian vessels, at the level of the cardinal ligament (in this area the ureter dives under the uterine artery), at the level of the uterosacral ligaments along the pelvic side wall, and at the level of the vaginal cuff while securing the angles for hemostasis

1.8.2 Fascial Ligaments

Together, the cardinal and uterosacral ligaments provide Level 1 support for the uterus, cervix, and upper vagina [14].

The cardinal ligament is the dense connective tissue located lateral to the cervix. It is abutted by the broad ligament anteriorly, posteriorly, and inferiorly by the pelvic floor. It is continuous with the paracervix, a thick fibrous sheath around the lower cervix and the upper vagina. It is attached to the pelvic walls laterally and contains major branches of the uterine vessels.

The uterosacral ligaments are bands of connective tissue and smooth muscle that stretch from the posterior paracervix to the sacrum and rectum.

1.8.3 Gubernacular Ligaments

The ovarian ligament runs within the broad ligament and attaches the medial pole of the ovary to the posterolateral uterine surface beneath the fallopian tube. The round ligament is a fibromuscular structure that runs from the anterolateral surface of the uterus and continues through the deep, external, inguinal ring and terminates in the connective tissue of the labium majora.

References

1. Nezhat F, Brill AI, Nezhat CH, Nezhat A, Seidman DS, Nezhat C. Laparoscopic appraisal of the anatomic relationship of the umbilicus to the aortic bifurcation. J Am Assoc Gynecol Laparosc. 1998;5:135–40.
2. Hurd WW, Bude RO, DeLancey JO, Pearl ML. The relationship of the umbilicus to the aortic bifurcation: implications for laparoscopic technique. Obstet Gynecol. 1992;80:4851.
3. Hurd WW, Bude RO, DeLancey JOL, Gauvin JM, Aisen AM. Abdominal wall characterization by magnetic resonance imaging and computed tomography: the effect of obesity on laparoscopic approach. J Reprod Med. 1991;36:473–6.
4. Stultz P. Peripheral nerve injuries resulting from common surgical procedures in the lower abdomen. Arch Surg. 1982;117:324–7.
5. Whiteside J, Barber M, Walters M, Falcone T. Anatomy of ilioinguinal and iliohypogastric nerves in relation to trocar placement and low transverse incisions. Am J Obstet Gynecol. 2003;189:1574–8.
6. Hurd WW, Amesse LS, Gruber JS, Horowitz GM, Cha GM, Hurteau JA. Visualization of the epigastric vessels and bladder before laparoscopic trocar placement. Fertil Steril. 2003;80:209–12.
7. Park AJ, Barber MD. Anatomy of the uterus and its surgical removal. In: Walters MD, Barber MD, editors. Hysterectomy for benign disease: female pelvic surgery video atlas series. Philadelphia: WB Saunders; 2010.
8. Hurd WW, Bude RO, DeLancey JOL, Newman JS. The location of abdominal wall blood vessels in relationship to abdominal landmarks apparent at laparoscopy. Am J Obstet Gynecol. 1994;171:642–6.
9. Hurd WW, Pearl ML, DeLancey JO, Quint EH, Garnett B, Bude RO. Laparoscopic injury of abdominal wall blood vessels: a report of three cases. Obstet Gynecol. 1993;82(4 Pt 2 Suppl):673–6.
10. Patsner B. Laparoscopy using the left upper quadrant approach. J Am Assoc Gynecol Laparosc. 1999;6:323–5.
11. Tulikangas PK, Nicklas A, Falcone T, Price LL. Anatomy of the left upper quadrant for cannula insertion. J Am Assoc Gynecol Laparosc. 2000;7:211–4.
12. Hurd WW, Chee SS, Gallagher KL, Ohl DA, Hurteau JA. Location of the ureters in relation to the uterine cervix by computed tomography. Am J Obstet Gynecol. 2001;184:336–9.
13. Patel DA, Xu X, Thomason AD, Ransom SB, Ivy JS, DeLancey JO. Childbirth and pelvic floor dysfunction: an epidemiologic approach to the assessment of prevention opportunities at delivery. Am J Obstet Gynecol. 2006;195:23–8.
14. DeLancey JO. Anatomic aspects of vaginal eversion after hysterectomy. Am J Obstet Gynecol. 1992;166:1717–24.

Laparoscopic Myomectomy

2

M. Brigid Holloran-Schwartz and Patrick P. Yeung Jr.

Leiomyomas are the most common benign pelvic tumors. They can be asymptomatic but frequently cause symptoms of abnormal uterine bleeding, anemia, pelvic pressure, urinary frequency, and impaired fertility. Based on improved perioperative outcomes, myomectomy, using a minimally invasive approach, is the preferred treatment modality for symptomatic women desiring future fertility. Detailed imaging can be done preoperatively and even intraoperatively to maximize removal of all accessible myomas. A laparoscopic approach is preferred for myomas not accessible through the hysteroscope. Myomectomy can significantly improve the quality of life for symptomatic women, and in many cases it can improve reproductive outcomes.

Uterine leiomyomas are the most common benign pelvic tumors, occurring in up to 70 % of white women and 80 % of African American women [1]. Depending on the size and location of the tumor, they may cause adverse pregnancy outcomes, bleeding, and pressure. Treatment options are based on the symptoms that they cause and can include continuing observation or medical or surgical options. Surgical options may include hysterectomy, uterine artery embolization, myomectomy, magnetic resonance–guided focused ultrasonography, and the newer US Food and Drug Administration approved procedure Acessa (Halt Medical, Inc.; Brentwood, CA). Myomectomy remains the surgical option of choice for those who wish to retain their fertility. It is also an option for those who have completed child-bearing but wish to retain their uterus.

It is well established that compared to open laparotomy, laparoscopic myomectomy is preferred and produces less blood loss, shorter hospital stays, faster recovery rates, decreased pain, and better cosmesis.

M.B. Holloran-Schwartz, MD (✉) • P.P. Yeung Jr., MD
Department of Obstetrics,
Gynecology, and Women's Health,
St. Louis University, 6420 Clayton Road,
St. Louis, MO 63117, USA
e-mail: holloran@slu.edu; yeungpjr.md@gmail.com

P.F. Escobar, T. Falcone (eds.), *Atlas of Single-Port, Laparoscopic, and Robotic Surgery*,
DOI 10.1007/978-1-4614-6840-0_2, © Springer Science+Business Media New York 2014

2.1 Preoperative Evaluation

2.1.1 Imaging

Symptomatic fibroids are usually seen by the gynecologist with abnormal bleeding or pressure-like symptoms. The diagnosis is typically made with pelvic ultrasound. For women ultimately desiring myomectomy, magnetic resonance imaging (MRI) is the recommended imaging modality of choice. MRI has a greater sensitivity and specificity in terms of the number, size, and location of myomas than ultrasound. It can help identify lesions suspicious for sarcoma and provides superior visualization of the endometrial cavity [1, 2]. MRI results for myomectomy can be reviewed before surgery with the intent of retrieving as many fibroids as possible by compensating for the relatively decreased tactile sensation compared with an open laparotomy.

If there is still uncertainty about the integrity of the endometrial cavity, ultrasound with saline infusion or office hysteroscopy should be considered preoperatively.

Preliminary studies with intra-abdominal ultrasound, as used in the Acessa procedure (Table 2.1), demonstrated significantly improved detection of submucosal, subserosal, and intramural myomas [3]. Future use of this intraabdominal ultrasound during myomectomy may show improved identification and evacuation of myomas. This, in turn, may lead to greater symptom reduction and reduced rates of recurrence.

A preoperative pelvic examination is crucial to alert the surgeon to uterine mobility and potential access to each myoma. If limited mobility or extremely large fibroids are present, plans should be made to have a skilled assistant present, or consideration can be given to pretreatment with a gonadotropin-releasing hormone agonist (GnRHa).

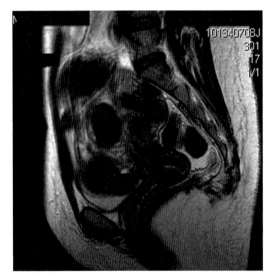

Fig. 2.1 Sections of a magnetic resonance image of a patient with a large uterine fibroid desiring myomectomy. Ultrasound study in this patient could not delineate the endometrium

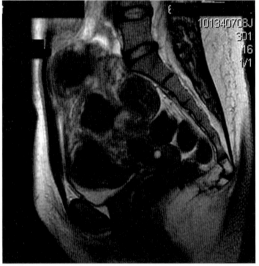

Fig. 2.2 Magnetic resonance imaging shows small intracavitary myoma

Table 2.1 Halt study

Halt study	Intramural	Subserosal	Submucosal	Transmural	Combination
Laparoscopic ultrasound	386	184	110	27	89
Magnetic resonance imaging	292	121	80	16	22
Transvaginal ultrasound	197	92	42	23	33

Modified from Halt Fibroid Study [3]

2.1.2 GnRHa Pretreatment

A subject of some discussion has been whether or not pretreatment with a GnRHa before laparoscopic myomectomy is beneficial. Some advocate the potential benefit of shrinkage in size of the fibroids with GnRHa pretreatment and on hemostasis [4], whereas others have been concerned with a blurring of the cleavage plane between the myoma and the myometrium [5]. A recent systematic review and meta-analysis [6] has clarified the issue that pretreatment with GnRHa does not increase the operative time associated with laparoscopic myomectomy, a finding consistent with the most recent similar Cochrane review [7] related to the topic. Operative time can be thought of as a surrogate for operative ease, which would incorporate several surgical factors including myoma size, hemostasis, and the cleavage plane between the myoma and the myometrium.

Systematic reviews [6, 7] of the three randomized trials on GnRHa pretreatment before laparoscopic myomectomy did demonstrate a statistically significant reduction in intraoperative blood loss (60 mL) and postoperative hemoglobin (1.15 g/dL). It is debatable whether these findings have clinical significance. It is also interesting to note that there is a discrepancy between the very minimal decrease in intraoperative blood loss and the decrease in postoperative hemoglobin. It is possible, too, that a potential benefit of pretreatment (for 3–6 months) with GnRHa of surgical bleeding is outweighed by the adverse effects of cost and the delay in receiving treatment. This discrepancy may be attributable to an inaccurate estimate of intraoperative blood loss but also may be because of continued postoperative bleeding or oozing. If the latter is true, pretreatment with GnRHa may

Table 2.2 Pros and Cons of GnRHa pretreatment

PROS:
May lead to shrinkage in the size of the fibroids
Has been shown to produce a significant reduction in intraoperative blood loss (60 mL)
Pretreatment with GnRHa has not been shown to increase operative time
Has been shown to lead to significant reduction in postoperative hemoglobin (1.15 g/dL)
CONS:
Potential blurring of the cleavage plane between the myoma and the myometrium
Requires time for pretreatment (usually 3 months) and may lead to delay in surgery

have a benefit on reducing peritoneal inflammation and postoperative adhesion formation given less postoperative blood loss. Further multicenter and long-term trials are needed.

2.2 Surgical Procedure

Consideration should be given to treating the most symptomatic fibroids first. In the patient with submucosal fibroids and heavy menstrual bleeding, a hysteroscopic resection should be performed first, followed by laparoscopic myomectomy. These procedures may be performed during the same operation.

Attempts should be made to remove all visible or palpable fibroids to prevent future growth and recurrence of symptoms.

Preoperative laboratory work should include a complete blood count, human chorionic gonadotropin type, and screening. For patients with significant anemia or large intramural fibroids, a type and cross of two units of blood should be available. For procedures for which significant blood loss is a risk, the patient may consider having autologous blood available, or the surgeon can arrange to have cell saver technology available.

2.2.1 Consent

Once the surgeon has reviewed all imaging results, the patient should be extensively counseled about the risks of the procedure. Standard risks of bleeding, infection, adhesion formation, laparotomy, transfusion as well as organ injury should be discussed. Additionally, risks inherent in myomectomy, such as myoma recurrence, should be discussed. Up to 25 % of women may require additional surgery in the future for symptomatic myoma recurrence [8]. The risks of possible uterine rupture with future pregnancy and the need for cesarean section birth should be discussed.

Limited studies are available on the risks of uterine rupture. Generally speaking, the risk of rupture during pregnancy or during labor is 2.4 per 1,000 between 29 and 35.5 weeks [9]. To minimize this risk, it is recommended that the pseudocapsules of excised myomas be preserved for uterine anatomic and functional integrity, especially in women desiring future pregnancy. This can be done by limiting the use of diathermocoagulation and excessive suturing [9]. The surgeon may individualize his or her recommendation for delayed conception based on the extent and size of the fibroids. For example, a patient with a large pedunculated myomectomy may only wait 3 months for a procedure, whereas a patient requiring an extensive repair of the myometrium may wait 6 months [10].

2.2.2 Equipment

Needed instruments, sutures, and solutions in the operating room are key to a successful myomectomy. These necessary items include a single tooth tenaculum, myoma screw, and V-Loc suture (V-Loc, Covidien; Dublin, Ireland) or the surgeon's suture preference. A dilute vasopressin solution of 20 U in 100 mL of normal saline

Table 2.3 Optional equipment

Dilute vasopressin solution
Red rubber catheter to use as a tourniquet
Single tooth tenaculum
Myoma screw
Suture (polydioxone, polyglactin, or an absorbable barbed suture on a CT 1 or GS 21 needle)
Morcellator or self-retaining retractor for minimally invasive morcellation (see Fig. 2.11)

is helpful to decrease intraoperative blood loss [11, 12]. The surgeon should plan a method of morcellation and have needed equipment available.

2.2.3 Patient Positioning and Port Placement

The patient is placed in the dorsal lithotomy position in Allen stirrups, arms tucked, and a Foley catheter is placed. A uterine manipulator that can antiflex and retroflex the uterus is helpful to assist with exposure when suturing. We use the reusable Valtchev uterine manipulator (Conkin Surgical Instruments; Toronto, Canada).

Use of the umbilical port is optimal for the camera, as this is cosmetically most appealing and serves as an excellent site to extend through the base for morcellation. This technique will be described later in this chapter. We typically place a 10-mm trocar in the umbilicus using the Hasson approach and use a 10-mm, 30-degree angled laparoscope. Other options include a flexible laparoscope or a variable-view laparoscope to allow more flexibility in available views. For straightforward fibroids, a 10-mm, zero degree laparoscope can be used. If the uterus extends above the umbilicus, placing the camera port above the level of the umbilicus in the midline may give greater exposure.

Additional port placement may be individualized based on the size and location of the myoma. Depending on the surgeon's training and preference, three accessory ports are generally needed. Options include placing two 5-mm ports on the primary surgeon's side and one on the assistant's side. It is important when placing two ports on

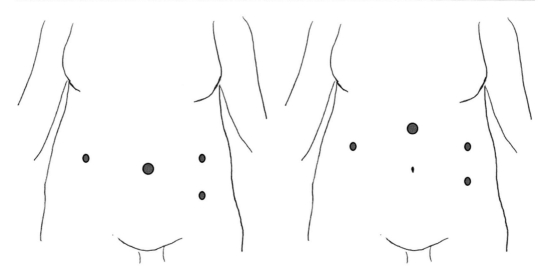

Fig. 2.3 Port placement for most uteri with myomas extending up to the umbilicus

Fig. 2.4 Alternative port placement for large myomas extending above the umbilicus

the same side to place them at least a hands width (approximately 5–6 cm) apart from each other to prevent instrument clashing. The assistant's side port must be placed above the level of the uterus, since this is the port will be used to elevate and enucleate the fibroid out of the uterus.

CT-1 or GS 21 (V-Loc) needles are best for uterine repair and can be introduced and removed through the 10- to 12-mm trocar at the umbilicus.

Other options include dragging the needle into the abdominal cavity on the swedge through a 5-mm skin incision. Another choice is replacing the suprapubic 5-mm trocar with a 10- to 12-mm trocar and introducing the needle directly through this port. This larger port site could also then be utilized for a disposable or reusable morcellator. It is important to close the fascia of any port that is 10 mm or larger.

2.3 Surgical Technique

Once pneumoperitoneum and port placement are obtained, the abdominopelvic cavity is explored. The uterus is carefully assessed and a comparison made with its appearance in preoperative imaging. The relationship of the myomas to the fallopian tubes and ovaries is assessed. In uteri with multiple fibroids, the most symptomatic myoma may be targeted first. There may be cases where the uterus must be debulked by removing smaller, less symptomatic fibroids to achieve better access to the primary fibroid. Generally, removing fundal fibroids first will afford greater access to lower uterine segment fibroids.

Formulating a plan for hemostasis is critical. Typically, bleeding from the myometrium adjacent to the myoma is anticipated until the entire defect is closed. The bleeding may be slow but constant. The nature of this slow, steady bleeding may be deceiving. Communication with the anesthesiologist is important to keep an accurate count of blood loss. A dilute vasopressin solution (20 U/100 mL normal saline) can help limit blood loss [9]. The site of injection depends on the type of myoma. For example, a pedunculated myoma should be injected at the myometrial base of the stalk of the myoma. An intramural fibroid can be injected through the uterine serosa, ideally in the plane just inside of the pseudocapsule, creating a "wheel" effect. This technique is more effective than deep myoma injection. With large intramural myomas, the deeper adjacent myometrium toward the base may be injected as it is exposed if excessive bleeding is encountered. Spot cautery with bipolar energy can be helpful for distinct vessels but its use is limited with bleeding from the raw surface of the myometrium. Excessive use of thermal energy for hemostasis is discouraged because this may increase destruction of healthy myometrial tissue and impair uterine healing and functionality [9].

For patients with extremely large intramural myomas (>10 cm) that would require multilayer closure, additional steps may be considered for preventing excessive blood loss. Some authors describe selective use of a laparoscopically

Table 2.4 Tips for hemostasis

1. Vasopressin: inject a dilute solution in the plane just inside the pseudo-capsule, creating a "wheel" effect. Always alert the anesthesiologist prior to injecting.
2. Avoid injecting large surface myometrial vessels. If bleeding occurs at injection sites, hold temporary pressure with laparoscopic grasper to control and prevent extravasation of vasopressin.
3. For large myomas, if needed repeat injection to the myometrium that is adjacent to the deeper base of the myoma, always alerting the anesthesiologist first.
4. Consider the use of a tourniquet for large (>10 cm) myomas.
5. Targeted spot cautery to distinct vessels and avoid excessive coagulation to myometrial tissue.
6. If child-bearing is completed, consider permanent uterine artery occlusion methods as adjuncts for hemostasis

placed tourniquet to compress the uterine arteries at the level of the cervix [10, 12]. This technique involves threading a red rubber catheter through bilateral windows created in the broad ligament encircling the cervix. The ends of the red rubber catheter are brought through the lateral trocar skin incisions on contralateral sides, outside of the trocar, and secured with Kelly clamps where they exit the port sites [10].

For women who have completed childbearing, permanent uterine artery occlusion, using clips, suture, or complete transection can be performed. Preliminary studies suggest that this technique can decrease intraoperative blood loss and may also help prevent fibroid recurrence [12].

2.3.1 Incision

The incision type should be individualized based on myoma type and location. Injection with a dilute vasopressin solution is made. A transverse incision facilitates suturing from lateral ports and runs parallel to the arcuate vessels of the myometrium, limiting blood loss [10]. This initial incision can be made with ultrasonic or monopolar energy and must be to the level of the fibroid capsule and over the entire diameter. Generally speaking, the closer the incision is to the fundus over the myoma, the easier it will be to repair with traditional laparoscopy.

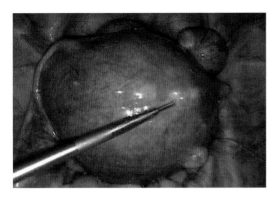

Fig. 2.5 Injection with a dilute vasopressin solution is made

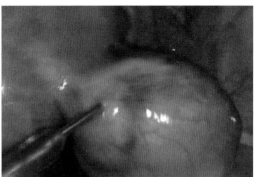

Fig. 2.7 Injection of pedunculated myoma at the base of the stalk

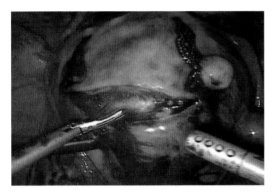

Fig. 2.6 Horizontal incision is made to the level of the pseudocapsule

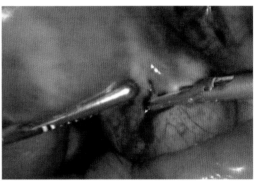

Fig. 2.8 Excision of pedunculated myoma preserving a small serosal edge of tissue

2.3.1.1 Pedunculated Myomas

When excising pedunculated myomas, do not excise the stalk at the base of uterine surface. Rather, save a portion of the serosa of the stalk and excise the myoma only. Typically, the preserved serosa will immediately start to retract. Spot cautery can be attempted to achieve hemostasis but in the event of persistent bleeding, the preserved serosa will assist with suture closure and avoid tearing.

2.3.1.2 Intramural or Subserosal Myomas

With intramural and subserosal myomas, a horizontal incision is made over the entire length of the myoma to the capsule. Occasionally, with large intramural myomas or those lying in an oblique plane within the uterus, the entire length of the fibroid may not clear. In this case, the capsule that has been identified can be grasped with a single-tooth tenaculum. Elevating the myoma away from the uterus while expanding the original incision can help delineate the exact size and location of the myoma.

2.3.1.3 Broad Ligament Myomas

With broad ligament myomas, the ureter should be identified and the relation to the operative sight noted. The incision is made over the length of the myoma to the capsule as described with an intramural fibroid. Once the capsule is exposed, grasping it with a single-tooth tenaculum and elevating the myoma away from the ureter and uterine artery with careful blunt dissection will keep the ureter safe. Care should be taken to limit the use of energy. Small vessels can easily be isolated with traction and countertraction while elevating the specimen out of the myoma bed and selectively sealing it.

2.3.1.4 Lower Uterine Segment

For intramural myomas in the lower anterior or posterior uterine segment, suture closure can be a challenge with traditional laparoscopy. The uterine arteries are also entering at this level. The initial horizontal incision is typically easier to repair if made toward the superior aspect of the myoma rather the center. As previously stated, the closer to the fundus an incision can be made, the more straightforward the repair will be while using traditional laparoscopy. As with any myomectomy, the dead space must be closed in a multilayered fashion. Use of a uterine manipulator that can anteflex and retroflex the uterus will be helpful for repair of these defects.

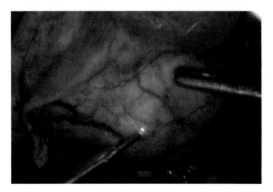

Fig. 2.9 Injection of a lower uterine segment fibroid above the midline diameter of the myoma, along the intended incision line

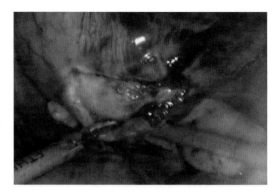

Fig. 2.10 Incision is made superior to the midline diameter of the myoma, and the myoma is lifted out of the incision to make suture repair more straightforward

2.3.2 Enucleation

Once the capsule of the myoma is exposed, one edge is firmly grasped with a single-tooth tenaculum or myoma screw. Myoma extraction is best accomplished through traction and countertraction. Traction and countertraction will delineate the natural tissue plane and identify vascular attachments that can then be selectively transected with energy. The removed myoma should be avascular and pearly white in appearance. The tenaculum or myoma screw should be replaced into the new edge of the myoma for successive enucleation. It is important never to "dig" or "carve" the myoma out of the uterus. The act of elevating the myoma out of the uterus will help avoid injury to the normal myometrial tissue and inadvertent entry into the endometrial cavity. This elevation is especially important with broad ligament myomas in order to avoid ureteral and uterine artery injury. All efforts should be made to remove all myomas detected to prevent future growth and recurrence of symptoms.

Few studies have examined the technique of laparoscopic myomectomy, and most surgeons have their own operative preferences. Some authors maintain that a myoma is anchored by a pseudocapsule that is formed by connective tissue bridges but lacks its own true vascular pedicle [9]. Macroscopic examination of this tissue reveals parallel arrays of extremely dense capillaries and shows that larger vessels are separated from the myometrium by a narrow avascular cleft. Some myomas have a central vascular network that forms a pedicle. This fibrovascular bundle has been described as the "fibroid neurovascular bundle." These authors maintain that preserving this neurovascular bundle by performing an "intracapsular" myomectomy will have a favorable impact on uterine healing and functionality postoperatively [9].

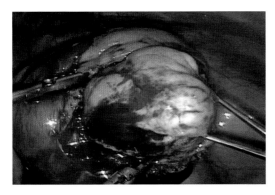

Fig. 2.11 Enucleation of the myoma is accomplished through traction and counter-traction

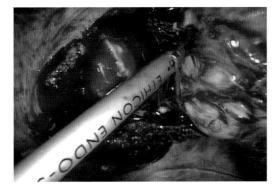

Fig. 2.12 Small vascular attachments are selectively ligated

2.3.3 Uterine Repair

Uterine defects should be closed in a multilayered fashion, eliminating all dead space. Use of a unidirectional, absorbable, barbed suture (V-Loc 180) on a GS-21 needle in a running fashion is extremely helpful. The barbed nature of the suture maintains tension evenly along the length of the defect and facilitates tissue reapproximation by compressing the uterine defect as it is closed, a task that was previously required of the surgical assistant. For large myometrial defects, the muscle fibers will immediately start to contract down. It is not advisable to trim what may seem like redundant tissue as this may be needed for closure to decrease tension on the suture line. Extreme tension may cause the suture to tear through the normal myometrial tissue with increased bleeding and impaired closure. The same multilayered closure that would be performed via open laparotomy should be performed laparoscopically. When closing the serosal layer, an effort should be made to minimize the amount of exposed serosal suture, as in open myomectomy.

If the endometrial cavity is entered, the endometrium is reapproximated with a rapidly dissolving suture like 2-0 Monocryl (Ethicon Inc., San Angelo, TX). Place successive layers over the endometrium with the barbed suture, taking care not to allow the needle to pass through the endometrium. Some surgeons recommend using a balloon stent in the intrauterine cavity that is removed 2 weeks postoperatively. Additionally, they recommend using estradiol 1 mg twice a day for 4 weeks followed by 10 days of progesterone. Postoperative hysteroscopy, sonohysterogram, or hysterosalpingogram can be performed to evaluate the endometrial cavity [10].

If the surgeon is just starting to perform laparoscopic myomectomies, suturing may be a challenge, particularly at lower uterine segment locations or with large defects. In the event of excessive blood loss, where the surgeon feels the suture repair should be expedited, a 3-cm suprapubic horizontal skin incision can be made. To maximize exposure, the fascia is transected in a vertical fashion, resulting in a "cruciate" incision, and a self-retaining retractor, like the Alexis (Applied Medical, Santa Margarita, CA), is placed. This incision can easily be displaced to expose the uterine defect, which can then be brought to the surface for open closure. For posterior lower uterine segment defects, this incision may need to be enlarged for greater exposure. By bringing the uterine incision up to the surface, the bowel does not need to be displaced mechanically. These patients typically recover on the same time line as those with laparoscopic repair.

Preserving the hypertrophied myometrial tissue does not always leave the most cosmetically acceptable surgical appearance at the conclusion of the case, but full preservation is important for future uterine functionality. Postoperative ultrasound studies have shown significant reduction of the uterine scar from 78 % of the previous myoma location on the first day, to 19 % on the 30th day, and less than 4 % on the 45th day [13]. However, depending on what type of suture is used in repair, imaging with ultrasound at 6 weeks often demonstrates artifact from partially dissolved sutures, especially if the patient had a multilayered closure. Therefore, postoperative imaging should be delayed until 3 months for a clearer picture of complete healing. Imaging at 3 months postoperatively will demonstrate the amazing contractile properties of the uterine muscle as it resembles a normal shape.

Myomas should be collected and counted either in the right upper quadrant or cul de sac to ensure complete evacuation from the peritoneal cavity. The use of an intraperitoneal drain removed postoperatively has not been well studied. Use of a drain is helpful in removing postoperative serous drainage. It could also alert the physician to the rare occurrence of significant postoperative bleeding. In our current practice, we use a Jackson-Pratt drain for our larger intramural myomectomies (>10 cm), exiting through one of the 5-mm lateral port sights; the drain is removed on postoperative day 1.

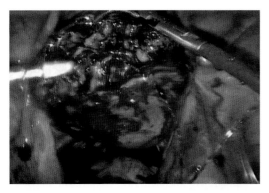

Fig. 2.13 Dead space is closed to prevent hematoma formation

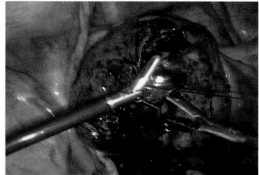

Fig. 2.15 Serosal edges are reapproximated

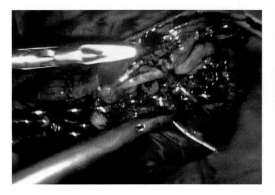

Fig. 2.14 Multilayered closure is performed

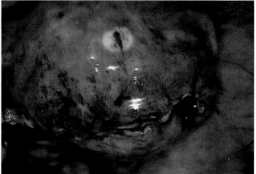

Fig. 2.16 Hemostasis is achieved with suture closure

2.3.4 Morcellation and Removal

A variety of techniques have been described for myoma removal. Removal can be accomplished with one of the disposable morcellators under direct vision. These often require extending one of the 5-mm trocar sights to a 12- to 15-mm incision. Alternatively, the umbilical port site may be extended to 2 cm through the natural creases of the umbilicus within the basin. This is the same technique often recommended for placement of a single-incision laparoscopic port and produces an excellent cosmetic result. Fascia and peritoneal layers are also extended, and a self-retaining retractor is placed for direct tissue extraction using a No. 10 blade on a long handled scalpel. This method is preferred in our practice for quick and efficient tissue removal. When using a cold knife, the No. 10 blades can easily and inexpensively be replaced when they dull, as is commonly encountered with calcified or large fibroids. Pneumoperitoneum is lost with this open morcellation technique, and therefore all fibroids must be accounted for before removal. Smaller fibroids, if multiple, can be placed into an endobag and retrieved through this same extended umbilical incision. Care should be taken to remove all myoma fragments, as postoperative disseminated leiomyomatosis has been extensively described [14].

Careful examination of the operative sight after morcellation should reveal excellent hemostasis. Spot cautery or additional sutures may be needed at the surgeon's discretion. Adjuvant agents, like Floseal (Baxter International Inc.; Deerfield, IL), may be helpful for oozing from the serosal suture lines.

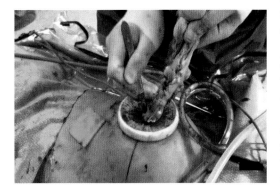

Fig. 2.17 Morcellation is accomplished efficiently using a 2-cm incision in the basin of the umbilicus with a self-retaining retractor

2.3.5 Adhesion Prevention

Adhesion formation after surgery should be considered the most common complication of gynecologic surgery, and myomectomy is well known to have a significant risk of postoperative adhesions formation [15]. Complications of postoperative adhesions include bowel obstruction, pelvic pain, and infertility. National [15, 16] and multinational [17] guidelines on best practices for reducing adhesion formation include the following recommendations: (1) surgeons should attempt to perform procedures using the least invasive method possible; (2) meticulous surgical technique should be employed, including minimizing tissue trauma and achieving optimal hemostasis; and (3) the use of adhesion prevention barriers should be considered after procedures at high risk for postoperative adhesions such as myomectomy.

Three barriers have been well studied in randomized trials [17] that are widely commercially available: polytetrafluoroethylene or Gore-Tex (W.L Gore & Associates; Flagstaff, AZ), oxidized regenerated cellulose or Interceed (Ethicon EndoSurgery Inc.; Blue Ash, OH), and modified sodium hyaluronate/carboxymethylcellulose or Seprafilm (Genzyme Corporation; Boston, MA). Gore-Tex was superior to no treatment and to Interceed in preventing adhesions, but its usefulness is limited by the need for suturing and later removal [16, 18]. Interceed was associated with a reduction in postoperative adhesions [7] but should not be used if there is ongoing risk of bleeding [16]. Seprafilm has been shown to reduce postoperative adhesions, especially after myomectomy [16]; however, there are few data on the benefits of long-term clinical outcomes such as bowel obstruction, pelvic pain, or fertility. No significant adverse events have been reported with these barriers, though none has emerged as a panacea for adhesion prevention.

Seprafilm has been used laparoscopically by creating a slurry [19], although its use in this form has not been well studied on adhesion prevention in gynecologic surgery. Further studies of commercial adhesion prevention and barrier methods that evaluate long-term clinical outcomes are needed.

Table 2.5 Advantages and disadvantages or adhesion prevention barriers

	Advantages	Disadvantages
Gore-Tex (polytetrafluoroethylene)	Most effective barrier when compared to others in laparoscopy or laparotomy.	Need for suturing in place and later removal.
Interceed (oxidized regenerated cellulose)	Shown to be effective in reducing adhesions and relative ease of use.	Should not be used if blood or bleeding risk is present.
Seprafilm (modified sodium hyaluronate/carboxymethycellulose)	Shown to reduce adhesion risk after myomectomy by laparotomy.	Not well studied laparoscopically in gynecologic surgery. Off-label use in slurry form.

Conclusion

Laparoscopic myomectomy has significantly improved patient morbidity and remains the ideal treatment for symptomatic patients desiring future fertility. Large studies are needed to accurately evaluate the advantages and disadvantages of the many variants in technique of each step. Again, no data exist on the amount of time a couple should wait to conceive after the surgery, but most surgeons would recommend waiting 6 months [10].

References

1. Laughlin S, Stewart E. Uterine leiomyomas: individualizing the approach to a heterogeneous condition. Obstet Gynecol. 2011;117:396–402.
2. Dueholm M. Evaluation of the normal uterine cavity with MRI, TV US, hysteroscopic examination and diagnostic hysteroscopy. Fertil Steril. 2001;76:350–7.
3. Halt Fibroid Study, NCT00874029, September 7, 2012, provided by Innovative Analytics, Kalamazoo, MI.
4. Friedman AJ, Lobel SM, Rein MS, Barbieri RL. Efficacy and safety considerations in women with uterine leiomyomas treated with gonadotropin-releasing hormone agonists: the estrogen threshold hypothesis. Am J Obstet Gynecol. 1990;163:1114–9.
5. De Falco M, Staibano S, Mascolo M, Mignogna C, Improda L, Ciociola F, et al. Leiomyoma pseudocapsule after pre-surgical treatment with gonadotropin-releasing hormone agonists: relationship between clinical features and immunohistochemical changes. Eur J Obstet Gynecol Reprod Biol. 2009;144:44–7.
6. Chen I, Motan T, Kiddoo D. Gonadotropin-releasing hormone agonist in laparoscopic myomectomy: systematic review and meta-analysis of randomized controlled trials. J Minim Invasive Gynecol. 2011; 18:303–9.
7. Lethaby A, Vollenhoven B, Sowter M. Pre-operative GnRH analogue therapy before hysterectomy or myomectomy for uterine fibroids. Cochrane Database Syst Rev. 2001;(2):CD000547.
8. Robinson J, Moawad G. Ins and outs of straight-stick laparoscopic myomectomy. OBG Manag. 2012;24: 37–44.
9. Frederick J, Fletcher H, Simeon D, Mullings A, Hardie M. Intramyometrial vasopressin as a haemostatic agent during myomectomy. Br J Obstet Gynaecol. 1994;101:435–7.
10. Burbank F, Hutchins Jr FL. Uterine artery occlusion by embolization or surgery for the treatment of fibroids: a unifying hypothesis-transient uterine ischemia. J Am Assoc Gynecol Laparosc. 2000;7 Suppl 4:S1–49.
11. Park BJ, Kim YW, Maeng LS, Kim TE. Disseminated peritoneal leiomyomatosis after hysterectomy: a case report. J Reprod Med. 2011;56:456–60.
12. Falcone T, Parker W. Surgical management of leiomyomas for fertility or uterine preservation. Obstet Gynecol. 2013;121:856–68.
13. De Wilde RL, Brolmann H, Koninckx PR, et al. Prevention of adhesions in gynaecological surgery: the 2012 European field guideline. J Gynecol Surg. 2012;9:365–8.
14. Robertson D, Lefebvre G, Leyland N, Wolfman W, Allaire C, Awadalla A, et al. SOGC clinical practice guidelines: adhesion prevention in gynaecological surgery: no. 243, June 2010. Int J Gynaecol Obstet. 2010;111:193–7.
15. Diamond MP, Wexner SD, diZereg GS, Korell M, Zmora O, Van Goor H, Kamar M. Adhesion prevention and reduction: current status and future recommendations of a multinational interdisciplinary consensus conference. Surg Innov. 2010;17:183–8.
16. Ahmad G, Duffy JM, Farquhar C, Vail A, Vandekerckhove P, Watson A, Wiseman D. Barrier agents for adhesion prevention after gynaecological surgery. Cochrane Database Syst Rev. 2008;(2):CD000475.
17. Ortiz MV, Awad ZT. An easy technique for laparoscopic placement of Seprafilm. Surg Laparosc Endosc Percutan Tech. 2009;19:e181–3.
18. Tinelli A, Hurst B, Hudelist G, Tsin D, Stark M, Mettler L, et al. Laparoscopic myomectomy focusing on myoma pseudocapsule: technical and outcome reports. Hum Reprod. 2012;27:427–35.
19. Tinelli A, Malvasi A, Hurst B, Tsin D, Davila F, Dominguez G, et al. Surgical management of the neurovascular bundle in uterine fibroid pseudocapsule. JSLS. 2012;16:119–29.

Laparoscopic Adnexal Surgery

3

Anna Fagotti and Giovanni Scambia

Any surgical technique involves the use of specific tools. A well-trained and adequately equipped operating room constitutes the fundamental element for the execution of a secure and effective surgery. The availability of more reliable and advanced technology makes procedures safer.

3.1 Placement of the Patient

The patient is placed flat on the table with her legs wide apart and thighs bent over the basin. For this purpose, leg stirrups are used (Allen Stirrups; Allen Medical Systems, Ashby Park, UK), which facilitate the several variations of approach at any time of the intervention and protect the sterile area. The buttocks are placed on the edge of the table and must be positioned to leave sufficient free space for the mobilization of the uterus, if needed. The arms are fixed along the body to reduce the risk of compression of the brachial plexus and at the same time to enhance and provide flexibility to the movements of the surgeon

and assistant. The patient must rest in a horizontal position until the positioning of all trocars is completed, because the Trendelenburg position accentuates the lumbar lordosis, bringing the great vessels close to the navel and increasing the risk of vascular lesions. Before each gynecologic laparoscopic surgery, it is essential to insert a Foley catheter to empty the bladder.

3.2 Placement of the Surgeons

Two surgeons are needed for this type of surgery. The first surgeon stands to the left of the patient, raised above on a platform for proper ergonomics to help reduce arm muscle fatigue (Fig. 3.1). The nurse stands at the side of the first surgeon to allow for the proper exchange of instruments without hindering the field of view of the surgeons. The second surgeon stands to the right of the patient. In some difficult cases (e.g., deep endometriosis), a third assistant may sit between the legs of the patient to manage the uterine manipulator.

A. Fagotti, MD (✉)
Division of Minimally Invasive Gynecologic Surgery,
St. Maria Hospital, University of Perugia,
Via Tristano di Joannuccio 1, 05100 Terni, Italy
e-mail: annafagotti@libero.it

G. Scambia
Department of Obstetrics and Gynecology,
Catholic University of the Sacred Heart,
Largo Agostino Gemelli 8, 100168 Rome, Italy
e-mail: giovanni.scambia@rm.unicatt.it

P.F. Escobar, T. Falcone (eds.), *Atlas of Single-Port, Laparoscopic, and Robotic Surgery*,
DOI 10.1007/978-1-4614-6840-0_3, © Springer Science+Business Media New York 2014

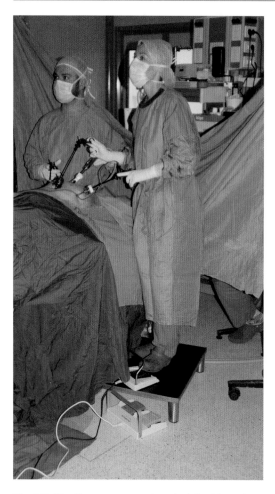

Fig. 3.1 The first surgeon stands to the left of the patient, raised above a platform for proper ergonomics in order to reduce arm muscle fatigue

3.3   Placement of the Trocars

Usually, the first trocar is placed through the umbilicus, but other positions may be explored according to the largest diameter of the adnexa or previous interventions. Different techniques may also be adopted for the insertion of the first trocar, such as the Verress needle, optic trocars, direct trocar, or open access. The diameter of the first trocar may vary between 5 and 10 mm; this is related both to the diameter of the optic and the need to use an endobag large enough to remove the adnexal cyst or adnexa.

Regarding ancillary trocars, we prefer to use three 5-mm trocars because the main instruments for all laparoscopic procedures are frequently 5 mm. Whatever the caliber, in each case the positioning of these trocars at the lateral side of the pelvis and the suprapubic position must always be controlled. At the time of accessory trocar placement, injury of the inferior epigastric vessels can cause bleeding that can be difficult to control. These deep vessels of large diameter cannot be viewed through the transillumination of the wall, which shows only the superficial epigastric vessels. Only palpation of the wall exposing the edge of the rectus abdominis muscle and laparoscopic visualization of this area allow the surgeon to choose the exact point for good trocar placement. The trocar should be introduced perpendicularly to the wall under visual control. The third trocar is introduced at the midline height of the two lateral trocar instruments.

3.4 Placement of Laparoscopic Instruments

There is a wide range of existing instruments for laparoscopic adnexal surgery. It is our opinion that only a few tools are reliable and therefore necessary. It is preferable to use an instrument with a handle and no clamping system in order to make the most dynamic movements. In our opinion, the essential instruments to perform laparoscopic adnexal surgery include

- Grippers: there are different types of grippers; those with a strong hold on the tip are preferable in the event of enucleation (stripping) of the cyst.
- Bipolar forceps: the development and constant search by medical engineering make currently available bipolar forceps completely different than those of the past. The latest generation of bipolar forceps, in fact, allows not only the ability to apply energy to the tissues for hemostatic purpose, but also allows the surgeon to exercise adequate traction. The ideal grasp is one that can be used for the duration of the intervention without the need for replacement and can also be useful to coagulate the ovarian vessels and bed of the cyst.
- Forceps: any type of scissors can be used if they ensure continued reliable cutting.
- Suction/irrigation system: any model can be used that provides adequate visualization of the surgical field and hydrodissection.

Many other new generation instruments are available for both coagulating, cutting, and handling. The choice depends on the surgeon, the type of surgery, and financial capabilities.

3.5 Surgical Technique

The first steps in laparoscopy involve the creation of the pneumoperitoneum and placement of trocars. When done properly, this greatly facilitates the smooth running of the surgery. After trocars are placed, an assessment of the pelvis, abdomen, and external surface of the cyst is performed for possible evidence of malignancy. Peritoneal fluid or washing is collected for cytologic examination. If necessary, lysis of adhesions is performed to free the adnexa. Once surgery and control of bleeding have been completed, the abdomen is deflated, the ports can be removed, and the incisions closed.

3.5.1 Fallopian Tube Surgery

3.5.1.1 Anatomy

The fallopian tubes are paired and symmetric tubular organs, connecting the body of the uterus with the adnexal region and providing a wide area for ovum catch. They can measure from 7 to 12 cm in length and up to 3 mm in thickness. These organs are covered by two layers of peritoneum, forming the mesosalpinx. Each tube can be divided into four portions going from the body of the uterus to the peritoneal cavity: the interstitial, the isthmic, the ampullary, and the fimbriated portions. The tubal branches of the uterine and ovarian arteries anastomose in the round ligament, providing branches for the different portions of the tubes passing through the mesosalpinx. The venous and lymphatic drainage follows the uterine and ovarian vessels. Laparoscopy, or in select cases robotic surgery, is currently the gold standard for tubal surgery.

3.5.1.2 Laparoscopic Salpingectomy
Indications

Monolateral salpingectomy is generally indicated in ectopic pregnancy and for salpingo-ovarian abscess. Bilateral salpingectomy is usually indicated in sterilization and in the prevention of ovarian cancer in high-risk patients.

Surgical Procedure

Once the tube has been isolated, it must be lifted and gently held with atraumatic graspers, without injuring adjacent structures. In order to minimize blood loss, all vessels in the mesosalpinx need to be coagulated. Using a bipolar grasp, it is possible to coagulate the proximal portion until no bleeding is noted. Scissors can be used to cut the coagulated portion. This process needs to be repeated serially in order to move from the proximal to the distal portion of the mesosalpinx. In the case of ectopic pregnancy, an endoscopic loop ligation can be performed, followed by cutting the distal tube to the looped portion. Once the distal portion is cut, the tube is freed and can be removed. Instead, it is also possible to use only monopolar scissors electrosurgically, thus coagulating the tube and then cutting it. If available, multifunctional devices can be used to reduce operative time. Irrigation and suctioning of free blood may help check the bleeding control before closing up the incision..

3.5.1.3 Laparoscopic Salpingostomy
Indications

Monolateral salpingostomy is mainly employed in the surgical conservative management of ectopic pregnancy. Patients need to be informed of the approximate 8 % risk of persistent trophoblastic tissue after the procedure and of possible permanent damage to the Fallopian tube. Chances of these adverse outcomes are increased in cases of high levels of beta-human chorionic gonadotropin (usually more than 6,000 IU/L) or large masses (>3.5–4 cm). Only patients with a strong desire for fertility and/or acceptance of only one functioning tube should undergo this type of procedure.

Surgical Procedure

For the removal of an ectopic pregnancy, a solution of vasopressin should be injected. A 1- to 2-cm longitudinal incision at the level of the tube along the ectopic pregnancy opposite the mesosalpinx is then performed using scissors, bipolar or monopolar, or a carbon dioxide laser. Widening the margins of the incisions, the pregnancy can be removed either with suction-irrigation followed by hydrodissection or with smooth grasping forceps. Any specimen must be extracted, preferably through an endobag. Hemostasis should be accurately checked. Irrigation and suction of free blood and tissue debris are recommended in order to prevent persistent trophoblastic tissue.

3.5.1.4 Tubal Reanastomosis
Indication

Desire for fertility after bilateral tubal ligation.

Surgical Procedure

This complex procedure is currently performed robotically because it provides a three-dimensional magnified view of the operating field, a great degree of freedom in the use of surgical instruments, and suppression of physiologic tremor, thereby enhancing precision. Pregnancy and delivery rates, however, are not encouraging in women over 40 years old.

3.5.2   Ovarian Surgery

3.5.2.1 Anatomy

The ovaries are paired endocrine pelvic organs, lying on either side of the uterus behind the broad ligament. They are attached to the posterior aspect of the broad ligament by the mesovarium, to the ipsilateral uterine cornu by the utero-ovarian ligament, and to the lateral pelvic wall by the infundibulopelvic ligament. The ovarian artery, a branch of the aorta, runs in the infundibulopelvic ligament and anastomoses with the ovarian branch of the uterine artery at the level of the mesovarian border. Here, approximately ten arterial branches originate, penetrating the ovarian hilus and forming a plexus at the corticomedullary junction. Arterioles penetrate the cortex in a radial fashion perpendicular to the ovarian surface. The veins within the ovaries accompany the arteries. The left and right ovarian veins drain into the left renal vein and the inferior vena cava, respectively. Three ill-defined zones are visible on the sectioned surface: an outer cortex, an inner medulla, and the hilus.

The current gold standard for benign ovarian surgery is laparoscopy.

3.5.2.2 Laparoscopic Adnexectomy
Indications

Laparoscopic adnexectomy is indicated when no residual ovarian parenchyma is thought to remain as a result of multilocular endometriotic cysts or large dermoids reaching the hilus vessels, or during the menopausal period, or for prophylactic purposes.

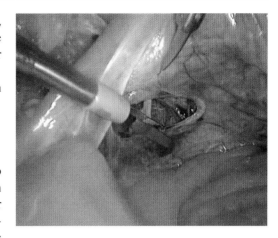

Fig. 3.4 Sequence for adnexectomy. Extension of the fenestration of the broad ligament

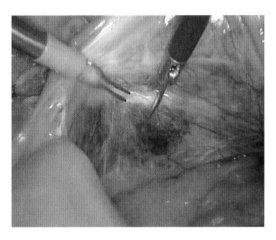

Fig. 3.2 Sequence for adnexectomy. Coagulation of the broad ligament

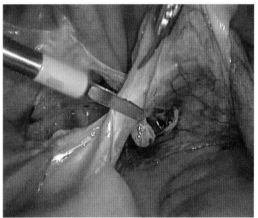

Fig. 3.5 Sequence for adnexectomy. Coagulation of the infundibulopelvic ligament

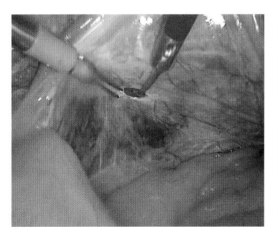

Fig. 3.3 Sequence for adnexectomy. Fenestration of the broad ligament

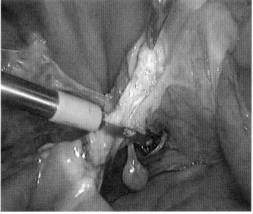

Fig. 3.6 Sequence for adnexectomy. Cut of the infundibulopelvic ligament

Surgical Procedure

To perform adnexectomy, bipolar grasping forceps and scissors are used. The technique consists of opening the wide ligament back to the round ligament, visualizing the ureter, and opening a window between the ovarian vessels and the ureter. In this way a safe coagulation and cut of the ovarian vessels is possible without any injury to the ureter. Then, the utero-ovarian, mesosalpinx, and meso-ovarium are resected and the adnexa can be removed within an endobag to avoid spillage. The bag may be inserted through a 10-mm trocar in the umbilicus to avoid any additional scarring. In the case of large cysts without any preoperative oncologic risk factors, suction of the cyst may be performed to reduce the volume (Figs. 3.2, 3.3, 3.4, 3.5, and 3.6).

3.5.2.3 Laparoscopic Cystectomy
Indications

Any type of ovarian cyst has the potential to be removed by laparoscopy. A clear and open discussion between patient and surgeon still remains the key to a successful procedure.

Surgical Procedure

When possible, the cyst is removed intact, without spillage. If this is not possible, the cyst is opened and drained, and the internal wall is inspected for excrescences or irregular thickening. In the case in which an unexpected endocystic lesion is identified, the cyst is entirely excised (or the adnexa is completely removed) and sent for frozen section examination. The *stripping technique* is performed, utilizing at least three atraumatic grasping forceps (one for the assistant and two for the first surgeon) after having mobilized the adnexa and located the plane of cleavage by cold scissors. Then the cyst capsule is separated from the ovarian tissue by means of repeated diverging tractions. Hemostasis is achieved with bipolar coagulation under irrigation control. The ovarian cortex is left open without suturing. Again, the cyst wall is removed from the abdomen through one of the 5-mm suprapubic trocar sleeves, if feasible; otherwise by an 11-mm trocar in the umbilicus. Recently, different techniques other than stripping have been proposed in order to reduce the trauma at the level of the ovarian parenchyma, thus preserving ovarian function [1–7]. Among these techniques are hydrodissection, laser vaporization, or plasma energy and procoagulating factors [1–7]. However, the recurrence rate and risk of leaving tissue not assessed histologically has not been calculated at this time. According to a recent meta-analysis [8], cystectomy of endometriomas provides better outcomes than fenestration/coagulation or laser ablation in terms of recurrence of symptoms, cyst recurrence, and pregnancy rates (fenestration/coagulation only), but further studies are warranted to clarify the effect of these surgical approaches on ovarian reserve (Figs. 3.7, 3.8, 3.9, 3.10, 3.11, 3.12, and 3.13).

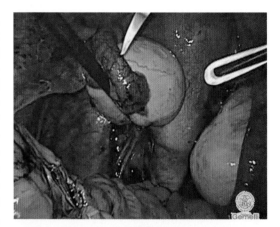

Fig. 3.7 Endometriosis: sequence for enucleating endometriomas. Mobilization of the adnexa

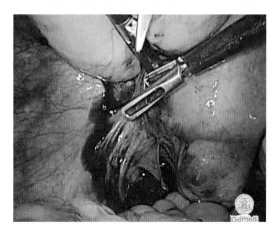

Fig. 3.8 Endometriosis: sequence for enucleating of endometriomas. Rupture of the cyst

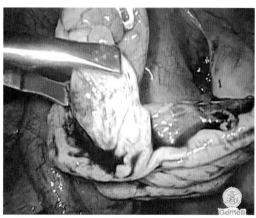

Fig. 3.11 Endometriosis: sequence for enucleating of endometriomas. Extraction of the cyst (part 1)

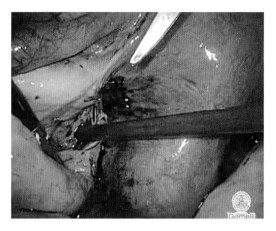

Fig. 3.9 Endometriosis: sequence for enucleating of endometriomas. Suction of the cyst

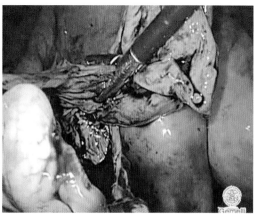

Fig. 3.12 Endometriosis: sequence for enucleating of endometriomas. Extraction of the cyst (part 2)

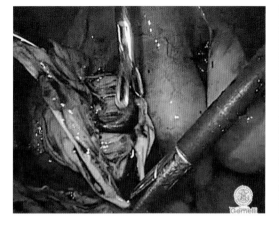

Fig. 3.10 Endometriosis: sequence for enucleating of endometriomas. Location of the plane of the cleavage

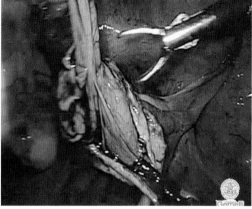

Fig. 3.13 Endometriosis: sequence for enucleating of endometriomas. Extraction of the cyst (part 3)

Conclusions

Laparoscopic adnexal surgery represents the basis of laparoscopic surgery, and in the robotic era it still remains relevant to minimize costs and provide procedural benefits.

References

1. Ferrero S, Venturini PL, Gillott DJ, Remorgida V, Leone Roberti Maggiore U. Hemostasis by bipolar coagulation versus suture after surgical stripping of bilateral ovarian endometriomas: a randomized controlled trial. J Minim Invasive Gynecol. 2012;19:722–30.
2. Morelli M, Mocciaro R, Venturella R, Imperatore A, Lico D, Zullo F. Mesial side ovarian incision for laparoscopic dermoid cystectomy: a safe and ovarian tissue-preserving technique. Fertil Steril. 2012;98:1336.e1–40.e1.
3. Coric M, Barisic D, Pavicic D, Karadza M, Banovic M. Electrocoagulation versus suture after laparoscopic stripping of ovarian endometriomas assessed by antral follicle count: preliminary results of randomized clinical trial. Arch Gynecol Obstet. 2011;283:373–8.
4. Celik HG, Dogan E, Okyay E, Ulukus C, Saatli B, Uysal S, Koyuncuoglu M. Effect of laparoscopic excision of endometriomas on ovarian reserve: serial changes in the serum antimüllerian hormone levels. Fertil Steril. 2012;97:1472–8.
5. Daniell JF, Kurtz BR, Lee JY. Laparoscopic oophorectomy: comparative study of ligatures, bipolar coagulation, and automatic stapling devices. Obstet Gynecol. 1992;80(3 Pt 1):325–8.
6. Saeki A, Matsumoto T, Ikuma K, Tanase Y, Inaba F, Oku H, Kuno A. The vasopressin injection technique for laparoscopic excision of ovarian endometrioma: a technique to reduce the use of coagulation. J Minim Invasive Gynecol. 2010;17:176–9.
7. Angioli R, Muzii L, Montera R, Damiani P, Bellati F, Plotti F, et al. Feasibility of the use of novel matrix hemostatic sealant (FloSeal) to achieve hemostasis during laparoscopic excision of endometrioma. J Minim Invasive Gynecol. 2009;16:153–6.
8. Dan H, Limin F. Laparoscopic ovarian cystectomy versus fenestration/coagulation or laser vaporization for the treatment of endometriomas: a meta-analysis of randomized controlled trials. Gynecol Obstet Invest. 2013;76:75–82.

Laparoscopic Total and Supracervical Hysterectomy

4

Stephen E. Zimberg

Although described as a medical procedure since the second century, the concept of removing the uterus, or hysterectomy, for medical indications has undergone a profound journey from a shunned operation with almost 100 % mortality to one of the most common, nonobstetric operations performed today. Advances in instrumentation and minimally invasive techniques, described in this chapter, have made this a virtually outpatient procedure, with many indications and minimal complication rates. This chapter describes step-by-step techniques to achieve a minimally invasive approach to hysterectomy as well as indications and caveats to minimize medical mishaps. Mastery of the technique is transferable to other minimally invasive pelvic procedures.

Hysterectomy, surgery to remove the uterus, is the most common nonobstetric operation performed in the United States at this time, with 602,457 procedures performed in 2003 alone [1]. In Western countries as a whole, it is the most common surgical procedure performed on women; 23.3 % of women, 18 years or older have a hysterectomy in one form or another [2]. The main indication listed for hysterectomy are fibroids (31 %), uterine prolapse (14.5 %), endometriosis (11 %), abnormal uterine bleeding

(14 %), and cancers of the female genital tract (10 %) [3]. The sentinel event in hysterectomy is attributed to Soranus, the Greek obstetrician practicing in Alexandria and subsequently Rome around 120 AD, who removed a prolapsing uterus through the vagina [4]. In general, the initial attempts were disastrous, with the procedure usually ending in death. Ellis Burnham is credited with performing the first successful hysterectomy in the United States, with the patient surviving, in 1853 in Lowell, Massachusetts [4]. He thought he was operating on an ovarian cyst but when the patient vomited, a large fibroid was delivered into the wound. He tied off both uterine arteries and did a supracervical hysterectomy [4]. Patrick Steptoe introduced the English-speaking world to laparoscopy, although it had been used in Europe in the 1940s [5]; and Harry Reich, in 1988, reported on the first total laparoscopic hysterectomy by completing the hysterectomy laparoscopically, removing it through a colpotomy incision, and closing it laparoscopically [6]. This was followed rapidly by reports of "outpatient laparoscopic-assisted vaginal hysterectomy" [7] and laparoscopic classic intrafascial Semm hysterectomy (CISH) subtotal [8]. Refinements in technique and instrumentation have propelled the laparoscopic approach to account for 14 % of hysterectomies in 2005 (up from 0.8 % in 1990) versus 64 % abdominal and 22 % vaginal [9]. A recent study out of Magee-Womens Hospital in Pittsburgh, PA, looking at 13,973 patients, documented the laparoscopic hysterectomy rate in 2010 of 43.4 %, with abdominal hysterectomy

S.E. Zimberg, MD, MSHA
Department of Gynecology,
Women's Health Institute, Cleveland Clinic Florida,
2950 Cleveland Clinic Boulevard,
Fort Lauderdale, FL 33331, USA
e-mail: zimbers@ccf.org

P.F. Escobar, T. Falcone (eds.), *Atlas of Single-Port, Laparoscopic, and Robotic Surgery*,
DOI 10.1007/978-1-4614-6840-0_4, © Springer Science+Business Media New York 2014

accounting for 36.3 % and vaginal hysterectomy accounting for 17.2 % [10]. Hysterectomy for gynecologic malignancy accounted for 24.4 % of these cases [10].

Laparoscopic hysterectomy would include total laparoscopic hysterectomy (TLH), laparoscopic supracervical hysterectomy (LSH), robotic assisted hysterectomy (RA), and laparoscopic assisted vaginal hysterectomy (LAVH). The basic technique for the laparoscopic portion of all of the subgroups is essentially similar and will be described below as either the total laparoscopic hysterectomy or laparoscopic supracervical hysterectomy.

There are few contraindications for total laparoscopic hysterectomy because this technique can be used in both benign and malignant conditions. Large benign fibroids can be adequately handled with LSH and TLH by an experienced surgical team. We have found that moving the trocar port sites cephalad gives the best advantage to these cases. Large malignant tumors are probably better handled by conventional laparotomy, but smaller lesions can be well addressed via the minimally invasive route. Malignancy of the uterus, cervix, or ovary is certainly a contraindication for laparoscopic supracervical hysterectomy because the morcellation process will spread the tumor and probably upstage the patient. Additionally, endometriosis in the cul-de-sac and lower uterine segment is best handled by removal of the cervix (TLH), since chronic pain may occur if it is left in.

4.1 Getting Started

The laparoscopic approach at its most basic requires adequate visualization of the pelvis and the uterus and the adnexal structures. As basic as it sounds, having an operating room table with adequate ability to achieve a steep patient Trendelenburg position is of paramount importance. Steep Trendelenburg is often 30° or greater to allow the intestine to migrate cephalad, thereby exposing the pelvic contents. The patient is placed in the dorsal lithotomy position and the legs are placed in Allen or similar stirrups. Securing the patient safely on the table is often a challenge, particularly with obese patients. We have been placing the patient directly on an egg crate mattress secured to the operating table as described by Klauschie and coworkers [11]. This allows for the use of steep Trendelenburg with minimal slippage and has the advantage of working even with the morbidly obese patient without extra straps or shoulder braces that can predispose to neurologic and other injuries in longer procedures. One particular axiom is that the larger the patient, the greater the Trendelenburg angle that is required for adequate visualization.

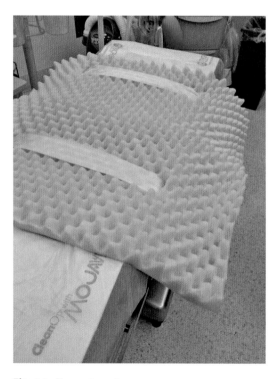

Fig. 4.1 Egg crate mattress

The patient is then fitted with a uterine manipulator to allow for greater movement and fewer ports to achieve the desired angles at which to operate. For the laparoscopic supracervical hysterectomies, we have been using a reusable Hulka tenaculum, and for the total laparoscopic hysterectomy, a VCare uterine manipulator (ConMed Endosurgery; Utica, NY) to outline the vaginal cuff. Other manipulators are on the market and can work equally well for these procedures.

Entry into the abdomen is gained through the use of trocars with the initial placement of a 5-mm trocar into the umbilicus for uteri up to 14 weeks in size and above the umbilicus for uteri larger than 14 weeks. This allows for adequate visualization of the pelvic structures. Accessory trocars are placed on the right and left sides traditionally 2 cm superior and medial to the anter-superior iliac spine under direct vision. We have found that this placement is often not

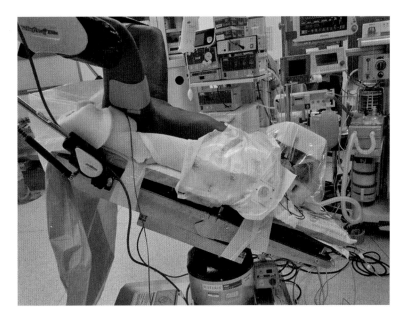

Fig. 4.2 Trendelenburg position

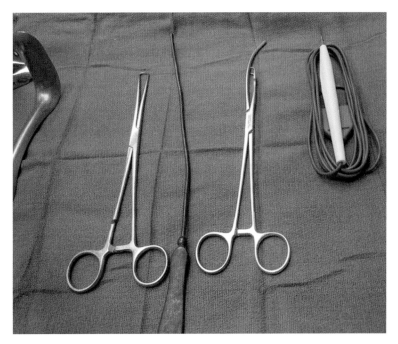

Fig. 4.3 Hulka tenaculum

adequate for good operating angles, and we prefer to determine placement at the time of insufflation with CO_2 gas once the patient is placed in
the Trendelenburg position. The size of the
uterus and the pelvic pathology, such as adhesions and endometriosis, determine the placement, with a 5-mm trocar placed on the patient's
right side and a 10-mm one placed on the
patient's left side for laparoscopic supracervical
hysterectomy. Larger uteri, such as those greater
than 18 weeks in size, require a 5-mm trocar for
the camera above the umbilicus and 10-mm trocars on each side, since 10-mm instruments are
needed for movement of the large uterus secondary to the torque (smaller instruments may

bend). Placement is decided at the time of insufflation once the angles needed for surgery are
determined.

For total laparoscopic hysterectomy, 3-mm,
5-mm, and one 10-mm port are used with a
5-mm port placed either in or above the umbilicus and 5-mm ports placed in the right and
left lower quadrants as determined by the
anatomy. A 10-mm port is then placed on the
patient's left side in the middle quadrant for
suture introduction and sewing. These ports
are moved cephalad if the uterus is larger.
The insufflation tubing is placed on one of
the lateral 5-mm ports, and smoke evacuation
is placed on one of the ports on the opposite

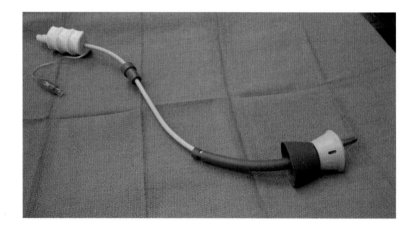

Fig. 4.4 VCare uterine
manipulator (Courtesy
of ConMed Endosurgery,
Utica, NY)

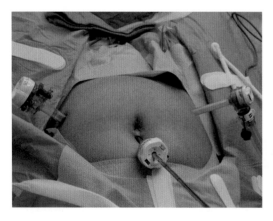

Fig. 4.5 Standard trocar placement

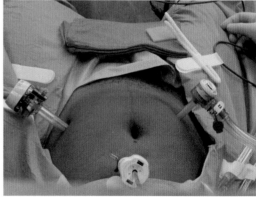

Fig. 4.6 Trocar placement for large uteri

side. Removal of smoke or water vapor from lysed tissue is essential for good visualization. The recent introduction of the AirSeal insufflator (Surgiquest; Millford, CT), allows heated insufflation and smoke evacuation from a single port and protects the pneumoperitoneum, which is an advantage in total laparoscopic hysterectomy and obese patients.

The general instrumentation for the standard laparoscopy is available in most operating rooms. Graspers such as bowel graspers and Maryland forceps as well as tenacula and laparoscopic scissors are used to manipulate the tissue and move the bowel. Electrosurgical devices are used to coagulate the blood vessels and cut the tissue. We tend to use the Sonicision Shears (Covidien Ltd.; Boulder, CO) for most dissection, vessel sealing, and cutting, as this one instrument can be used rather than several for tasks such as removing the uterus from the cervix in LSH and removing the cervix from the vagina in TLH. Large pedicles such as the infundibulo-pelvic ligament or uterine vessels are coagulated first with standard reusable bipolar cautery forceps with an impedance generator as an added precaution. Other vessel sealing and ligation devices are also available such as EnSeal (Ethicon Endo-Surgery Inc.; Somerville, NJ) and LigaSure (Covidien Ltd.; Boulder, CO).

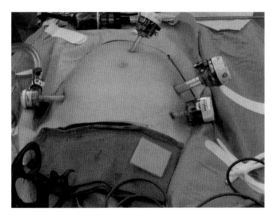

Fig. 4.7 Total laparoscopic hysterectomy trocars

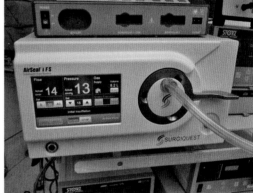

Fig. 4.8 AirSeal insufflator (Courtesy of SurgiQuest, Milford, CT)

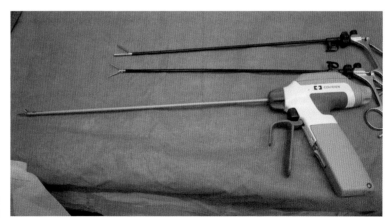

Fig. 4.9 Sonicision (Courtesy of Covidien Ltd., Boulder CO)

4.2 Procedure for Total Laparoscopic Hysterectomy

When the patient is asleep and in the lithotomy position, a bimanual examination is performed to evaluate the size of the uterus and any additional disease that may be present. Standard prophylactic preoperative antibiotics are given for hysterectomy. A standard Foley catheter is placed to drain the bladder during the procedure, although a two-port catheter may be useful if lower uterine segment adhesions are anticipated in order to inject dye to delineate the borders of the bladder in a scarred environment. We use a paracervical block with bupivicane and epinephrine to decrease pain post-procedure. If using a VCare uterine manipulator, the cup should be sutured to the cervix to aid in retrieval of the specimen. Once the uterine manipulator is placed, a 5-mm laparoscope is placed in the camera port. With the patient in the steep Trendelenburg position, full inspection of the abdomen and pelvis is performed. The uterus and adnexal structures are evaluated. Placement of the accessory ports is then done once in the Trendelenburg position with a 5-mm port in the right and left lower quadrants and a 10-mm port in the left middle quadrant for TLH and a 5-mm port on the right and a 10-mm port on the left for supracervical hysterectomy.

Step 1

The harmonic scalpel is then used to take the round ligament, utero-ovarian ligament, and tube on the left side as the first step in the procedure. If the ovary is to be taken, the infundibulopelvic ligament is coagulated first and then taken using the harmonic scalpel or another vessel-sealing device.

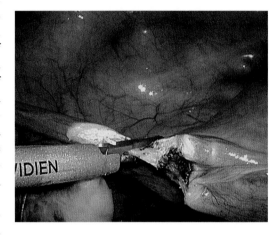

Fig. 4.11 Taking round and utero-ovarian ligament

Step 2

The broad ligament is opened, and the uterine vessels are exposed. This is done with harmonic energy to delineate the leaves using the cavitation effect of the harmonic scalpel. Alternatively, other vessel-sealing devices or plain monopolar scissors may be used for this step.

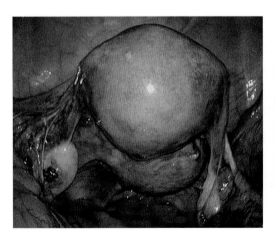

Fig. 4.10 Inspection of the pelvis

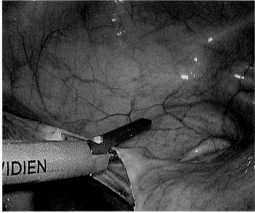

Fig. 4.12 Opening for broad ligament

Step 3

The bladder flap is then opened to expose the lower uterine segment and cervix as well as to move the bladder out of the way for the cervical dissection. Adhesions in this area are common, and sharp dissection is done to remove the bladder from the lower uterine segment. Injury to the bladder is common in this location, and if it occurs, it has been our experience to complete the dissection of the bladder from the cervix with adequate margins prior to repairing the bladder using a simple two-layer closure with polydioxanone (PDS) or Vicryl suture, usually 3-0 gauge.

Step 4

The posterior peritoneum at the level of the lower uterine segment is opened using harmonic energy, a vessel-sealing energy source, or scissors with monopolar energy. Following this, the uterine vessels should be exposed and are coagulated with a bipolar cautery prior to incising the vessels using the harmonic scalpel. Technically, the harmonic scalpel should handle up to 7-mm vessels, which is appropriate for most uterine arteries, but our experience has been that bipolar cautery is often needed as a backup.

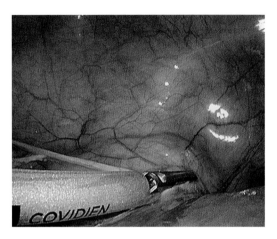

Fig. 4.13 Bladder flap

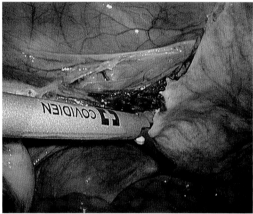

Fig. 4.14 Isolate and take uterine vessels

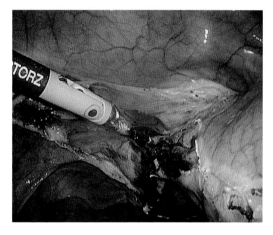

Fig. 4.15 Coagulation of the uterine artery

Step 5

This is a repeat of step 1, but on the right side, which involves taking the round ligament, utero-ovarian ligament (or infundibulopelvic ligament), and tube. The pedicles can either be taken with the harmonic scalpel or a vessel-sealing device or cauterized first with a bipolar cautery if the vessels are very large. Steps 2 and 3 are repeated on this side, as previously noted.

Step 6

The uterine vessels are isolated on the right side and coagulated with a bipolar cautery. The vessels are then moved laterally using the harmonic scalpel to move them over the cervical cup and well away from the vagina, leaving a 1- to 2-cm cuff for dissection. The ureters should be off to the side and well out of harm's way. The blood supply to the uterus should now be completely isolated, and no further bleeding should occur.

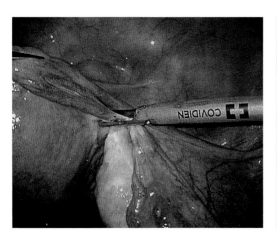

Fig. 4.16 Taking contralateral side

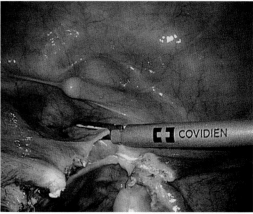

Fig. 4.17 Isolation of the uterine vessels

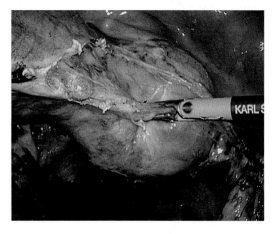

Fig. 4.18 Taking and moving of the cervical cup

Step 7

The cervix is then dissected free of the vagina using the harmonic scalpel or monopolar scissors or hook. The dissection occurs over the VCare cup, Rumi uterine manipulator (CooperSurgical; Trumbull, CT), McCartney transvaginal tube (LiNA; Glostrup, Denmark), a sponge on a sponge-stick, or other device that is being used in the vagina. The uterus is pulled into the vagina and the fundus is used to occlude the vagina and maintain the pneumoperitoneum. Alternatively, the uterus can be removed and a wet sponge placed in a glove or a similar device can be used to occlude the vagina. In the case of an excessively large uterus, vaginal morcellation can be accomplished in the standard fashion using a coring or bivalve technique to remove the uterus from the vagina.

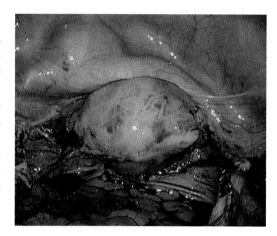

Fig. 4.21 Pulling of the uterus into the vagina

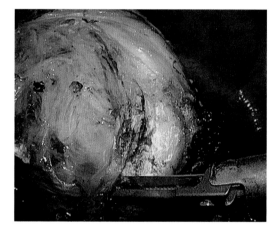

Fig. 4.19 Dissection of the cervix

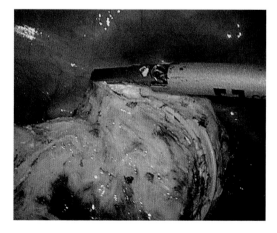

Fig. 4.20 Removal of the cervix

Step 8

Once removed from its vaginal attachments, the pedicles are inspected for bleeding. We have been using a modified Richardson stitch at the vaginal angles incorporating the uterosacral ligaments as originally described for open hysterectomy by Richardson in 1929 [12]. This involves placement of a stitch in a figure-of-eight fashion at the vaginal angles and taking the uterosacral ligament, being careful not to involve the vaginal mucosa when using a permanent stitch. Care must also be taken not to kink the ureter if using this stitch. We use number 1 prolene for this.

The remaining portions of the vagina are closed using absorbable suture in interrupted figure-o-eight fashion, providing a watertight vaginal closure. Our practice is to use 0 PDS or Vicryl suture for this. Alternatively, one of the new barbed sutures such as VLoc can be used for this purpose. Care must be taken to get beyond the thermal damage to the cuff in closing the vagina. Care must also be taken to avoid the bladder, thereby preventing the possibility of a later fistula. The finished cuff is well suspended. To help with pain management postoperatively, we have been using 5 cc of 2 % lidocaine jelly intravaginally at the end of the procedure. This can also be used postoperatively in this form or 5 mL in injectable form every 4–6 h to help with low pelvic pain that patients often have postoperatively.

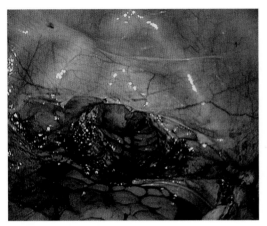

Fig. 4.22 Inspection of cuff pedicles

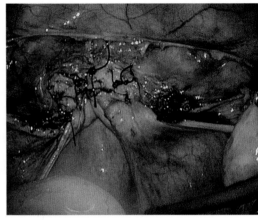

Fig. 4.25 Well-suspended finished cuff

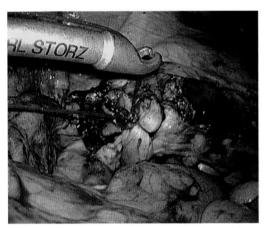

Fig. 4.23 Modified Richardson stitch

Step 9

If the ovaries are left in situ, we have been removing the fallopian tubes prophylactically to decrease the risk of tubal or adnexal malignancy later in life [13]. This is done using the harmonic scalpel, bipolar cautery and scissors, or other vessel-sealing device. It adds little time to the procedure and may have dramatic benefits over time.

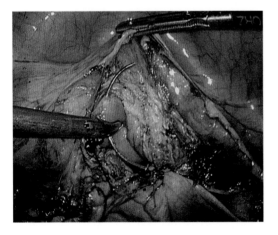

Fig. 4.24 Vaginal closure with absorbable suture

4.3 Procedure for Laparoscopic Supracervical Hysterectomy

To accomplish the LSH, Steps 1–6 remain the same. Once the uterus is devascularized above the level of the lower uterine segment, it is amputated from the cervix at the level of the lower uterine segment. Because the cervix is being left in situ, a normal Papanicolaou smear within the last year is advisable as well as an endometrial biopsy confirming that no malignant or premalignant change in the endometrium or endocervix has occurred. In the case of a supracervical hysterectomy, we have been cauterizing the endocervix from the vaginal side prior to placement of the uterine manipulator by using the cautery and ablating the cervical os. We then use a reusable Hulka tenaculum or VCare uterine manipulator.

Step 7

The uterus is amputated using the harmonic scalpel at the level of the internal os. Alternatively, monopolar scissors or a monopolar wire loop can be used. Once this is performed, the endocervix is cauterized from above using a bipolar cautery to ablate the endocervix and lessen the chance of cyclic bleeding. The combination of cauterization of the vaginal portion of the endocervix from below and the endocervix from above has lowered our incidence of cyclic bleeding to 3 %. Most remaining spotting postoperatively can be treated in the office by using silver nitrate or Monsels solution in the endocervix. The cervix is then closed with a stitch of number 1 PDS suture to prevent peritoneal fluid from leaking through the open cervical os.

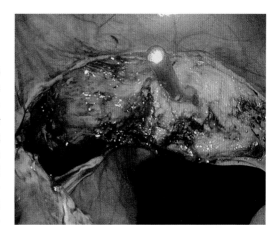

Fig. 4.26 Amputation of the uterus

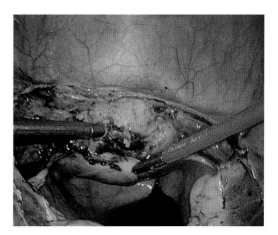

Fig. 4.27 Cautery of endocervix

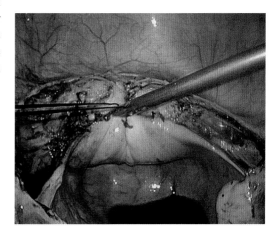

Fig. 4.28 Closure of the cervix

Step 8

The uterus is then morcellated by placing a mechanical morcellator through the left-sided 10-mm port site or the umbilicus. It is our practice to use the left lower quadrant port site because visualization and the tracking of any loose fragments of uterus from the morcellation are easier, although an umbilical or right-sided approach is acceptable, depending on the case. We have been using the Karl Storz morcellator (Karl Storz; El Segundo, CA, USA) for morcellation owing to its variable power settings. This is a reusable motor and trocar with a disposable blade. There are numerous other morcellators on the market, both reusable and disposable. Individual preference dictates which is best for each surgeon. All fragments of the uterus and endometrium should be removed prior to closure, owing to well-documented cases of parasitic myomas and iatrogenic endometriosis [9].

Step 9

As in the previous section, the fallopian tubes are removed prophylactically for ovarian cancer risk reduction. See the previous Step 9 for hysterectomies done via a single port and robotically.

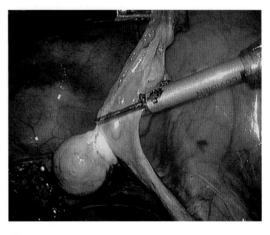

Fig. 4.30 Prophylactic salpingectomy

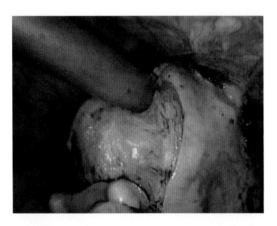

Fig. 4.29 Morcellation

4.4 Postoperative Care

The Foley catheter is removed in the operating room unless bladder repair has been performed, and the patient undergoes standard postanesthesia care. Once the patient's postoperative pain is under control and she is able to urinate, she is discharged from the outpatient center and followed in 2 weeks in the office. A hemoglobin and hematocrit reading is checked 2 h postoperatively prior to discharge. For those patients unable to urinate, which is an occasional issue secondary to dissection, anesthesia, or concomitant procedures, the catheter is left in for 2 days and removed in the office to avoid overdistension and damage. The patient is sent home with narcotic analgesics and in the case of TLH, vaginal lidocaine jelly, as previously described.

When the patient goes home, she is encouraged to achieve early ambulation prior to leaving the outpatient unit. A large part of a successful transition from the outpatient unit to home is preoperative management of expectations: the patient and the family know that the patient is being discharged on the same day and what her limitations might be. The use of an abdominal binder is also helpful in ambulation during the postoperative period, as it provides support to the patient's core.

4.5 Complications

As with any procedure, complications related to laparoscopy by itself and complications unique to the type of surgery may occur. Bojahr and colleagues looked at this in 1,706 consecutive patients (Berlin) in 2006 [14], and the results are illustrative. The mean uterine weight was 226 g with a mean operative time of 91 min. Fifty two percent had previous laparotomy. Of the 1,706 procedures performed, 14 patients were converted to laparotomy owing to their size and immobility and one because of adhesions. There were two bladder injuries and one ureter injury in an 818-g uterus. Overall, there was a 1.2 % postoperative complication rate (infection, bleeding). Kafy and coworkers looked at 1,792 patients

comparing abdominal, vaginal, and laparoscopic hysterectomy [15]. The overall morbidity was 6.1 % with one bowel injury in the laparoscopic and abdominal hysterectomy groups, two bladder injuries in the laparoscopic and abdominal hysterectomy groups, and one ureter injury in the abdominal hysterectomy group. Vaginal hysterectomy was associated with more urinary retention and hematoma formation. Conversion rates were 1.7 % in the laparoscopic group and 0.4 % in the vaginal hysterectomy group. Reoperation rate was 0.4 % in the abdominal group; overall morbidity was low in all groups, and no deaths occurred.

Laparoscopic removal of large uteri represents a particular challenge and barrier for many surgeons. Alpern did a retrospective analysis of Kaiser Permanente's experience of 446 consecutive cases with uteri over 500 g [16]. The median uterine weight was 786 g (500–4,500). Life-threatening complications occurred in 0.7 % of cases with re-operation in 0.45 % of cases. There were six cystotomies, and 92.8 % of cases were discharged on postoperative day 0 with a 1.1 % readmission rate. There was no association between perioperative complications and morbidity and patient/surgical characteristics.

Total laparoscopic hysterectomy, done conventionally or with the robot (as well as total abdominal and vaginal), has a unique complication in the form of vaginal cuff dehiscence. It is a matter of debate as to whether this is secondary to the suturing technique or is caused by thermal injury to the cuff, particularly with the use of monopolar energy. In a 2012 Italian study, Uccella and associates did a multi-institutional analysis of 12,398 patients who underwent hysterectomy for both benign and malignant disease, examining the rate of cuff dehiscence with different types of closure [17]. Total laparoscopic hysterectomy was associated with the highest number of cuff separations (23 or 0.64 %), versus 9 abdominal (0.2 %) and 6 vaginal (0.13 %). Laparoscopic suturing of the vaginal cuff had the highest rate of separation (0.86 %) over transvaginal suturing (0.24 %). Reducing the monopolar current from 60 to 50 W did not alter the cuff separation rates. Blikkendaal and coworkers, in a retrospective cohort Dutch study in 2012, compared techniques of laparoscopic cuff closure [18]. They compared the incidence of vaginal cuff dehiscence after closure with transvaginal interrupted, laparoscopic interrupted, and laparoscopic running suture with conventional or bidirectional barbed suture. Their data did not show superiority of one technique over the other.

Laparoscopic supracervical hysterectomy has three unique associated complications that are procedure-specific. The first is continued cyclic bleeding after surgery, as the cervix is left in situ. This appears to be in the range of 17–19 %. The study by Ghomi and colleagues in 2005 is representative [19]. The objective was to estimate the incidence of bleeding when the cervix is amputated at or below the level of the internal os. They confirmed this with tissue biopsy and found a total incidence of any bleeding at 19 % and the incidence of cyclic bleeding to be 17 % regardless of the age, body mass index, presence of endometriosis, adenomyosis, endocervical fulguration, or a history of previous cesarean section. Interestingly, we have found that cauterization of the endocervix with monopolar cautery from the vagina prior to hysterectomy, followed by cauterization of the endocervix from above after the uterus is amputated at the level of the endocervix, has dropped our bleeding rate at The Cleveland Clinic to 3.5 %. Postoperatively, much of this can be reduced by the use of silver nitrate in the os in the office for refractory cases, with a 0.25 % trachelectomy rate for nonresponsive cases.

Case reports of iatrogenic leiomyomatosis and endometriosis from the morcellation process have been reported but can be mitigated by careful search of the abdomen for fragments after morcellation [20]. This has been reported from months to years after a procedure and is now well recognized. We try to eliminate this possibility by washing down the morcellating trocar prior to withdrawal, thereby preventing port site contamination as well as careful searching of the abdomen prior to closure.

The complication of LSH of most concern is the inadvertent morcellation of a gynecologic malignancy or de novo cervical cancer in a retained cervical stump. The risk of cancer of the cervix following a subtotal hysterectomy is 0.11 % with cautery of the endocervix [21]. Standard guidelines for Pap smear surveillance are indicated in these patients.

The risk of sarcoma in our population is 1.7/100,000 and represents less than 1 % of gynecologic malignancies. Parker reported on 1,332 patients operated on for symptomatic leiomyomata, with half being done for "rapid growth" [22]. Only one patient had a leiomyosarcoma in the group and none met the published criteria for "rapid growth." This report gave an incidence of sarcoma in patients operated on for leiomyomas of 0.23 and 0 % for rapid growth. Theben and coworkers in 2012 analyzed 1,584 laparoscopic supracervical hysterectomy German patients for unexpected malignancy [23]. All of the patients were screened for malignancy with cytologic examination (Pap smear) and preoperative ultrasound or dilatation and curettage. Unexpected malignancies were found in four patients (0.25 %) screened in the above manner and two endometrial carcinomas were found and two sarcomas were found. This showed a very small probability of unexpected malignancies in patients who were appropriately screened and remains a good procedure for presumed benign disease. Once found, surgical staging is imperative as soon as possible. Memorial Sloan-Kettering Hospital retrospectively reviewed all of their cases of malignancy found at supracervical hysterectomy or after morcellation from 2000 to 2006 [24]. Seventeen patients were identified, with 15 having presumed stage 1 disease and two with stage 3 disease. Approximately 15 % will be upstaged with completion surgery, but in the remaining 85 % who undergo completion surgery and are not upstaged, the prognosis is good.

Conclusion

Both LSH and TLH represent minimally invasive alternatives to conventional abdominal and sometimes vaginal procedures. This chapter describes our technique for successful achievement of both techniques. Reoperation rates are equivalent in the two procedures with no differences in intraoperative and postoperative complications noted, with a trend toward lower complications in the LSH group [25]. A method-specific procedure after the LSH was trachelectomy, which occurred in 2.7 % of patients, and repair of vaginal cuff dehiscence, which occurred after TLH in 0.7 % of patients. In addition, both procedures offer documented increases in quality of life. Einarsson and associates completed a prospective evaluation of quality of life in TLH versus LSH using validated quality of life questionnaires [26]. Laparoscopic supracervical hysterectomy appears to provide greater improvement in short-term quality of life compared with TLH. No significant differences were noted in postoperative pain or return to daily activities. Mastering both techniques will allow for continued conversion to minimally invasive alternatives for most gynecologic procedures.

References

1. Wu JM, Wechter ME, Geller EJ, Nguyen TV, Visco AG. Hysterectomy rates in the United States, 2003. Obstet Gynecol. 2007;110:1091–5.
2. Merrill RM. Hysterectomy surveillance in the United States, 1997 through 2005. Med Sci Monit. 2008;14: CR24–31.
3. US Department of Health and Human Services Centers for Disease Control and Prevention National Center for Health Statistics. Health, United States 2006 with chartbook on trends in the health of Americans. Table 99. Hyattsville; 2006.
4. Sutton C. Hysterectomy: a historical perspective. Baillieres Clin Obstet Gynaecol. 1997;11:1–22.
5. Steptoe PC. Gynecological endoscopy-laparoscopy and culdoscopy. J Obstet Gynaecol Br Commonw. 1965;72:535–43.
6. Reich H, de Cipro J, McGlynn F. Laparoscopic hysterectomy. J Gynecol Surg. 1989;5:213–5.
7. Summitt Jr RL, Stovall TG, Lipscomb GH, Washburn SA, Ling FW. Outpatient hysterectomy: determinants of discharge and rehospitalization. Am J Obstet Gynecol. 1994;17:1480–4; discussion 1484–7.
8. Semm K. Endoscopic subtotal hysterectomy without colpotomy; classic intrafascial Semm hysterectomy. A new method of hysterectomy by pelviscopy, laparotomy, per vaginam or functionally by total uterine mucosal ablation. Int Surg. 1996;81:362–414.
9. Sepillian V, Della Badia C. Iatrogenic endometriosis caused by uterine morcellation during a supracervical hysterectomy. Obstet Gynecol. 2003;102(5 pt 2): 1125–7.
10. Turner LC, Shepherd JP, Wang L, Bunker CH, Lowder JL. Hysterectomy surgical trends: a more accurate depiction of the last decade. Am J Obstet Gynecol. 2013;208:277.e1–e7.
11. Klauschie J, Wechter ME, Jacob K, Zanagnolo V, Montero R, Magrina J, Kho R. Use of anti-skid material and patient-positioning to prevent patient shifting during robotic-assisted gynecologic procedures. J Minim Invasive Gynecol. 2010;17:504–7.
12. Richardson EH. A simplified technique for abdominal panhysterectomy. Surg Gynaecol Obstet. 1929;48: 248–51.
13. Anderson CK, Wallace S, Guiahi M, Sheeder J, Behbakht K, Spillman MA. Risk-reducing salpingectomy as preventative strategy for pelvic serous cancer. Int J Gynecol Cancer. 2013;23:417–21.
14. Bojahr B, Raatz D, Schonleber G, Abri C, Ohlinger R. Perioperative complication rate in 1706 patients after a standardized laparoscopic supracervical hysterectomy technique. J Minim Invasive Gynecol. 2006; 13:183–9.
15. Kafy S, Huang JY, Al-Sunaidi M, Wiener D, Tulandi T. Audit of morbidity and mortality rates of 1792 hysterectomies. J Minim Invasive Gynecol. 2006;3: 55–9.
16. Alpern M, Kivnick S, Poon KY. Outpatient laparoscopic hysterectomy for large uteri. J Minim Invasive Gynecol. 2012;19:689–94.
17. Uccella S, Ceccaroni M, Cromi A, Malzoni M, Berretta R, De Iaco P, et al. Vaginal cuff dehiscence in a series of 12,398 hysterectomies: effect of different types of colpotomy and vaginal closure. Obstet Gynecol. 2012;120:516–23.
18. Blikkendaal MD, Twijnstra AR, Pacquee SC, Rhemrev JP, Smeets MJ, de Kroon CD, Jansen FW. Vaginal cuff dehiscence in laparoscopic hysterectomy: influence of various suturing methods of the vaginal vault. Gynecol Surg. 2012;9:393–400.
19. Ghomi A, Hantes J, Lotze EC. Incidence of cyclical bleeding after laparoscopic supracervical hysterectomy. J Minim Invasive Gynecol. 2005;12: 201–5.
20. Hilger WS, Magrina JF. Removal of pelvic leiomyomata and endometriosis 5 years after supracervical hysterectomy. Obstet Gynecol. 2006;108:772–4.
21. Johns A. Supracervical hysterectomy vs total abdominal hysterectomy. Clin Obstet Gynecol. 1997;40: 903–13.
22. Parker WH, Fu YS, Berek JS. Uterine sarcoma in patients operated on for presumed leiomyoma and rapidly growing leiomyoma. Obstet Gynecol. 1994;83:414–8.
23. Theben JU, Schellong AR, Altgassen C, Kelling K, Schneider S, Große-Drieling D. Unexpected malignancies after laparoscopic-assisted supracervical hysterectomy (LASH): an analysis of 1584 LASH cases. Arch Gynecol Obstet. 2013;287:455–62.

24. Einstein MH, Barakat RR, Chi DS, Sonoda Y, Alektiar KM, Hensley ML, Abu-Rustum NR. Management of uterine malignancy found incidentally after supracervical hysterectomy or uterine morcellation for presumed benign disease. Int J Gynecol Cancer. 2008;18:1065–70.

25. Boosz A, Lermann J, Mehlhorn G, Loehberg C, Renner SP, Thiel FC, et al. Comparison of re-operation rates and complication rates after total laparoscopic hysterectomy (TLH) and laparoscopy-assisted supracervical hysterectomy (LASH). Eur J Obstet Gynecol Reprod Biol. 2011; 158:269–73.

26. Einarsson JI, Suzuki Y, Vellinga TT, Jonsdottir GM, Magnusson MK, Maurer R, et al. Prospective evaluation of quality of life in total versus supracervical laparoscopic hysterectomy. J Minim Invasive Gynecol. 2011;18:617–21.

Laparoscopic Excision of Endometriosis

5

Rebecca Rossener, Luiz Fernando Pina Carvalho,
Juan Luis Salgado, and Mauricio S. Abrao

Endometriosis is a gynecologic disease that affects more than 150 million women around the world. The disease is usually found in the pelvic cavity, affecting the ovaries, the fallopian tubes, the peritoneum, and the rectovaginal septum; it is less commonly found in the abdominal cavity affecting the small bowel, the large bowel, and other abdominal organs. It has been established that the best examination to evaluate endometriosis is transvaginal ultrasonography with bowel preparation. The laparoscopic ablation or excision of endometriotic lesions has as its objectives pain relief or fertility improvement and increasing the patient's quality of life. It is essential to remove all visible lesions and to biopsy the doubtful ones in order to reduce the chances of recurrences and repeat surgery. Therefore, it is important to keep in mind that the laparoscopic treatment should always be a diagnostic procedure as well, regardless of the previous imaging evaluation. The appearance of peritoneal endometriotic lesions in laparoscopy is widely variable. They can have the typical black appearance or atypical red, white, or yellow lesions, or they can form adhesions and anatomic distortions. Ovarian endometriosis can present as hemorrhagic superficial lesions or hemorrhagic cysts. The surgery for endometriomas must minimize the ovarian tissue trauma in all possible situations and concurrently remove all unhealthy tissue. The deep infiltrative lesions, on the other hand, are focused on a clinical presentation centered on pain. The operation comprises liberation of the adhesions or, less commonly, bowel resection. Endometriotic lesions in the urinary tract usually have cyclical urinary alterations as symptoms. The surgery is done aiming at minimal damage to the tissues. Laparoscopic surgery has a fundamental role in the management of endometriosis. In conclusion, surgical planning must be aligned with each patient's pathologic condition. It is still the gold standard for diagnosis, and excision of lesions can reduce pain symptoms and increase the fertility rate, contributing to improving patient quality of life.

R. Rossener • L.F.P. Carvalho • M.S. Abrao, MD (✉)
Department of Obstetrics and Gynecology,
University of São Paulo, São Paulo, SP, Brazil
e-mail: rebecca.rossener@gmail.com;
luizcarvalho.dr@me.com; msabrao@mac.com

J.L. Salgado, MD
Department of Obstetrics and Gynecology,
Universidad Central Caribe School of Medicine,
Bayamon, PR 00956, USA
e-mail: salgadomd@migsec.com

P.F. Escobar, T. Falcone (eds.), *Atlas of Single-Port, Laparoscopic, and Robotic Surgery*,
DOI 10.1007/978-1-4614-6840-0_5, © Springer Science+Business Media New York 2014

5.1   Introduction

Endometriosis is a gynecologic disease that affects more than 150 million women around the world. It does not discriminate based on ethnicity or social background. Several studies have shown that the prevalence of the disease affects approximately 10 % of women in the reproductive age group, meaning that one 1 of every 10 women will have endometriosis [1].

Endometriosis is defined as the occurrence of endometrial stroma and glands outside the endometrial cavity. The ectopic implants can induce a chronic inflammatory reaction that leads to adhesions and distortion of the tissues and pelvic anatomy [2].

The disease is usually found in the pelvic cavity affecting the ovaries, fallopian tubes, peritoneum, rectovaginal septum; less commonly it is found in the abdominal cavity, the small bowel, the large bowel, and other abdominal organs [2]. In addition, there are reports of endometriosis affecting distal organs, such as the lungs, brains, and eyes [3].

Endometriosis is very commonly diagnosed several years after initial symptoms appear [4, 5] owing to lack of patients' awareness about the significance of their symptoms, assuming that some of them, like dysmenorrhea and dyspareunia, are normal. A lack of knowledge about the disease may also delay physician diagnosis [4].

Consequently, many patients are found with an advanced stage of endometriosis at the time of initial diagnosis. Several organizations worldwide are working to create awareness so that diagnosis is made earlier. Early diagnosis and treatment can prevent complications. Even though endometriosis is not cancer, it behaves similarly by invading and not respecting the boundaries of the organs.

5.2   Clinical Aspects

There are many ways to classify endometriosis and the distribution of lesions found at each stage, but none have been fully accepted. The most commonly used classification is from the American Society for Reproductive Medicine (ASRM) [6], in which Stage I disease is minimal, Stage II is mild, Stage III is moderate, and Stage IV is severe as seen in Fig. 5.1). Therefore, the classification of disease can only be determined after surgical pelvic evaluation [6].

Owing to the difficulties found in the use of the existing methods of classification, the American Association of Gynecological Laparoscopists (AAGL) is formulating a new classification for the disease based on pain, infertility, and surgical difficulty, which are criteria that are not considered by the ASRM classification [7]. The main symptoms of endometriosis are dysmenorrhea, chronic pelvic pain, dyspareunia, cyclical intestinal alterations, cyclical urinary alterations, and infertility, with the latter occurring in 40 % of women with endometriosis [2, 8]. Pain is usually assessed by a visual scale analysis. The clinical examination, including the gynecologic examination, can be normal or unspecific. Some of the alterations that can be found are visible lesions on external genital organs, pain during the mobilization of the cervix, nodules, and thickenings on palpable ligaments.

Many scientists have attempted explanations Physiopathology for the development of endometriosis, such as endometrial tissue and cell reflux during menstruation as described by Sampson [9], the differentiation of other cells from endometrial cells (metaplasia), and the hematogenous and lymphatic spread of endometrial cells [9, 10]. However, the disease has been evidenced in patients with the absence of a uterus or in men who have taken high doses of estrogen for prostatic cancer, showing that no theory fully explains the physiopathology of endometriosis [9, 10].

**AMERICAN SOCIETY FOR REPRODUCTIVE MEDICINE
REVISED CLASSIFICATION OF ENDOMETRIOSIS**

Patient's Name _____ Date_____

Stage I   (Minimal)   · 1-5
Stage II (Mild)   · 6-15   Laparoscopy_____ Laparotomy_____ Photography_____
Stage III (Moderate) · 16-40   Recommended Treatment_____
Stage IV (Severe)   · >40   _____
Total_____   Prognosis_____

PERITONEUM	**ENDOMETRIOSIS**	<1cm	1-3cm	>3cm
	Superficial	1	2	4
	Deep	2	4	6
OVARY	R Superficial	1	2	4
	Deep	4	16	20
	L Superficial	1	2	4
	Deep	4	16	20

	POSTERIOR CULDESAC OBLITERATION	Partial		Complete
		4		40

	ADHESIONS	<1/3 Enclosure	1/3-2/3 Enclosure	>2/3 Enclosure
OVARY	R Filmy	1	2	4
	Dense	4	8	16
	L Filmy	1	2	4
	Dense	4	8	16
TUBE	R Filmy	1	2	4
	Dense	4*	8*	16
	L Filmy	1	2	4
	Dense	4*	8*	16

*If the fimbriated end of the fallopian tube is completely enclosed, change the point assignment to 16.

Denote appearance of superficial implant types as red [(R), red, red-pink, flamelike, vesicular blobs, clear vesicles], white [(W), opacifications, peritoneal defects, yellow-brown], or black [(B) black, hemosiderin deposits, blue]. Denote percent of total described as R___%, W___% and B___%. Total should equal 100%.

Additional Endometriosis: _____ | Associated Pathology: _____
_____ | _____
_____ | _____
_____ |

To Be Used with Normal | To Be Used with Abnormal
Tubes and Ovaries | Tubes and/or Ovaries
L   R | L   R

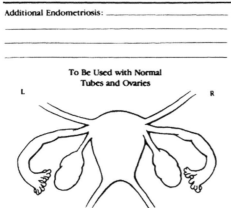

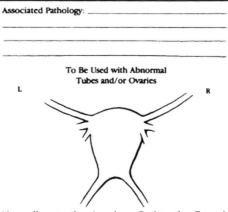

Fig. 5.1 Revised classification of endometriosis by American Society for Reproductive Medicine. The localization and size of the endometriotic lesions are the main markers used to provide classification of the disease (According to the American Society for Reproductive Medicine, classification can only be determined after surgery)

Table 5.1 Main symptoms of endometriosis

Symptom	Peritoneal	Ovarian	Deep	P
Severe dysmenorrhea	22 (51.8 %)	126 (48.5 %)	229 (62.9 %)	0.005
Chronic pain	96 (50.3 %)	143 (54.8 %)	233 (63.5 %)	0.006
Infertility	56 (28.7 %)	66 (25.2 %)	124 (34.1 %)	0.03
Cyclic dyschezia	21 (11.4 %)	33 (13 %)	120 (33.5 %)	<0.001
Cyclic dysuria	27 (14.1 %)	34 (13 %)	56 (15.3 %)	0.71
Dyspareunia	97 (51.6 %)	138 (52.9 %)	227 (63.4 %)	0.007

A study of 819 patients helped define main symptoms and their variance of the disease [8]

What is known is that genetics plays an important role in its development. Patients who have first-degree relatives who have or have had the disease have a six times higher possibility of developing endometriosis than those without such a relative. The prevalence is 4–9 % in first-degree relatives [11]. Diagnosis histology is still the gold standard to diagnose endometriosis. Biopsy is done by laparoscopy. However, surgical diagnosis is considered an invasive procedure, and efforts are being made to develop less invasive techniques with high sensibility and specificity, such as transvaginal ultrasonography and the CA 125 test.

The CA 125 blood levels measurement is a laboratory test commonly used as an ovarian cancer marker of epithelial origin and also to evaluate patient response to chemotherapy. But it can also be used as a predictor of endometriosis [12]. However, many studies demonstrate that it is not as good a predictor for early stages such as I and II (mild and moderate endometriosis) as it is for severe endometriosis [13].

It has been established that the best examination to evaluate endometriosis is transvaginal ultrasonography (TV-USG) with bowel preparation. It can detect lesions that are larger than 2 cm. For deep infiltrating endometriosis (DIE), studies have demonstrated that the TV-USG has 98 % sensibility and 100 % specificity, which are better than the results of magnetic resonance imaging (MRI) [14]. Therefore, it is important and feasible to diagnose the disease early in life in order to prevent long-term complications.

Likewise, ovarian endometriosis has been well documented with TV-USG as well as with MRI. Both show the same results, but the former is less expensive. On the other hand, lesions involving ureters are better evaluated by MRI than by TV-USG for a more accurate identification of the site of the lesion.

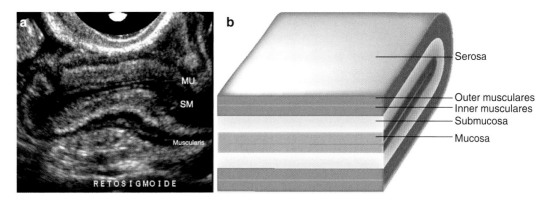

Fig. 5.2 Transvaginal ultrasound showing intestinal layers. (**a**) A rectosigmoid section showed by ultrasound with all layers delimited. (**b**) With careful analysis of each layer, endometriotic lesions can be diagnosed by ultrasound. *MU* musculares, *SM* submucosas

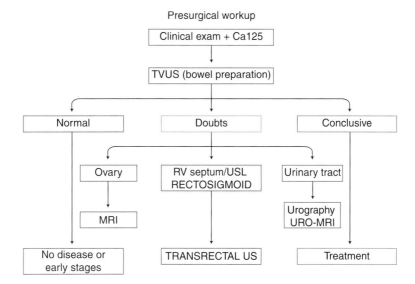

Fig. 5.3 Flow chart for diagnosis of endometriosis. The investigation starts with the clinical history and the physical examination; although the measure of CA 125 levels can be used as well, it has low sensibility and specificity. The next step is to perform a transvaginal ultrasound (*TV-US*) with bowel preparation by professionals specializing in finding lesions of endometriosis in ultrasound images. If these steps are conclusive for endometriosis, then treatment should be planned. With a normal image examination, there is probably no disease or it is in very early stages. If the initial investigation is inconclusive, other imaging examinations can be indicated according to the probable location of the lesions. *MRI* magnetic resonance imaging, *URO-MRI* urologic magnetic resonance imaging

5.3   Treatment

Treatment for endometriosis should be individualized for each patient. Management of the disease should only be initiated after careful analysis of symptoms and image examinations, after thorough discussion with the patient regarding the consequences of each procedure and reason for treatment (pain, pregnancy). Furthermore, endometriosis is frequently a multisystem disease, and this is the reason why treatment requires a multidisciplinary team to provide the best care for patients [15]. This often includes other areas of medicine, such as proctology and urology, as well as other health care areas, such as psychology and physiotherapy.

Treatment of endometriosis consists mainly of three procedures: pharmacologic ovarian suppression, painkillers, and video-assisted laparoscopic surgery. The pharmacologic treatment involves any agent that blocks ovarian hormone production and theoretically reduces pain, as endometriotic lesions are responsive to hormone levels [16].

5.4   Laparoscopic Surgery

The benefits of laparoscopic surgery versus laparotomy for endometriosis have been established in the literature [17]. Laparoscopic surgery provides better visualization of the pelvic cavity, less formation of adhesions, faster discharge of the patient, lower costs, and less postoperative pain, the last being essential for a patient who already suffers pain owing to the disease.

The objectives of laparoscopic ablation or excision of endometriotic lesions include pain relief, improved fertility, and improved patient quality of life [18]. It is imperative to remove all visible lesions and to biopsy any doubtful lesions to reduce the chance of recurrence and reoperation [19]. However, even with complete resection, the recurrence rate is high [19]. Fibrotic tissue surrounding the lesions should be removed as well because the tissue is reactive to hormones and can lead to recurrence of disease [19].

The main indications for laparoscopic surgery are pain, pelvic pain refractory to pharmacologic treatment, severe disease with anatomic distortion, large endometriomas, bowel involvement, urinary obstructions, contraindication for hormone therapy, and potential malignant disease. There is also scientific evidence supporting the benefits of laparoscopic surgery in infertile endometriosis patients who have previously failed to conceive spontaneously or by in vitro fertilization (IVF). Laparoscopic surgery has been shown to increase pregnancy outcome [20].

The first step of laparoscopic treatment should always be a diagnostic procedure, despite previous image evaluation. Careful analysis of pelvic anatomy during surgery can help with more precise excision of lesions and in classification of disease stage. Many implants are called "iceberg lesions," when the deep level of the disease is not consistent with its superficial laparoscopic appearance, another reason to insist on a complete examination of pelvic lesions.

There are two possible surgical approaches: conservative and complete. Conservative surgery consists of maintaining the uterus and as much of the ovarian tissue as possible in order to preserve fertility. On the other hand, complete surgery is characterized by total removal of the uterus with or without removal of the ovaries. According to the ASRM, the indications for a complete surgery are recurrent conservative surgeries, disabling pain without reproductive desire, and associated uterine diseases that must be treated with hysterectomy [21].

A low-residue diet is recommended before all surgeries, and bowel preparation is necessary when lesions are in the rectovaginal septum or when there is need for a hysterectomy. The anesthesia is general and can be associated with peridural blockage. The patient is put in a Trendelenburg position between a 10-degree and 45-degree incline in order to keep the intestinal loops away from field of vision [22].

Laparoscopy is initiated with a vertical incision in the inferior portion of the umbilical scar and insufflation of carbon dioxide with a Veress needle to deliberately create a pneumoperitoneum. A 10-mm trocar is inserted into the umbilical incision, and two other auxiliary punctures are made in the suprapubic area to insert 5-mm trocars. In some cases, another 5-mm port can be placed for better triangulation [22]. If the content to be removed is larger, one of the auxiliary trocars can be substituted for a 12-mm port.

The appearance of peritoneal endometriotic lesions in laparoscopy is widely variable. They can have a typical black or atypical red, white, or yellow appearance, or form adhesions and anatomic distortions [6]. Removal of lesions is usually done by excision or cauterization. Excision includes carbon dioxide laser or monopolar current for bigger lesions. Cauterization is used to treat more punctiform lesions with a bipolar current laser until normality is restored.

Ovarian endometriosis can present as hemorrhagic superficial lesions or hemorrhagic cysts. Those lesions hardly respond to treatment and is the reason that the presence of large endometriomas is an important indication for surgery. It has already been demonstrated that ovarian endometriosis is

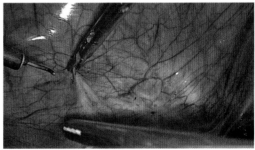

Fig. 5.5 Peritoneal endometriotic lesions. In this image of a laparoscopic surgery, red lesions of peritoneal endometriosis can be seen

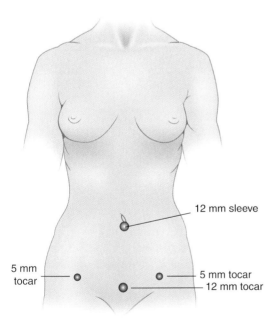

5 mm tocar

12 mm sleeve

5 mm tocar
12 mm tocar

Fig. 5.4 Position of trocars in a laparoscopic procedure. Generally, a 12-mm trocar is inserted into the umbilical incision, and two 5-mm trocars are inserted in the suprapubic area. Depending on the surgeon, another 5-mm trocar can be inserted in the suprapubic area

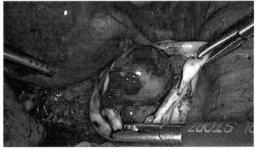

Fig. 5.6 Endometrioma. A large endometrioma looking like a hemorrhagic (or chocolate, in current language) cyst that is leaking

associated with an increased risk of ovarian cancer [23]. Therefore, it is absolutely necessary to look for malignant aspects of the ovaries during surgery. When performing a conservative procedure, trauma to the ovarian tissue must be minimized, with concurrent removal of all unhealthy tissue [24].

There are many different ways to remove an endometrioma. The two most common procedures are drainage of the cysts or cystectomy. There is a great deal of discussion about the advantages and detriments of each technique [25]. If the cyst is smaller than 3 cm, incision, drainage, aspiration, and capsule cauterization can be performed. If the endometrioma is larger than 3 cm, implying greater ovarian damage, a cystectomy with complete removal of the capsule is recommended [26].

Deep infiltrative lesions are responsible for clinical presentation of pain. It can affect the rectovaginal septum and the ureters and bowel, and preoperative care involves bowel preparation and antibiotics. The disease can be total or partial and is determined during the surgery. If the cul-de-sac is normal, impairment is partial. If the rectum is adhered to the rectovaginal septum or the uterus, there is total impairment. The operation comprises the liberation of the anterior wall of the rectum and the uterosacral ligaments with laser, electrosurgery, or scissors. According to Koninckx and coworkers [27], bowel resections are rare in these surgeries unless the nodule is in the bowel.

The laparoscopic segmental resection of the rectum affected by endometriosis includes the following successive steps:

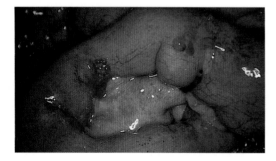

Fig. 5.7 Deep infiltrative endometriosis. Laparoscopic image showing the anatomic pelvic distortion caused by deep infiltrative disease

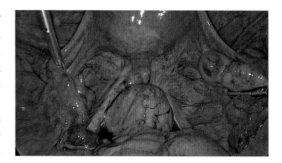

Fig. 5.8 Bowel endometriosis. Laparoscopic image of small bowel endometriotic lesions

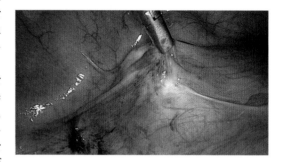

Fig. 5.9 Endometriosis of the urinary tract. Laparoscopic image of endometriosis in the bladder

1. Placement of an umbilical incision and insufflation of CO_2 through the Veress needle to obtain proper pneumoperitoneum and subsequent insertion of a 10-mm trocar and optics.
2. Insertion of three auxiliary trocars, two at the iliac fossa (10–12 mm on the right and 5 mm on the left) and a 5-mm trocar in the left flank.
3. Examination of the abdominal and pelvic cavities and identification of all the sites affected by endometriosis.
4. Lysis of the any adhesions affecting the adnexal regions, uterine fundus, posterior cul-de-sac, and uterosacral ligaments and relevant bowel adhesions.
5. Release of the sigmoid from the left lateral abdominal wall and from the retroperitoneum and identification of the left ureter up to the level of the pelvic brim.
6. Opening of the mesosigmoid.
7. Mobilization of the rectum by dissecting its anterior wall from the posterior surface of the

cervix, followed by a linear stapler applied distal to the area affected by the disease.

8. The 10–12-mm incision on the right iliac fossa is enlarged sufficiently to exteriorize the divided bowel enclosing the diseased portion. The proximal stump is sutured to form a pouch; the ogive of the circular stapler is placed inside the stump.

9. The bowel containing the ogive is reintroduced into the abdominal cavity; the abdominal incision is closed.

10. The circular stapler is introduced through the anus, connected to the ogive, and activated to form the end-to-end anastomosis.

The next step is to ascertain the integrity of the ureters and the anastomotic site. The latter is checked under laparoscopic control by injecting 120 cc of air into the rectum, which is submerged in irrigation fluid to ensure that there is no leakage. In addition, a dilute solution of methylene blue is introduced into the rectum to confirm the absence of leakage.

Endometriotic lesions in the urinary tract usually present cyclical urinary alterations as symptoms. The surgery is done aiming at minimal damage to the tissues. However, in cases with ureteral obstruction, a more aggressive approach is needed with extensive resection of the endometriosis, uretero-ureteral reanastomosis, and ureteral reimplantation. It is important to remember that in all cases of endometriosis in the bladder, a cystoscopic examination is necessary in order to observe the anatomy of the bladder.

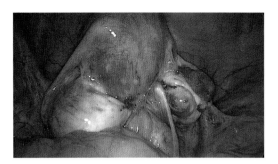

Fig. 5.10 Frozen pelvis in advanced deep infiltrating endometriosis

Conclusion

Laparoscopic surgery plays a central role in the management of endometriosis. It is still the gold standard for diagnosis of the disease, excision of the lesions, reduction of the pain, and increasing fertility—all of which contribute to improving patient quality of life. Thus, some essential principles of laparoscopic treatment should be kept in mind, such as the principle of the "one-shot" surgery, which involves careful analysis of the pelvic cavity with excision and biopsy of all confirmed and suspected lesions. In addition, surgical planning must be aligned with each patient's individual needs, especially concerning fertility preservation after surgery, which determines the surgeon's choice of a complete or conservative approach.

References

1. Burney RO, Giudice LC. Pathogenesis and pathophysiology of endometriosis. Fertil Steril. 2012;98: 511–9.
2. Giudice LC. Clinical practice. Endometriosis. N Engl J Med. 2010;362:2389–98.
3. Huang H, Li C, Zarogoulidis P, Darwiche K, Machairiotis N, Yang L, et al. Endometriosis of the lung: report of a case and literature review. Eur J Med Res. 2013;18:3.
4. Arruda MS, Petta CA, Abrão MS, Benetti-Pinto CL. Time elapsed from onset of symptoms to diagnosis of endometriosis in a cohort study of Brazilian women. Hum Reprod. 2003;18:756–9.
5. Nnoaham KE, Hummelshoj L, Webster P, d'Hooghe T, de Cicco Nardone F, et al. World Endometriosis Research Foundation Global Study of Women's Health Consortium. Impact of endometriosis on quality of life and work productivity: a multicenter study across ten countries. Fertil Steril. 2011;96:366–73.
6. Revised American Society for Reproductive Medicine classification of endometriosis: 1996. Fertil Steril. 1997;67:817–21.
7. Chapron C, ABrao MS, Miller CE. Endometriosis classification need to be revied: A new one is arriving. NewsScope.2012; 26:9.
8. Bellelis P, Dias Jr JA, Podgaec S, Gonzales M, Baracat EC, Abrão MS. Epidemiological and clinical aspects of pelvic endometriosis – a case series [in English and Portuguese]. Rev Assoc Med Bras. 2010;56:467–71.
9. Sampson JA. Metastatic or embolic endometriosis, due to the menstrual dissemination of endometrial tissue into the venous circulation. Am J Pathol. 1927;3: 93–110.
10. Carvalho L, Podgaec S, Bellodi-Privato M, Falcone T, Abrão MS. Role of eutopic endometrium in pelvic endometriosis. J Minim Invasive Gynecol. 2011;18: 419–27.
11. Nouri K, Ott J, Krupitz B, Huber JC, Wenzl R. Family incidence of endometriosis in first-, second-, and third-degree relatives: case–control study. Reprod Biol Endocrinol. 2010;8:85.
12. Abrão MS, Podgaec S, Pinotti JA, de Oliveira RM. Tumor markers in endometriosis. Int J Gynaecol Obstet. 1999;66:19–22.
13. Patrelli TS, Berretta R, Gizzo S, Pezzuto A, Franchi L, Lukanovic A, et al. CA 125 serum values in surgically treated endometriosis patients and its relationships with anatomic sites of endometriosis and pregnancy rate. Fertil Steril. 2011;95:393–6.
14. Abrao MS, Gonçalves MO, Dias Jr JA, Podgaec S, Chamie LP, Blasbalg R. Comparison between clinical examination, transvaginal sonography and magnetic resonance imaging for the diagnosis of deep endometriosis. Hum Reprod. 2007;22:3092–7.
15. Dell'oro M, Collinet P, Robin G, Rubod C. Multidisciplinary approach for deep endometriosis: interests and organization [article in French]. Gynecol Obstet Fertil. 2013;41:5864.
16. Triolo O, Laganà AS, Sturlese E. Chronic pelvic pain in endometriosis: an overview. J Clin Med Res. 2013;5:153–63.
17. Chapron C, Dubuisson JB, Fernandez B, Dousset B. Surgical treatment of endometriosis [article in French]. Rev Prat. 1999;49:276–8.
18. Bianchi PH, Pereira RM, Zanatta A, Alegretti JR, Motta EL, Serafini PC. Extensive excision of deep infiltrative endometriosis before in vitro fertilization significantly improves pregnancy rates. J Minim Invasive Gynecol. 2009;16:174–80. Erratum in J Minim Invasive Gynecol. 2009;16:663.
19. Paka C, Miller J, Nezhat C. Predictive factors and treatment of recurrence of endometriosis. Minerva Ginecol. 2013;65:105–11.
20. Chapron C, Fritel X, Dubuisson JB. Fertility after laparoscopic management of deep endometriosis infiltrating the uterosacral ligaments. Hum Reprod. 1999;14:329–32.
21. Practice Committee of American Society for Reproductive Medicine. Treatment of pelvic pain associated with endometriosis. Fertil Steril. 2008;90(5 Suppl):S260–9.
22. Khan J, Gill M, Clarke H. Onset of benign paroxysmal positional vertigo after total laparoscopic hysterectomy in the Trendelenburg position. J Minim Invasive Gynecol. 2012;19:798–800.
23. Vargas-Hernández VM. Endometriosis as a risk factor for ovarian cancer [in Spanish]. Cir Cir. 2013;81:163–8.
24. Donnez J, Squifflet J, Jadoul P, Lousse JC, Dolmans MM, Donnez O. Fertility preservation in women with ovarian endometriosis. Front Biosci (Elite Ed). 2012;4:1654–62.
25. Somigliana E, Benaglia L, Vigano P, Candiani M, Vercellini P, Fedele L. Surgical measures for endometriosis-related infertility: a plea for research. Placenta. 2011;32 Suppl 3:S238–42.
26. Sugita A, Iwase A, Goto M, Nakahara T, Nakamura T, Kondo M, et al. One-year follow-up of serum anti-müllerian hormone levels in patients with cystectomy: are different sequential changes due to different mechanisms causing damage to the ovarian reserve? Fertil Steril. 2013;100(2):516–22.e3.
27. Koninckx PR, Ussia A, Adamyan L, Wattiez A, Donnez J. Deep endometriosis: definition, diagnosis, and treatment. Fertil Steril. 2012;98:564–71.

Techniques in Gynecologic Oncology

Michael Frumovitz

Gynecologic oncologists have been performing various minimally invasive procedures for some time for both uterine and cervical cancer. For apparent early-stage ovarian cancer, a minimally invasive approach also seems adequate; however, for advanced disease, an open exploration and maximal effort at tumor debulking still remains the standard of care. Minimally invasive procedures may be used for radical hysterectomy, pelvic and para-aortic lymphadenectomy, and omentectomy. Although most associate radical hysterectomy with cervical cancer, para-aortic lymphadenectomy with uterine cancer, and omentectomy with ovarian cancer, these procedures may be used for any gynecologic malignancy. Some patients may undergo more than one of these minimally invasive techniques. Minimally invasive procedures unique to gynecologic oncology are described in this chapter.

6.1 Introduction

In the 1960s, gynecologists developed laparoscopy as a means to visualize pelvic anatomy and quickly innovated from diagnostic to operative laparoscopy by performing tubal ligations in the 1970s. However, in the 1980s, urologists led the development of the approach for the treatment of cancer, with gynecologic oncologists trailing the uptake with minimal utilization throughout the 1990s. In 2003, a minority of gynecologic oncologists felt that a minimally invasive approach was appropriate for treating any pelvic malignancy [1]. However, less than 5 years later, the majority of gynecologic oncologists recognized the value of patient care and oncologic equivalence in relation to minimally invasive surgery [2]. As frequently happens with new technologies and procedures, widespread adoption into clinical care often occurs based on retrospective studies, clinical judgment, and expert opinion. This, too, has been the case in gynecologic oncology, in which minimally invasive surgery is now routinely employed to treat women with uterine, cervical, and ovarian cancers.

For women with uterine cancer, many gynecologic oncologists were performing minimally invasive hysterectomy and staging long before the data showed it was oncologically equivalent to open surgery. In 2012, however, results from the LAP2 study were published [3]. This randomized study of 2,616 women with uterine cancer confirmed what all had assumed: open and minimally invasive approaches to uterine cancer had equivalent disease-free and overall survival rates [3]. Furthermore, women who underwent laparoscopy had better short-term quality of life and shorter hospital stays than those who had laparotomy. Interestingly, long-term (6 months) quality of life characteristics were equivalent [4].

M. Frumovitz, MD, MPH
Department of Gynecologic Oncology,
Unit 1362, M. D. Anderson Cancer Center,
1515 Holcombe Boulevard, Houston, TX 77030, USA
e-mail: mfrumovitz@mdanderson.org

P.F. Escobar, T. Falcone (eds.), *Atlas of Single-Port, Laparoscopic, and Robotic Surgery*,
DOI 10.1007/978-1-4614-6840-0_6, © Springer Science+Business Media New York 2014

Similar to the treatment of women with uterine cancer, a majority of patients with cervical cancer are being offered a minimally invasive approach for treatment. Typically, radical hysterectomy and bilateral pelvic lymphadenectomies are performed for stage IA2/IB1 disease as well as for stage IA1 disease with high-risk features such as lymphovascular space invasion. However, the oncologic equivalency of this approach in these tumors is supported by retrospective studies that demonstrate equivalent pathologic parameters and recurrence rates, not survival [5, 6]. A prospective validation study similar to LAP2 is currently under way [7].

Unlike uterine and cervical cancers, the appropriateness of a minimally invasive approach for women with ovarian cancer remains controversial [2] because the goal of surgery for women with ovarian cancer is complete cytoreduction to microscopic disease. For women with stages III and IV disease, we believe strongly that optimal cytoreductive surgery can only be achieved through a laparotomy via a vertical incision, and we do not perform minimally invasive surgery for tumor debulking in these patients. However, some have advocated a diagnostic laparoscopy in patients with obvious metastatic disease to assess for resectability of tumors [8, 9]. This use of minimally invasive surgery may be appropriate in women with widely metastatic disease. For women with clinical stage I disease, a minimally invasive surgery and staging are reasonable. The necessary staging surgery for ovarian cancer, including exploration, peritoneal biopsies, omentectomy, and pelvic and para-aortic lymphadenectomies can be done laparoscopically [10, 11]. For these patients with disease limited to the ovaries, a minimally invasive surgery seems equivalent to a laparotomy [12].

In this chapter, minimally invasive procedures that are unique to gynecologic oncology are described and include radical hysterectomy, pelvic and para-aortic lymphadenectomy, and omentectomy. Although most associate radical hysterectomy with cervical cancer, para-aortic lymphadenectomy with uterine cancer, and omentectomy with ovarian cancer, these procedures may be used for any gynecologic malignancy. For example, a patient with clinical stage II uterine serous carcinoma may undergo a radical hysterectomy, pelvic and para-aortic lymphadenectomies, and omentectomy.

6.2 Total Laparoscopic Radical Hysterectomy

6.2.1 General Considerations

A radical hysterectomy removes not only the uterine fundus and cervix (as in a simple hysterectomy) but also a portion of the upper vagina and parametrium en bloc. Removal of these additional margins are what classifies the procedure as "radical" and what increases the operative morbidity and technical difficulty beyond those of a simple hysterectomy. For women with early stage cervical cancer, however, this extra dissection is necessary to determine disease status beyond the cervix, since the tumor may have already spread to the vagina or the parametrium by either direct extension or through the lymphatics into the parametrial nodes.

The radicality of the procedure may be tailored to tumor factors such as size and location. The most commonly used classification for radical hysterectomy was originally proposed in 1974 by Piver, Rutledge, and Smith (Table 6.1) [13]. In 2008, Querleu and Morrow proposed an updated classification that considered parasympathetic nerve preservation and paracervical tissue involvement (Table 6.2) [14].

For patients with cervical cancer, radical hysterectomy is almost always accompanied by pelvic lymphadenectomy. Pelvic lymphadenectomy is important because 15–20 % of patients with stage I disease may have disease that has spread to draining nodes and lymphatic channels, and tumors carrying emboli may bypass the parametrium and directly implant in the pelvic nodal basins [15]. Currently, data are emerging that lymphatic mapping and sentinel node biopsy may be adequate for women with early stage cervical cancer (tumors <2 cm) [16, 17]; however, this approach is not yet the standard of care. Removal of aortocaval nodes is done at the discretion of the surgeon.

Removal of the ovaries is not necessarily required as part of radical hysterectomy. Performance of salpingo-ophorectomy should be personalized to patients based on age, reproductive history, and tumor histology. If adnexectomy is to be performed, we recommend leaving the infundibulopelvic ligament intact until after complete mobilization of the parametrium because the additional tension created by this ligament greatly assists in the parametrial dissection.

Finally, for a minimally invasive laparoscopic radical hysterectomy, a good uterine manipulator is of utmost importance. A variety of manipulators exist, each with their strengths and weaknesses. For the most part, these devices will improve visualization, create proper countertension during bladder, ureteral, and parametrial dissections, and delineate the appropriate margins for vaginal colpotomy.

Table 6.1 Piver-Rutledge-Smith classification of radical hysterectomy

Name (type)	Point of uterine vessels transection	Amount of vagina removed	Point of uterosacral ligament transection
Simple (I)	At insertion into cervix (level of the internal os)	Minimal	At insertion into cervix
Modified radical (II)	At level of the ureter	1–2 cm	Midway between cervix and rectum
Radical (III)	At their origin from the internal iliac vessels	Upper half	At their origin
Extended radical (IV)	At their origin from the internal iliac vessels	Upper three-fourths with paravaginal tissue	At their origin
Partial exenteration (V)	At their origin and en bloc with ureters (and possibly bladder)	Entire vagina above levator muscles	At their origin (and possibly en bloc with rectum)

Modified from Piver et al. [13]

Table 6.2 Querleu–Morrow classification of radical hysterectomy

Type	Extent of resection	Ureter	Comment
Type A	The paracervix is transected medial to the ureter but lateral to the cervix. Uterosacral and vesicouterine ligaments are not transected at a distance from the uterus. Vaginal resection is minimal without removal of the paracolpos	Ureter palpated or directly visualized without freeing from bed	
Type B1	Paracervix is transected at the level of the ureteral tunnel. Partial resection of ureterosacral and vesicouterine ligaments. No resection of caudal (deep) neural component of the paracervix (caudal to the deep uterine vein). Vaginal resection of at least 10 mm of the vagina from the cervix or tumor	Unroofing of ureter. Ureter rolled laterally	**Type B2**: Type B1 + removal of the lateral lymph nodes
Type C	Transection of paracervix at junction with internal iliac vascular system, uterosacral ligaments at the rectum, and vesicouterine ligaments at the bladder. Resection is 15–20 mm of the vagina from the tumor or cervix and corresponding paracolpos	Ureter completely mobilized	**Type C1**: with autonomic nerve sparing/preservation. **Type C2**: without autonomic nerve sparing/preservation
Type D1	Resection of the paracervix at the pelvic side with vessels arising from internal iliac system, exposing the roots of the sciatic nerve	Ureter completely mobilized	
Type D2	Resection of the paracervix at the pelvic side, with hypogastric vessels plus adjacent fascial or muscular structures (laterally extended endo-pelvic resection)	Ureter completely mobilized	

Modified from Querleu et al. [14]

6.2.2 Procedure

What follows is a description of the Piver-Rutledge-Smith type III radical hysterectomy. Once mastered, this procedure can easily be modified for more (type IV) or less (type II) radical procedures. The order of the steps listed may differ slightly from surgeon to surgeon. Although this surgery can be performed with monopolar electrocautery, we recommend using one of the many advanced vessel sealing devices because they tend to have better hemostasis and, more importantly, less lateral thermal spread. The latter is particularly important when dissecting near the ureter.

The surgery begins with a careful exploration of the entire peritoneal cavity for evidence of intraperitoneal spread. This includes inspection of the upper abdomen and all peritoneal surfaces. For women with cervical cancer, if metastatic disease is encountered, the surgery should be terminated and the patient reassigned to chemotherapy and/or radiation.

The round ligament is then divided and the retroperitoneal space is entered. Gentle blunt dissection in this avascular space is performed, and the external iliac vessels, internal iliac artery, and ureter are identified. A careful examination of the pelvic lymph nodes should be made, and any enlarged or abnormal-appearing nodes should be removed and sent for frozen section evaluation. One of the few limitations of the minimally invasive radical hysterectomy is the decreased tactile sensitivity for palpating lymph node basins.

A bladder flap is then created using a combination of the advanced vessel sealing device and blunt dissection. Early in the surgery only a small bladder flap is necessary. However, throughout the procedure, the surgeon returns to the bladder, further dissecting it from the pubovaginal fascia to achieve the desired vaginal margins.

The pararectal and paravesical spaces are then opened. We favor opening the pararectal space first, although this varies based on the surgeon's preference. The pararectal space is entered by bluntly dissecting between the ureter and internal iliac artery along the curve of the sacrum. This is another avascular space bordered by the internal

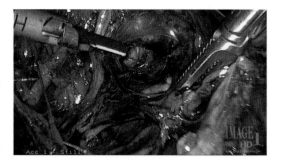

Fig. 6.1 The uterine artery is seen at its origin from the internal iliac (hypogastric) artery

iliac artery/levator ani laterally, the rectum medially, the sacrum posteriorly, and the cardinal ligament (parametrium) anteriorly.

Once the pararectal space is opened to the pelvic floor, the paravesical space should be opened. With anterior retraction of the proximal portion of the severed round ligament and using the superior vesicle artery as a landmark, this space can be entered either medially or laterally to that vessel (although we favor lateral entry). Again, blunt dissection is used to open this avascular space bordered by the obturator internus muscle laterally, the bladder medially, the pubis symphysis anteriorly, and the cardinal ligament posteriorly. Care must be taken not to create an inadvertent cystotomy. Historically, after opening these spaces, the surgeon would place one finger in each space, palpating the cardinal ligament to rule out tumor infiltration. With a minimally invasive approach, this is not possible. However, opening these two spaces does help identify the uterine artery and its surrounding parametrial tissue (Fig. 6.1).

Once identified, the uterine artery is dissected and ligated at its origin using an advanced vessel sealing device. With gentle traction upward, the surrounding parametrial tissue is taken en bloc with the uterine vessels. As the parametrial tissue is freed laterally and deeply, the ureter is tunneled from underneath it as the parametrial tissue is brought up over it (Fig. 6.2). The tunneling of the ureter continues until its insertion into the bladder is reached. Along the way, the ureter is freed from its medial attachments and "rolled" laterally. When dissecting the deep portion of the parametrium, care must be taken not to disrupt

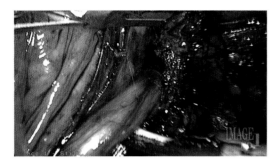

Fig. 6.2 The ureter is untunneled as it courses through the parametrial tissue

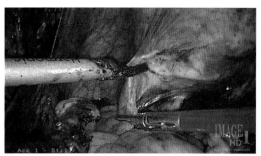

Fig. 6.4 The uterosacral ligaments are transected

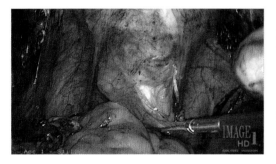

Fig. 6.3 The recotvaginal space is opened, exposing the uterosacral ligaments

the sympathetic nerve fibers innervating the bladder and rectum.

The vesicouterine peritoneal fold is now transected using the advanced vessel sealing device. This often requires further mobilization of the bladder downward. Care must be taken not to perform an inadvertent cystotomy during this portion of the procedure. Backfilling the bladder may assist in helping to decide the best surgical plane to take.

The uterus is now anteflexed, and the rectovaginal space is developed. Another avascular space, this can be entered by retracting the sigmoid colon caudally and posteriorly and incising the fold between the bowel and the posterior cervix (Fig. 6.3). This incision is extended laterally, and the rectovaginal space is developed bluntly. This mobilizes the rectum away from the vagina and exposes the uterosacral ligaments. With good visualization of the lateralized ureters, the uterosacral ligaments can now be transected at their origin using an advanced vessel sealing device (Fig. 6.4).

With the bladder, the vesicouterine fold, the parametrium, and the uterosacral ligaments now freely dissected and the ureters mobilized laterally, a circumferential colpotomy incision can be made, taking care to achieve the desired vaginal margins. The radical hysterectomy specimen is removed through the vagina, and the vaginal cuff is closed either vaginally or laparoscopically based on the preference of the surgeon.

6.3 Pelvic and Para-aortic Lymphadenectomy

6.3.1 General Considerations

The most important key to safely perform lymphadenectomies for gynecologic malignancies is mastery of the anatomy and careful dissection to identify aberrant vessels and structures. For example, an accessory obturator vein may be present in up to 25 % of women and accessory renal arteries in 3 %. In addition, the bilateral ureters cross the dissection fields in multiple locations and should always be identified. Transecting tissue and nodal bundles without dissecting and identifying both known anatomic landmarks and unknown anomalies puts the patient at risk for major complications.

For pelvic and para-aortic lymphadenectomies, we favor a four-port diamond configuration with 5-mm trocars in the umbilicus, one in the lateral lower quadrant, and suprapubic locations and a 12-mm trocar in the contralateral lateral lower quadrant. This larger port allows for placement of a specimen bag for removal of nodal bundles.

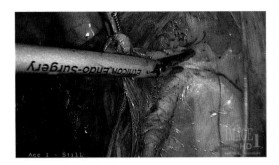

Fig. 6.5 The nodal tissue overlying the external iliac artery is gently retracted medially as the incision over the artery is extended distally

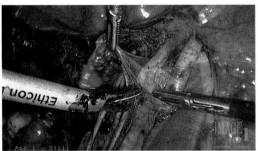

Fig. 6.6 The nodal tissue is carefully dissected from the external iliac vein

As previously described, these procedures are best performed with an advanced vessel sealing device (bipolar or ultrasonic). These devices allow for rapid coagulation and transection of tissue and vessels with minimal lateral thermal spread.

6.3.2 Procedures

6.3.2.1 Pelvic Lymphadenectomy

To begin the pelvic lymphadenectomy, the camera starts in the umbilical port. The tissue overlying the external iliac artery is grasped and the peritoneal surface is incised just lateral to the vessel. The surgeon can then enter the avascular space between the external iliac artery and the psoas muscle. With medial tension on the nodal bundle and after identification of the genitofemoral nerve as it runs on the medial aspect of the psoas muscle, the incision over the external artery is extended distally (Fig. 6.5). The assistant grasps the cut round ligament and elevates it toward the anterior abdominal wall to allow for this distal dissection. The dissection continues until the circumflex iliac vein is visualized.

The nodal bundle is then freed from the external iliac vein by gently pulling medially on the bundle and bluntly dissecting the avascular space between the vein and the nodes (Fig. 6.6). In order to avoid tearing the nodal bundle and the subsequent oozing from the nodes, it is important to grasp a large amount of nodal tissue as opposed to a small bite at the edge. Because the vein is

much less resilient than the artery, care must be taken to visualize the edge of the vein and avoid any accidental venotomy. During this portion of the procedure, the assistant can use a blunt instrument to retract the vein along its route to aid in visualization and countertraction.

After the nodal bundle is medialized from the external iliac vein, the obturator space is entered bluntly, and the obturator nerve is identified. This structure is the deep margin of the dissection, and care must be taken not to inadvertently transect this nerve. The nodal bundle can typically be released from the nerve by bluntly running an instrument on top of the nerve and in a parallel direction. Minimal bleeding may be encountered, but this typically can be halted by utilizing the nodal bundle for direct pressure. A more hemostatic approach can be performed by creating pedicles above the nerve by spreading with a blunt instrument parallel to the nerve and then using an advanced energy device to coagulate and transect these pedicles.

The internal iliac artery/superior vesicle artery, the medial border of the dissection, is then identified, and the nodal bundle is freed from it either bluntly or with the advanced energy device. This is best achieved with the assistant grasping the vessel and providing countertraction (Fig. 6.7). Care is taken not to go deep into this vessel because the ureter runs close to it and this risks injury. This part of the dissection is continued proximally along the internal iliac artery until the bifurcation of the common iliac artery is encountered. At this point the bundle is removed.

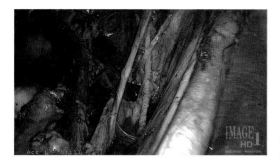

Fig. 6.7 The final aspect of the pelvic lymphadenectomy with the external iliac artery and vein, internal iliac/superior vesicle artery, and obturator nerve cleared of the nodal tissue

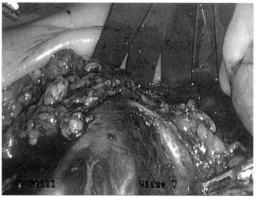

Fig. 6.8 A laparoscopic retractor is used to expose the bifurcation of the aorta

Remember that the ureter crosses at the bifurcation of the common iliac artery into the internal and external arteries, and visualization of the ureter is important to protect it from transection or thermal injury.

6.3.2.2 Para-aortic Lymphadenectomy

After the pelvic nodal bundles are removed, the dissection continues proximal along the common iliac artery. Getting proper set-up and visualization of the entire nodal basin to be dissected is not only the most difficult part of this procedure but also the most important. If this set-up is completed correctly and good visualization of the superior border is achieved first (whether it is the inferior mesenteric artery or the renal vessels), the actual dissection and removal of the nodal basins are somewhat straightforward.

The peritoneum over the common iliac artery is incised and elevated. The underlying nodal tissue is initially left adherent to the vessels as this peritoneal "tent" is raised. With graspers raising this tent, the small bowel may be retracted behind it out of the surgical field. Often visualization of the great vessels owing to the position of the small bowel is the greatest challenge of a laparoscopic para-aortic lymphadenectomy and as patient body mass index increases, so does the level of difficulty of retracting these organs. Many surgeons maintain the camera in the umbilicus throughout the para-aortic lymphadenectomy; however, we find that switching the camera to the suprapubic port and moving the monitors to the head of the

patient often help with visualization and precision in instrument placement. This configuration with the camera held by the assistant using the suprapubic port and the bilateral lower quadrant trocars utilized by the primary surgeon standing between the patient's legs is particularly helpful if the renal vessels are the upper limit of the dissection (as opposed to the inferior mesenteric artery favored by some surgeons). One other technique to assist in visualization is to place a laparoscopic retractor through the umbilical port. We often exchange the 5-mm umbilical port for a 12-mm trocar to allow for placement of a large laparoscopic fan retractor to assist in holding the small bowel in the upper abdomen out of the surgical field (Fig. 6.8). Finally, if needed a fifth trocar may be introduced in the upper quadrant to allow for another assistant to help with retraction.

Once the peritoneum is open to the superior border of the dissection (inferior mesenteric artery or renal vessels), dissection is begun at the distal portion over the common iliac artery. The avascular plane between the nodal bundle and the artery is entered. The nodal bundle is grasped and elevated gently so as not to tear the inferior vena cava underneath it. The nodal bundle is mobilized along the common iliac artery and over the lower portion of the abdominal aorta. The advanced energy device is used to spread parallel to the vessels, creating pedicles that can then be taken with the device. This technique is particularly important over the vena cava at the level of the aortic bifurcation as this is commonly where the surgeon will encounter the fellow's vein. As the surgeon moves cephalad, the lateral portion of the vena cava should be identified and the nodal bundle should be separated from its lateral attachments. It is imperative at this point that the right ureter is identified and lateralized away from the dissection. The anatomic borders of this nodal bundle are the common iliac inferiorly and the lateral portion of the vena cava, the aorta, and the inferior mesenteric artery/renal vessels superiorly.

After this portion of the aortocaval nodes is removed, the nodes along the left side of the aorta can be removed. We find this more easily done separately from those nodes overlying the aorta and vena cava described above. When working in this area just lateral to the aorta, care must be taken to identify the left ureter because it courses close to the dissection. In addition, the surgeon should continue to gently create pedicles, since this will help visualize and avoid the lumbar vessel where they originate on the posterior portion of the aorta.

6.4 Infracolic Omentectomy

6.4.1 General Considerations

Laparoscopic omentectomy may be performed as part of the staging surgery for presumed early stage ovarian cancer in addition to certain types of high-risk endometrial cancers. If gross disease is visualized in the omentum or on other upper abdominal organs, we strongly recommend conversion to laparotomy for careful exploration and optimal tumor debulking. For staging of patients without evidence of metastatic disease, most surgeons perform an infracolic omentectomy.

Like all of the procedures described in this chapter, this procedure is best performed with an advanced vessel sealing device (bipolar or ultrasonic). We do not recommend using monopolar electrosurgical instruments because the dissection plane between the omentum and transverse colon can be small, and use of this technology risks a thermal bowel injury.

6.4.2 Procedure

We recommend placing the camera in the suprapubic port and moving the monitors toward the head of the patient. The surgeon stands between the legs of the patient and uses the bilateral lower quadrant trocars to operate. The assistant stands on the side of the patient holding the camera and utilizing the umbilical assistant port.

Utilizing the left lower quadrant and umbilical ports, graspers are used to raise the omentum toward the anterior abdominal wall allowing for visualization of the transverse colon. For a large omentum, this may require grasping the omentum toward its base close to the transverse colon. A fifth trocar may be introduced into the left upper quadrant (Palmer point) for an additional grasper if needed. We do not recommend pulling the omentum down into the pelvis and performing the procedure from above the omentum. This risks damage to both the transverse colon and the small bowel underneath the draping omentum. It is important to ensure visualization of the small bowel and transverse colon throughout the procedure. Slightly reducing the steep Trendelenburg position may help with visualization.

Using an advanced vessel sealing device placed in the right lower quadrant trocar, we start at the hepatic flexure and transect the edge of the omentum heading toward the transverse colon to enter the avascular space between the omentum and colon. We then head across the omentum toward the left side of the patient, mobilizing the omentum from the colon (Fig. 6.9). During the procedure, it is important to be mindful and avoid the bowel mesentery. As the omentum is released from its connections to the colon, the freed portion is placed into the left upper quadrant and the omentum is regrasped closer to the area still attached to the colon. As the splenic flexure is approached, the omentum becomes thicker and bunches up toward the spleen. While remaining in the same trajectory and coming across the base of the omentum, it is completely freed. We typically remove the omentum through the opened vagina.

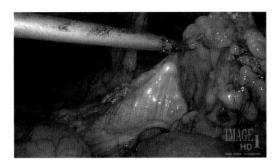

Fig. 6.9   The omentum is dissected from the transverse colon

References

1. Frumovitz M, Ramirez PT, Greer M, Gregurich MA, Wolf J, Bodurka DC, Levenback C. Laparoscopic training and practice in gynecologic oncology among Society of Gynecologic Oncologists members and fellows-in-training. Gynecol Oncol. 2004;94: 746–53.

2. Mabrouk M, Frumovitz M, Greer M, Sharma S, Schmeler KM, Soliman PT, Ramirez PT. Trends in laparoscopic and robotic surgery among gynecologic oncologists: a survey update. Gynecol Oncol. 2009;112:501–5.

3. Walker JL, Piedmonte MR, Spirtos NM, Eisenkop SM, Schlaerth JB, Mannel RS, et al. Recurrence and survival after random assignment to laparoscopy versus laparotomy for comprehensive surgical staging of uterine cancer: Gynecologic Oncology Group LAP2 Study. J Clin Oncol. 2012;30:695–700.

4. Kornblith AB, Huang HQ, Walker JL, Spirtos NM, Rotmensch J, Cella D. Quality of life of patients with endometrial cancer undergoing laparoscopic international federation of gynecology and obstetrics staging compared with laparotomy: a Gynecologic Oncology Group study. J Clin Oncol. 2009;27:5337–42.

5. Frumovitz M, dos Reis R, Sun CC, Milam MR, Bevers MW, Brown J, et al. Comparison of total laparoscopic and abdominal radical hysterectomy for patients with early-stage cervical cancer. Obstet Gynecol. 2007;110:96–102.

6. Spirtos NM, Eisenkop SM, Schlaerth JB, Ballon SC. Laparoscopic radical hysterectomy (type III) with aortic and pelvic lymphadenectomy in patients with stage I cervical cancer: surgical morbidity and intermediate follow-up. Am J Obstet Gynecol. 2002; 187:340–8.

7. Obermair A, Gebski V, Frumovitz M, Soliman PT, Schmeler KM, Levenback C, Ramirez PT. A phase III randomized clinical trial comparing laparoscopic or robotic radical hysterectomy with abdominal radical hysterectomy in patients with early stage cervical cancer. J Minim Invasive Gynecol. 2008;15:584–8.

8. Deffieux X, Castaigne D, Pomel C. Role of laparoscopy to evaluate candidates for complete cytoreduction in advanced stages of epithelial ovarian cancer. Int J Gynecol Cancer. 2006;16 Suppl 1:35–40.

9. Fagotti A, Vizzielli G, Fanfani F, Costantini B, Ferrandina G, Gallotta V, et al. Introduction of staging laparoscopy in the management of advanced epithelial ovarian, tubal and peritoneal cancer: impact on prognosis in a single institution experience. Gynecol Oncol. 2013;131(2):341–6.

10. Leblanc E, Querleu D, Narducci F, Occelli B, Papageorgiou T, Sonoda Y. Laparoscopic restaging of early stage invasive adnexal tumors: a 10-year experience. Gynecol Oncol. 2004;94:624–9.

11. Chi DS, Abu-Rustum NR, Sonoda Y, Ivy J, Rhee E, Moore K, Levine DA, Barakat RR. The safety and efficacy of laparoscopic surgical staging of apparent stage I ovarian and fallopian tube cancers. Am J Obstet Gynecol. 2005;192:1614–9.

12. Lecuru F, Desfeux P, Camatte S, Bissery A, Blanc B, Querleu D. Impact of initial surgical access on staging and survival of patients with stage I ovarian cancer. Int J Gynecol Cancer. 2006;16:87–94.

13. Piver MS, Rutledge F, Smith JP. Five classes of extended hysterectomy for women with cervical cancer. Obstet Gynecol. 1974;44:265–72.

14. Querleu D, Morrow CP. Classification of radical hysterectomy. Lancet Oncol. 2008;9:297–303.

15. Frumovitz M, Euscher ED, Deavers MT, Soliman PT, Schmeler KM, Ramirez PT, Levenback CF. "Triple injection" lymphatic mapping technique to determine if parametrial nodes are the true sentinel lymph nodes in women with cervical cancer. Gynecol Oncol. 2012;127:467–71.

16. Altgassen C, Hertel H, Brandstadt A, Kohler C, Durst M, Schneider A. Multicenter validation study of the sentinel lymph node concept in cervical cancer: AGO Study Group. J Clin Oncol. 2008;26:2943–51.

17. Lecuru F, Mathevet P, Querleu D, Leblanc E, Morice P, Darai E, et al. Bilateral negative sentinel nodes accurately predict absence of lymph node metastasis in early cervical cancer: results of the SENTICOL Study. J Clin Oncol. 2011;29:1686–91.

Techniques in Urogynecology and Pelvic Reconstructive Surgery

7

Cecile A. Unger and Beri Ridgeway

Our fastest growing population is the elderly, and the incidence and prevalence of uterovaginal prolapse and urinary incontinence increase with age. Because of the significant impact on quality of life, patients continue to seek surgical management for treatment of these disorders. While there are three approaches to surgery that exist for pelvic floor disorders, laparoscopy has emerged as a minimally invasive option for appropriate candidates. Many perioperative considerations must be examined before performing laparoscopic operations, including patient positioning, trocar placement, and prevention of infectious and venous thrombotic events.

Patients who have undergone prior hysterectomy and suffer from vaginal vault prolapse may be good candidates for laparoscopic uterosacral ligament suspension of the vagina, which has yielded favorable results. However, sacrocolpopexy remains the gold standard for vaginal vault suspension, as patients attain very high cure rates. Successful outcomes have been shown with

the laparoscopic approach to this procedure. For patients who have not undergone previous hysterectomy, there is the option for hysterectomy at the time of vault suspension. For patients without risk factors for cervical dysplasia or malignancy, the option for uterine preservation exists, and this can be achieved either with laparoscopic uterosacral hysteropexy or sacrohysteropexy. These operations have also yielded excellent results for management of pelvic organ prolapse. Patients with stress urinary incontinence may also be candidates for laparoscopic surgery, as the Burch colposuspension is a procedure that continues to be performed in certain patients.

There are many advantages to laparoscopic surgery; however, there are perioperative complications that are related to this surgical approach. Most complications are the result of trocar entry or instrument-related injury involving the pelvic and abdominal vasculature, the small and large bowels, the ureters, and the bladder. Complications involving synthetic mesh placement also exist, and these include infection at the site of mesh attachment as well as mesh erosion.

As advances in minimally invasive surgery are made, more surgeons will perform laparoscopic procedures to treat pelvic floor disorders and urinary incontinence. And as the population continues to age, the need for surgical management of these disorders will increase. Reconstructive surgeons should strive to learn the important principles of laparoscopy, avoid the complications that can be associated with certain procedures, and determine which operations are appropriate for their patients.

C.A. Unger, MD, MPH (✉)
Division of Female Pelvic Medicine
and Reconstructive Surgery,
Department of Obstetrics and Gynecology,
Cleveland Clinic, 9500 Euclid Avenue, A81,
Cleveland, OH 44195, USA
e-mail: ungerc@ccf.org

B. Ridgeway, MD
Department of Obstetrics, Gynecology,
Women's Health Institute, Cleveland Clinic,
9500 Euclid Avenue, A81,
Cleveland, OH 44195, USA
e-mail: ridgewb@ccf.org

P.F. Escobar, T. Falcone (eds.), *Atlas of Single-Port, Laparoscopic, and Robotic Surgery*,
DOI 10.1007/978-1-4614-6840-0_7, © Springer Science+Business Media New York 2014

7.1 Introduction

Pelvic organ prolapse and urinary incontinence are common problems in women that can cause substantial morbidity and negatively affect quality of life. The management of pelvic organ prolapse and incontinence can be challenging, as several support defects often coexist. To achieve the goals of pelvic reconstruction, the surgeon must understand normal anatomic support as well as physiologic function of the organs involved. The goals of surgery are to reconstruct anatomy, maintain or restore normal bowel and bladder function, and preserve vaginal length.

Three modes of surgery exist in pelvic reconstructive surgery: vaginal, open abdominal, and laparoscopic (conventional and robot-assisted). Advances in minimally invasive surgery have led to the widespread adoption of laparoscopic techniques in pelvic reconstruction. Laparoscopy has many practical and economic advantages compared with traditional open procedures. These advantages include improved visualization of pelvic anatomy, decreased postoperative pain, less operative blood loss, shortened hospital stay, rapid recovery rate and return to daily activities by patients [1].

7.2 Perioperative Considerations

Selecting appropriate patients for laparoscopic procedures is very important. The pneumoperitoneum needed during these cases causes important systemic changes in the body, including decreased venous return, increased systemic and pulmonary vascular pressures, and increased ventilation pressures [2]. These changes are amplified in the setting of the Trendelenburg position, which is often used in gynecologic procedures. These physiologic changes are not tolerated by patients with pre-existing cardiopulmonary disease. Therefore, appropriate preoperative tests, such as chest x-ray, pulmonary function tests, electrocardiogram and echocardiogram, may be necessary in patients with suspected cardiac and pulmonary comorbidities. These procedures should be avoided in patients with known and severe disease.

Visualization of all pelvic structures up to the level of the sacrum is very important for urogynecologic procedures, and therefore proper patient positioning before commencing surgery is essential. The patient should be positioned in the low lithotomy position using Allen stirrups with care to avoid hyperflexion or extension at the level of the hips and knees. All bony prominences should be padded. Placing an anti-slip device such as an egg crate underneath the patient to limit movement when the operating table is moved is very helpful. Additionally, positioning the patient so that the buttocks are slightly beyond the end of the table will help facilitate placement of vaginal and rectal manipulators. The arms should be tucked and padded adequately to relieve any pressure on the elbows, and the hands should be left in the proper anatomic position.

Patients should receive intravenous prophylactic antibiotics within 60 min of incision to reduce the risk of perioperative infection. The antibiotic of choice in all gynecologic surgery is a first-generation cephalosporin, usually cefazolin, or an alternative combination regimen such as ciprofloxacin and metronidazole if a patient has a documented allergy to penicillin [3].

All patients undergoing prolapse and/or incontinence surgery are at moderate risk for venous thromboembolic events (VTE) and require perioperative prophylaxis. A systematic review of VTE prophylaxis in gynecologic surgery concluded that application of intermittent pneumatic compression devices to the lower extremities before induction of anesthesia is sufficient for VTE prophylaxis [4]. Patients at higher risk for VTE (those with significant comorbidities, cancer history, morbid obesity, or history of prior VTE) should have intermittent pneumatic compression devices and low-dose unfractionated heparin or low-molecular-weight heparin administered before surgery [5].

The value of a mechanical bowel preparation for prevention of infectious complications or an

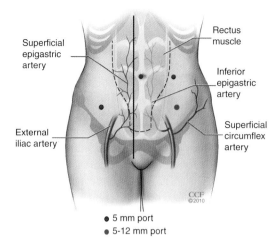

Superficial epigastric artery

Rectus muscle

Inferior epigastric artery

External iliac artery

Superficial circumflex artery

CCF ©2010

● 5 mm port
● 5-12 mm port

Fig. 7.1 Laparoscopic trocar placement. Trocar placement plays a key role in facilitating laparoscopic procedures performed for pelvic prolapse and incontinence. Proper positioning of each trocar allows reach of the laparoscopic instruments from the deep pelvis up to the level of the sacrum as well as adequate articulation for suturing and knot-tying. Sufficient distance between trocars is necessary to prevent instrument crossing. For surgeries such as laparoscopic sacrocolpopexy, which involves dissection over the sacrum and lower pelvis as well as extensive suturing of graft material to both regions, placement of at least four ports is usually necessary. Multiple port configurations are described in the literature. Placement of a 5- mm trocar is recommended in the umbilicus for the laparoscope, two ports placed 2 cm superior and medial to the anterior iliac spine on each side (typically a 10-mm port on the left and a 5- mm port on the right), and a 5-mm port placed in the midclavicular line at the level of the umbilicus on the side from which the surgeon will suture. The inferior epigastric vessels are the most commonly injured vessels at the time of lateral trocar placement [2]. Although these vessels are not easily visualized, placing the ports lateral to the rectus abdominis muscles usually ensures their avoidance. All trocars should be placed under direct visualization to avoid injury to the internal vasculature and surrounding soft tissues. When placing the initial port through the umbilicus, the table should be level to avoid injury to the greater vessels, and entry should be gained in the manner with which the surgeon is most comfortable. If the patient has a history of midline laparotomy or adhesions are expected, a left upper quadrant approach is recommended. After the entry site is inspected and the upper abdomen is surveyed, the patient should be placed in a steep Trendelenburg position to move the bowels cephalad for good visualization of the pelvis and for placement of the subsequent trocars (From Cleveland Clinic Center for Medical Art & Photography. Copyright © 2010–2013, with permission.)

intraoperative bowel leak or for reducing the rates of anastomotic leak if bowel surgery is performed has been challenged in a recent meta-analysis [6]. Therefore, it does not seem necessary to complete bowel preparation for all patients undergoing operations to treat prolapse or incontinence [6].

7.3 Uterovaginal Prolapse Procedures

While there is sparse literature on outcomes from laparoscopic uterosacral ligament suspension because most studies do not follow patients beyond 2 years, the reported cure rate ranges from 76 to 90 % [8, 9]. Additionally, the laparoscopic approach has also been shown to have a lower risk of ureteral injury than transvaginal uterosacral suspension [7] and therefore may be a safe alternative to transvaginal surgery.

The most commonly used material is a large-pore polypropylene mesh, which has proven to have fewer complications because of its favorable synthetic properties [11]. The technique of laparoscopic sacrocolpopexy using graft placement begins with proper positioning of the patient in the low lithotomy position using Allen stirrups so that there is access to the vagina during the operation. A sponge stick or end-to-end anastomosis (EEA) sizer should be placed in the vagina for manipulation of the apex. A Foley catheter is placed in the bladder for continuous drainage throughout the operation. After intraperitoneal access is gained and laparoscopic trocars are placed, the small bowel should be gently placed into the upper abdomen and the sigmoid colon deviated to the left pelvis as much as possible. If manual retraction of the sigmoid colon is not adequate, a temporary suture can be placed through the epiploica of the colon, passed through a trocar on the left side of the patient, and clamped to the drapes, with removal of the suture at the end of the procedure. The ureters are identified bilaterally; it is important to note their location throughout the duration of the case. Attention is then turned to the sacrum, and the sacral promontory is identified so that the presacral space may be entered.

A review of abdominal sacrocolpopexy reported the success rate when defined as lack of apical vaginal prolapse postoperatively from 78 to 100 % [12]. The median reoperation rates for pelvic organ prolapse and for stress urinary incontinence in the studies that reported these outcomes were 4.4 % (range, 0–18.2 %) and 4.9 % (range, 1.2–30.9 %), respectively. A randomized, controlled trial of sacrocolpopexy with and without concomitant Burch colposuspension at 2-year follow-up had reassuring anatomic outcomes, with 95 % of subjects having excellent objective outcomes for the vaginal apex (within 2 cm of total vaginal length), with 2 % of subjects demonstrating stage III prolapse, and 3 % of subjects undergoing reoperation for prolapse [13]. These subjects also demonstrated improved urinary, defecatory, and sexual function based on validated questionnaires. Although most of the literature has been focused on abdominal sacrocolpopexy, there are emerging data on the laparoscopic approach. A comprehensive review looking at over 1,000 patients in 11 series who underwent laparoscopic sacrocolpopexy revealed that the conversion rates and operative times had decreased substantially with increased experience in performing this procedure [10]. The mean follow-up for these series was 24.6 months with an average patient satisfaction rate of 94.4 % and a 6.2 % prolapse reoperation rate [10]. From this review, the authors concluded that a laparoscopic approach to sacrocolpopexy upholds the outcomes of the gold standard of abdominal sacrocolpopexy and is a very good minimally invasive option for patients with vaginal vault prolapse [10].

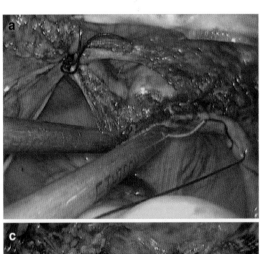
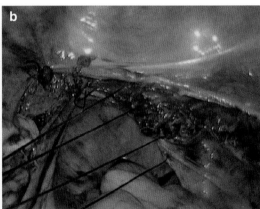
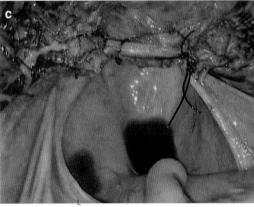

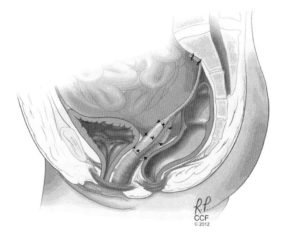

Fig. 7.3 Laparoscopic sacrocolpopexy. Laparoscopic sacrocolpopexy has become an alternative to open abdominal sacrocolpopexy for repair of vaginal vault prolapse. Abdominal sacrocolpopexy is considered the gold standard for vault prolapse and has demonstrated superior anatomic outcomes compared to transvaginal suspension procedures [10]; however, the operation is associated with a higher complication rate. A laparoscopic approach aims at bridging the gap between the advantages of vaginal surgery, namely, decreased morbidity and faster patient recovery, and the surgical success rates of abdominal sacrocolpopexy [10]. For young women who are sexually active with symptomatic pelvic organ prolapse, reconstruction with a sacrocolpopexy procedure is beneficial because the success rates are high because the procedure adequately restores normal pelvic anatomy and maintains vaginal length [11]. Laparoscopic sacrocolpopexy involves suspension of the vagina to the sacral promontory using a bridging graft that can be made of biologic or synthetic materials. The graft is sutured to the anterior as well as the posterior vagina and then to the anterior longitudinal ligament of the sacrum. We strongly believe that the minimally invasive approach to sacrocolpopexy should not have alterations from the open approach. The exact same steps, suture type and number, and graft should be used with open or laparoscopic surgery (From Cleveland Clinic Center for Medical Art & Photography. Copyright © 2012–2013, with permission)

Fig. 7.2 Laparoscopic uterosacral ligament vaginal vault suspension. Uterosacral ligament suspension is a procedure that is commonly performed at the time of hysterectomy for treatment of vaginal vault prolapse. The procedure involves attaching the vaginal vault to the midportion of the uterosacral ligament, which serves to restore the apical support of the vagina. When compared with the transvaginal approach, this type of suspension may decrease the risk of rectal and ureteral injury at the time of placement of the suspension sutures because these structures are easily identified in laparoscopic surgery [7]. Although laparoscopic uterosacral suspension after transvaginal hysterectomy is not very common, these benefits should be considered, especially if concomitant laparoscopic procedures are necessary. A laparoscopic approach can be taken at the time of laparoscopic hysterectomy, especially if no further vaginal reconstruction is needed at the end of the procedure. An Allis clamp can be used to elevate the vaginal cuff to delineate the uterosacral ligaments. Alternatively, a vaginal probe can be used to elevate the vagina, demarcating the uterosacral ligaments. Care is taken to avoid tenting the peritoneum close to the ureter on the ipsilateral side so as to not obstruct the ureter when the suspension sutures are tied down. A releasing peritoneal incision between the ligament and the ureter can be made in order to reduce peritoneal tension and subsequent ureteral kinking from suture placement. (**a**) A permanent or delayed absorbable suture is placed through the midportion of the uterosacral ligament (at the level of the ischial spine) with lateral to medial needle placement and then secured to the ipsilateral posterior and anterior vaginal cuffs. (**b**) One or two sutures can be placed on each side of the vagina, extracorporeal or intracorporeal knot-tying technique can be employed to suspend the vagina, (**c**) and the cuff is closed in an uninterrupted fashion

Table 7.1 Tips for performing minimally invasive sacrocolpopexy [11]

Patient positioning is critical

    Place egg crate or other anti-slip device directly below patient to prevent movement during operation.

    Position buttocks slightly beyond end of table so that vaginal manipulation is possible.

    Both arms are tucked and protected.

    Once intra-abdominal access is gained, steep Trendelenburg positioning helps move the small bowel into the upper abdomen,

Two knowledgeable assistants are necessary

    One works intra-abdominally and helps with retraction.

    One works vaginally and manipulates the vagina and rectum to optimize visualization.

Side dock the robot, either parallel or at a 45-degree angle, to the table.

Placement of ports is integral to procedure success.

Ensure there is enough space between the robot arms to prevent collision.

If the colon is redundant, an epiploica can be sutured temporarily to the left anterior abdominal wall to improve visualization.

If hysterectomy is planned, a supracervical hysterectomy should be considered because the cervix may help to decrease future mesh erosions. Alternatively, a vaginal hysterectomy can be performed prior to a laparoscopic repair.

Given the lack of tactile feedback in robotic surgery, identification of the sacral promontory can be challenging. Using laparoscopy initially, this area can be identified and marked with a cautery before docking the robot.

Care should be taken to avoid the intervertebral disc while placing the sacral sutures. Deep stitches through the disc and periosteum should be avoided because cases of osteomyelitis have been reported after robotic sacrocolpopexy.

A barbed suture can be used to close the peritoneum.

Convert to laparotomy when necessary. Patient safety is of utmost importance

From Walters and Ridgeway [11]; with permission

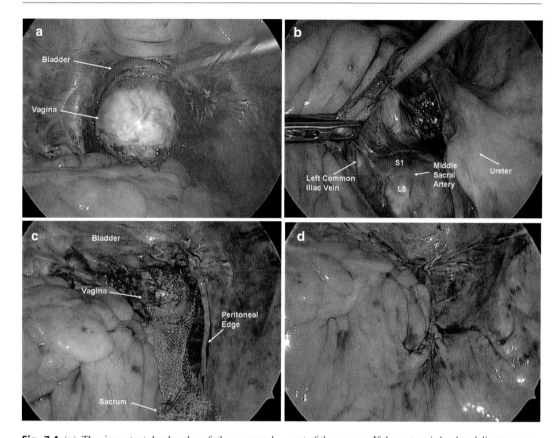

Fig. 7.4 (**a**) The important landmarks of the presacral space include the aortic bifurcation, the common and internal iliac vessels, the sigmoid colon, and the right ureter. Notably, the left common iliac vessel is located medial to the iliac artery and is particularly vulnerable to injury during this procedure, as are the internal iliac vessels, the right ureter, and the middle sacral artery. Once all structures are identified, a longitudinal peritoneal incision is made over the sacral promontory. Dissection is done carefully to reveal the bony promontory as well as the anterior longitudinal ligament, which will later serve as the attachment point for the graft. Approximately 4 cm of exposure is necessary, and this is achieved by using blunt dissection or electrocauterization of the subperitoneal fat. Caution should be taken to avoid the presacral venous plexus as well as the middle sacral vein and artery, which are often encountered during this dissection. Dissection caudally through the peritoneum and subperitoneal fat is carried down to the level of the posterior culde-sac. The rectum and right ureter are visualized at all times during this part of the procedure as the course of the dissection is located between these two structures. (**b**) The vagina is elevated cephalad using a sponge stick or EEA sizer, the peritoneum overlying the anterior vaginal apex is incised transversely, and the bladder is dissected off the anterior vagina using sharp dissection, creating a 4- to 5-cm pocket. If this plane is difficult to establish, the bladder can be filled in a retrograde fashion to find the correct dissection plane. Similarly, the peritoneum overlying the posterior vagina is incised, and dissection is done overlying the vagina and extending into the posterior cul-de-sac, creating a 4- to 5-cm pocket. Care must be taken to avoid injury to the rectum during this part of the surgery. If the rectum is hard to delineate, a second EEA sizer should be introduced into the rectum, and with manipulation of the vaginal and rectal EEA sizers, the correct dissection plane is identified. If the patient has concomitant defecatory dysfunction and/or rectal prolapse, the posterior dissection is sometimes carried down to the level of the perineal body. In most cases, however, the 4- to 5-cm pocket is sufficient. Once dissection is complete, the graft is prepared. A lightweight polypropylene mesh is currently most commonly used. The mesh is fashioned into two arms that are approximately 4 Å~ 15 cm in size. The graft is first attached to the posterior vaginal wall using 4–6 permanent or delayed-absorbable No. 0 or 2-0 sutures in an interrupted fashion, 1–2 cm apart from each other. Sutures are placed through the fibromuscular tissue of the vagina but not through the underlying epithelium. *S1* 1st sacral vertebral body, *L5* 5th lumbar vertebral body. (**c**) The graft extends approximately half-way down the posterior vaginal wall. The second arm of the graft is then attached to the anterior vaginal wall in a similar fashion. Delayed absorbable sutures should be used for the most distal stitches close to the bladder to avoid suture erosion and fistulization. The vagina is then elevated with the sponge stick or EEA sizer toward the sacral promontory. The graft is trimmed to the appropriate length and then sutured to the anterior longitudinal ligament using a stiff but small half-curved tapered needle with two to three permanent No. 0 monofilament sutures. (**d**) The peritoneum is then closed over the exposed graft with absorbable suture. After cystoscopy, a vaginal examination is performed, and a posterior colporrhaphy and perineorrhaphy are performed if needed

7.3.1 Laparoscopic Hysteropexy

Hysterectomy is often done at the time of surgical repair for uterine and uterovaginal prolapse. Uterine preservation techniques have largely been employed in women with uterovaginal prolapse desiring future fertility. However, there has been a small shift in this practice as more women are requesting uterine preservation for other important reasons, including issues of sexuality, body image, cultural preferences, and the concern for earlier-onset menopause after hysterectomy [11]. The risk of unanticipated pathology in asymptomatic women remains low [14]; however, it is important to determine which patients are appropriate candidates for uterine-preserving surgery. Uterine-preserving surgery is contraindicated in women with a history of cervical dysplasia, dysfunctional uterine bleeding, postmenopausal bleeding, and risk factors for endometrial carcinoma. Additionally, women who choose to undergo hysteropexy should be counseled about the need for continued cancer surveillance and potential risks associated with future pregnancies [15].

Most procedures that aim to suspend the vaginal apex are performed in a similar fashion to those performed with hysterectomy, with some necessary modifications [11]. The minimally invasive abdominal procedures most commonly described in the literature include laparoscopic uterosacral ligament suspension and laparoscopic sacrohysteropexy. Laparoscopic uterosacral ligament suspension is performed similarly to vaginal vault suspension to the uterosacral ligaments. The uterus is suspended to a portion of the ligament on each side, preferably using permanent suture. Additionally, the uterosacral ligaments can be shortened with sutures, providing additional support. This procedure is favorable because it restores normal anatomy while preserving the uterus. Furthermore, it carries little risk for subsequent pregnancy and delivery. The only study to compare laparoscopic hysteropexy via uterosacral ligament suspension to vaginal hysterectomy with subsequent vaginal vault suspension is a retrospective cohort study of 50 patients [16]. The authors found that hysteropexy patients had better vault suspension as measured by the Pelvic Organ Prolapse Quantification examination postoperatively and experienced fewer failures as measured by reoperation rates when compared to the vaginal vault suspension group [16].

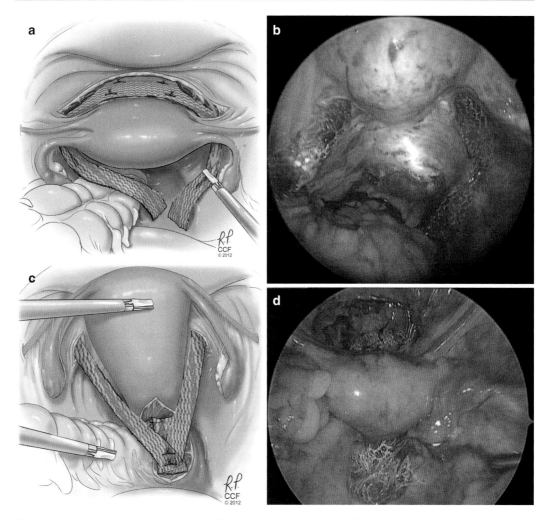

Fig. 7.5 Laparoscopic sacrohysteropexy. This can be done using different techniques but is similar to the technique used during sacrocolpopexy. Graft material can be sutured anteriorly and/or posteriorly, usually on the cervix, but can also be sutured to a portion of the proximal vagina. The graft is then suspended to the anterior longitudinal ligament of the sacrum using permanent sutures. (**a–b**) If anterior mesh is applied, windows are created through the broad ligament to allow the graft to pass through for attachment to the sacrum. (**c–d**) A posterior cervical graft has been placed, and this also has been sutured to the sacral promontory, thus suspending the uterus, cervix, and vagina to the sacrum. While outcomes data are sparse for laparoscopic sacrohysteropexy, results from abdominal sacrohysteropexy studies have shown similar high success rates when compared to open abdominal hysterectomy with subsequent sacrocolpopexy [17]. This procedure remains a viable option for patients with uterovaginal prolapse who desire uterine preservation. However, sacrohysteropexy with anterior mesh should not be offered to patients who desire future fertility. In these patients, placing a solitary posterior mesh can be considered (**a** and **c** from Cleveland Clinic Center for Medical Art & Photography. Copyright © 2012–2013, with permission)

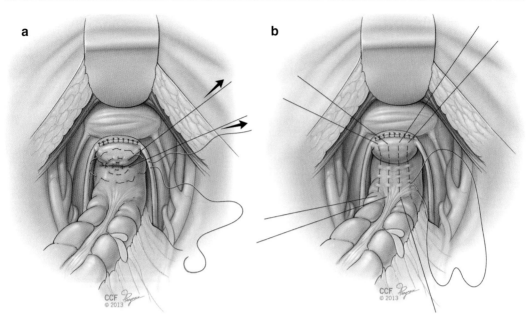

Fig. 7.6 Laparoscopic enterocele repair. An enterocele is a true hernia of the peritoneal pouch of Douglas and most often occurs in conjunction with additional uterovaginal prolapse or develops following vaginal or abdominal hysterectomy. The repair of an enterocele is traditionally done transvaginally or abdominally for larger enteroceles. However, there are times when laparoscopic repair is indicated, such as during concomitant surgery for other uterovaginal prolapse [18]. Two different laparoscopic techniques have been described to repair an enterocele: the Moschcowitz and Halban procedures. In both operations, a transvaginal manipulator or digital manipulation is necessary to apply transvaginal pressure for easy identification of the posterior vagina, rectum, and hernia sac. (**a**) In the Moschcowitz procedure, the enterocele sac is obliterated by reapproximating the pelvic peritoneum between the rectum and vagina, incorporating the uterosacral ligaments with a permanent No. 0 suture in a purse-string fashion (*arrows*). (**b**) The Halban culdoplasty is similar but involves placing permanent No. 0 sutures in an interrupted fashion, starting at the posterior vagina and proceeding longitudinally over the cul-de-sac peritoneum and then over the inferior sigmoid serosa; the sutures are tied as they are placed and should be approximately 1 cm apart [19]. Visualization of the ureters is important during both of these procedures to ensure that there is no obstruction or kinking of the overlying peritoneum when the cul-de-sac is closed (From Cleveland Clinic Center for Medical Art & Photography. Copyright © 2013, with permission)

7.4   Incontinence Procedures

The Burch colposuspension procedure remains an important technique for management of stress urinary incontinence in patients who have failed treatment with the midurethral sling, who decline synthetic mesh placement, or who are undergoing concomitant laparoscopic prolapse repair surgery and would prefer to have an abdominal approach for their incontinence procedure. Additionally, the paravaginal defect repair was once a routine procedure at the time of Burch colposuspension for treatment of stress urinary incontinence. While this procedure is no longer routinely performed, it remains indicated in certain patients.

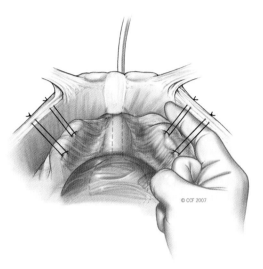

© CCF 2007

Fig. 7.7 Laparoscopic Burch colposuspension. Surgery for stress incontinence is recommended when conservative treatments fail. The open Burch colposuspension has been referred to as the gold standard for surgical management of urinary stress incontinence, with a reported cure rate higher than 80 % [20]. In recent years, the midurethral sling has become the most common method of surgical management of stress urinary incontinence owing to its minimally invasive approach and evidence that it has similar long-term efficacy to the Burch procedure [21]. However, the Burch colposuspension remains an important technique for management of stress urinary incontinence in patients who have failed treatment with the midurethral sling, who decline synthetic mesh placement, or who are undergoing concomitant laparoscopic prolapse repair surgery and would prefer to have an abdominal approach for their incontinence procedure. The laparoscopic Burch colposuspension was first described in the 1990s and while similar in technique to the open approach, has the same advantages as conventional laparoscopic surgery [20]. Miklos and Kohli provide a good description of how this procedure is performed [22]. The bladder is first filled in retrograde fashion to visualize the superior border of the bladder edge. The space of Retzius can be entered by creating a peritoneal incision above the bladder reflection, starting along the medial border of the right obliterated umbilical ligament. Confirmation of entry into the proper plane is made when the underlying loose alveolar tissue is encountered and the pubic rami are identified. The bladder is then drained and blunt dissection opens the space of Retzius until the bladder neck is identified. Important anatomic landmarks of this dissection include the pubic symphysis, Cooper's ligaments, and the arcus tendineus fascia pelvis. Once the bladder neck and midurethra are visualized, careful dissection exposes the underlying endopelvic fascia. A vaginal manipulator or digital manipulation elevates the vagina during placement of the sutures. Permanent No. 0 or 2-0 sutures are used, first placed lateral to and at the level of the midurethra, through the fibromuscular tissue of the vagina, with care not to incorporate the underlying epithelium. The suture is then passed through the Cooper's ligament on the ipsilateral side. A second suture is then placed at the level of the urethrovesical junction and again through the Cooper's ligament on the same side. The sutures are tied in an extracorporeal or intracorporeal fashion. The same procedure is repeated on the contralateral side. While the literature shows that midurethral sling procedures appear to offer greater benefits with better objective outcomes in the short term and similar subjective outcomes long term [23], the laparoscopic Burch procedure is still an important operation in pelvic reconstructive surgery and is appropriate for certain patients. Some studies have shown that that laparoscopic colposuspension is as efficacious as open colposuspension [20]; however, the 2010 Cochrane review on laparoscopic Burch colposuspension revealed that while women's subjective impression of cure was similar for both procedures, there was some evidence of poorer results for laparoscopic colposuspension on objective outcomes [23]. Additionally, while there were fewer postoperative complications and shorter hospital stays with laparoscopic Burch procedures when compared to open colposuspension, the laparoscopic approach was more costly (From Cleveland Clinic Center for Medical Art & Photography. Copyright © 2007–2013, with permission)

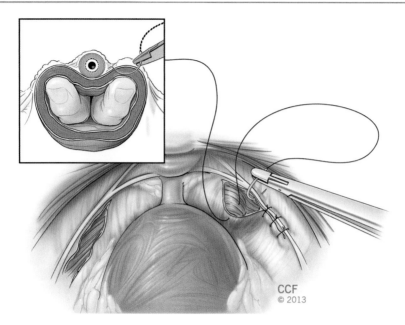

Fig. 7.8 Laparoscopic paravaginal defect repair. Lateral vaginal wall support defects may contribute to the development of stress urinary incontinence, and for this reason the paravaginal defect repair was once routine at the time of Burch colposuspension for treatment of stress urinary incontinence [22]. However, the rate of Burch colposuspension procedures continues to decrease with the increasing use of the midurethral sling. Additionally, the presence and degree of severity of paravaginal defects is challenging to diagnose as there is evidence that the clinical examination of these support defects displays poor interexaminer and intraexaminer agreement [24]. For these reasons, paravaginal defect repairs are performed much less frequently than in the past. However, a Cochrane review evaluating laparoscopic Burch colposuspension reported that paravaginal repair at the time of the Burch procedure appears to be beneficial with regard to postoperative outcomes. Therefore, understanding the steps of this procedure continues to be important [23]. These defects are identified when the space of Retzius is opened; the lateral attachments of the pubocervical fascia are detached from the side wall of the pelvis at the level of the arcus tendineus fascia pelvis. To repair these defects laparoscopically, a nonabsorbable suture can be used and passed through the fibromuscular layer of the vagina and then through the obturator internus muscle and its fascia around the arcus tendineus at its origin, approximately 2 cm from the ischial spine [22]. Several sutures are placed in an interrupted fashion from the ischial spine to the proximal portion of the vesicourethral junction until there is good restoration of vaginal anatomy. The procedure can be done unilaterally or bilaterally, depending on the nature of the defect (From Cleveland Clinic Center for Medical Art & Photography. Copyright © 2013, with permission)

7.5   Complications

The overall complication rate of gynecologic laparoscopic procedures has been reported to be approximately 0.46 % with a mortality rate of 3.3 per 100,000 laparoscopies [25]. As procedures become more complex, the risk of complication increases. Up to one-third of complications can be attributed to trocar entry or placement [2]. Vascular injuries, while rare, are associated with the highest rate of mortality from a laparoscopic injury. The reported incidence of laparoscopic vascular injury ranges from 0.01 to 0.64 % [25]. Morbidity from a vascular injury varies and is dependent on the vessel that is injured and time of recognition of the injury. The vessels most commonly injured during operative laparoscopy are the aorta, inferior vena cava, and iliac vessels [2]. Laparoscopic sacrocolpopexy adds additional risk to the vasculature of the presacral space, including the left common iliac vein, middle sacral artery, and sacral venous plexus [11].

Bowel injuries can account for almost one-third of laparoscopic complications during gynecologic procedures [25]. Injuries that occur at entry are usually associated with small bowel injuries and are the most common. Once entry has been achieved, injury to the rectosigmoid colon is the second most common type of injury [2]. Operative injuries with laparoscopic instruments, especially those using electrocautery, can also occur and can be very severe, as recognition of the injury can be delayed in these cases. Factors that increase the rate of bowel injury include complexity of the case, the presence of intra-abdominal adhesions, and the experience of the operating surgeon. A study by Warner and colleagues reported on the intraoperative and postoperative gastrointestinal complications specific to laparoscopic sacrocolpopexy [26]. Their intraoperative bowel injury rate was 1.3 %, and injury was not found to be associated with prior abdominal surgery, age, or body mass index. Their postoperative gastrointestinal complications included ileus and small bowel obstruction with a reported rate of 1 % in their patient population.

The incidence of ureteral injury (including transection, obstruction, fistula formation, and necrosis from thermal injury) during gynecologic laparoscopy ranges from less than 1–2 % [27]. The bladder is at risk of injury during its dissection at the time of hysterectomy and also during sacrocolpopexy. Injuries to the ureter occur most commonly at the level of the infindibulopelvic ligament and at the cardinal ligament, where the ureter passes underneath the uterine artery. Ureteral injury can also occur at the time of suspension suture placement during uterosacral ligament suspension if the sutures are placed in such a way that the peritoneum overlying the ureter receives too much tension or if the ureter itself is incorporated into the suspension. Cystoscopy after administration of indigo carmine dye should always be performed after laparoscopic reconstructive pelvic surgery because studies show that there is a higher injury detection rate seen when intraoperative cystoscopy is done [27].

Postoperative infection is rare after laparoscopic surgery. Spondylodiscitis of the L5 to S1 disc space is the most morbid infection associated with sacrocolpopexy and is very rare; only case reports have been written about this complication. *Staphylococcus aureus* is the most commonly reported organism, and cases were most commonly associated with concomitant hysterectomy at the time of prolapse repair [28]. When sacrocolpopexy is being performed, care should be taken to avoid the intervertebral disc space while placing the sacral sutures because deep stitches through the disc and periosteum may be the precipitating factors in the development of osteomyelitis. Patients with these infections require aggressive therapy with intravenous antibiotics and often reoperation for pelvic wash-out and removal of the infected graft.

Mesh erosion is also a complication related to laparoscopic sacrocolpopexy. A randomized clinical trial evaluating the outcomes of abdominal sacrocolpopexy with and without Burch colposuspension also looked at the risk of mesh and suture exposure following abdominal sacrocolpopexy and found the exposure rate to be 6 % in 322 study participants [29]. Results from a retrospective study of 188 subjects demonstrated a higher rate of mesh erosion in patients who had undergone concurrent total laparoscopic hysterectomy compared to those who were posthysterectomy or underwent supracervical hysterectomy at the time of surgery, with rates of 23, 5, and 5 %, respectively [30]. Performing a supracervical hysterectomy at the time of prolapse surgery rather than a total vaginal hysterectomy prior to sacrocolpopexy has become more common, and patients should be counseled regarding the risks and benefits of both options.

Conclusions

Currently, our fastest growing population is the elderly, and the incidence and prevalence of uterovaginal prolapse and urinary incontinence increase with age. Current data show that 23.7 % of women suffer from at least one pelvic floor disorder [31] and that the overall prevalence of these disorders is projected to increase by 56 % by 2050 [32]. While there are three approaches to surgery that exist for pelvic floor disorders, in this chapter we focused on the laparoscopic procedures that are used to treat prolapse and incontinence. There are many advantages to performing these surgeries in a minimally invasive fashion; however, the burden of postoperative complications remains. For this reason, it is imperative that the appropriate surgical candidates undergo the correct procedures for their surgical needs and that important perioperative precautions are taken. Surgical management of pelvic organ prolapse and incontinence remains complex. The principles for management of these disorders are not new, and the difference lies in the route by which the surgery is performed. Adequate training is necessary to perform these procedures laparoscopically; however, pelvic floor surgeons should strive to learn these techniques as the benefits of improved visualization of pelvic anatomy and easier recovery for patients remain very desirable.

References

1. Diwadkar GB, Chen CC, Paraiso MF. An update on the laparoscopic approach to urogynecology and pelvic reconstructive procedures. Curr Opin Obstet Gynecol. 2008;20:496–500.
2. Makai G, Isaacson K. Complications of gynecologic laparoscopy. Clin Obstet Gynecol. 2009;52:401–11.
3. ACOG Committee on Practice Bulletins—Gynecology. ACOG practice bulletin no. 104: antibiotic prophylaxis for gynecologic procedures. Obstet Gynecol. 2009;113:1180–9.
4. Rahn DD, Mamik MM, Sanses TV, Matteson KA, Aschkenazi SO, Washington BB, et al. Venous thromboembolism prophylaxis in gynecologic surgery: a systematic review. Obstet Gynecol. 2011;118:1111–25.
5. Guyatt GH, Akl EA, Crowther M, Gutterman DD, Schuünemann HJ. Executive summary: antithrombotic therapy and prevention of thrombosis, 9th ed. American College of Chest Physicians Evidence-Based Clinical Practice Guidelines. Chest. 2012;141(2 Suppl):7S–47.
6. Güenaga KF, Matos D, Wille-Jørgensen P. Mechanical bowel preparation for elective colorectal surgery. Cochrane Database Syst Rev. 2011;(9):CD001544.
7. Rardin CR, Erekson EA, Sung VW, Ward RM, Myers DL. Uterosacral colpopexy at the time of vaginal hysterectomy: comparison of laparoscopic and vaginal approaches. J Reprod Med. 2009;54:273–80.
8. Seman EI, Cook JR, O'Shea RT. Two-year experience with laparoscopic pelvic floor repair. J Am Assoc Gynecol Laparosc. 2003;10:38–45.
9. Behnia-Willison F, Seman EI, Cook JR, O'Shea RT, Keirse MJ. Laparoscopic paravaginal repair of anterior compartment prolapse. J Minim Invasive Gynecol. 2007;14:475–80.
10. Ganatra AM, Rozet F, Sanchez-Salas R, Barret E, Galiano M, Cathelineau X, Vallancien G. The current status of laparoscopic sacrocolpopexy: a review. Eur Urol. 2009;55:1089–103.
11. Walters MD, Ridgeway BM. Surgical treatment of vaginal apex prolapse. Obstet Gynecol. 2013;121(2 Pt 1):354–74.
12. Nygaard IE, McCreery R, Brubaker L, Connolly A, Cundiff G, Weber AM, Zyczynski H. Abdominal sacrocolpopexy: a comprehensive review. Obstet Gynecol. 2004;104:805–23.
13. Brubaker L, Nygaard I, Richter HE, Visco A, Weber AM, Cundiff GW, et al. Two-year outcomes after sacrocolpopexy with and without Burch to prevent stress urinary incontinence. Obstet Gynecol. 2008;112:49–55.
14. Frick AC, Walters MD, Larkin KS, Barber MD. Risk of unanticipated abnormal gynecologic pathology at the time of hysterectomy for uterovaginal prolapse. Am J Obstet Gynecol. 2010;202(507):e1–4.
15. Burgess KL, Elliott DS. Robotic/laparoscopic prolapse repair and the role of hysteropexy: a urology perspective. Urol Clin North Am. 2012;39:349–60.
16. Diwan A, Rardin CR, Strohsnitter WC, Weld A, Rosenblatt P, Kohli N. Laparoscopic uterosacral ligament uterine suspension compared with vaginal hysterectomy with vaginal vault suspension for uterovaginal prolapse. Int Urogynecol J Pelvic Floor Dysfunct. 2006;17:79–83.
17. Costantini E, Mearini L, Bini V, Zucchi A, Mearini E, Porena M. Uterus preservation in surgical correction of urogenital prolapse. Eur Urol. 2005;48:642–9.

18. Cadeddu JA, Micali S, Moore RG, Kavoussi LR. Laparoscopic repair of enterocele. J Endourol. 1996; 10:367–9.

19. Paraiso MFR. Laparoscopic surgery for stress urinary incontinence and pelvic organ prolapse. In: Walters MD, Karram MM, editors. Urogynecology and reconstructive pelvic surgery. 3rd ed. St. Louis: Mosby Inc; 2007. p. 213–26.

20. Carey MP, Goh JT, Rosamilia A, Cornish A, Gordon I, Hawthorne G. Laparoscopic versus open Burch colposuspension: a randomised controlled trial. BJOG. 2006;113:999–1006.

21. Jelovsek JE, Barber MD, Karram MM, Walters MD, Paraiso MF. Randomised trial of laparoscopic Burch colposuspension versus tension-free vaginal tape: long-term follow up. BJOG. 2008;115:219–25. discussion 225.

22. Miklos JR, Kohli N. Laparoscopic paravaginal repair plus Burch colposuspension: review and descriptive technique. Urology. 2000;56(6 Suppl 1):64–9.

23. Dean NM, Ellis G, Wilson PD, Herbison GP. Laparoscopic colposuspension for urinary incontinence in women. Cochrane Database Syst Rev. 2006;(3):CD002239.

24. Whiteside JL, Barber MD, Paraiso MF, Hugney CM, Walters MD. Clinical evaluation of anterior vaginal wall support defects: interexaminer and intraexaminer reliability. Am J Obstet Gynecol. 2004;191:100–4.

25. Chapron C, Querleu D, Bruhat MA, Madelenat P, Fernandez H, Pierre F, et al. Surgical complications of diagnostic and operative gynaecological laparoscopy: a series of 29,996 cases. Hum Reprod. 1998;13: 867–72.

26. Warner WB, Vora S, Alonge A, Welgoss JA, Hurtado EA, von Pechmann WS. Intraoperative and postoperative gastrointestinal complications associated with laparoscopic sacrocolpopexy. Female Pelvic Med Reconstr Surg. 2012;18:321–4.

27. Manoucheri E, Cohen SL, Sandberg EM, Kibel AS, Einarsson J. Ureteral injury in laparoscopic gynecologic surgery. Rev Obstet Gynecol. 2012;5: 106–11.

28. Grimes CL, Tan-Kim J, Garfin SR, Nager CW. Sacral colpopexy followed by refractory Candida albicans osteomyelitis and discitis requiring extensive spinal surgery. Obstet Gynecol. 2012;120(2 Pt 2):464–8.

29. Cundiff GW, Varner E, Visco AG, Zyczynski HM, Nager CW, Norton PA, et al. Risk factors for mesh/suture erosion following sacral colpopexy. Am J Obstet Gynecol. 2008;199:688.e1–5.

30. Tan-Kim J, Menefee SA, Luber KM, Nager CW, Lukacz ES. Prevalence and risk factors for mesh erosion after laparoscopic-assisted sacrocolpopexy. Int Urogynecol J. 2011;222:205–12.

31. Nygaard I, Barber MD, Burgio KL, Kenton K, Meikle S, Schaffer J, et al. Prevalence of symptomatic pelvic floor disorders in US women. JAMA. 2008;300:1311–6.

32. Wu JM, Hundley AF, Fulton RG, Myers ER. Forecasting the prevalence of pelvic floor disorders in U.S. women: 2010 to 2050. Obstet Gynecol. 2009; 114:1278–83.

Techniques in Reproductive Surgery

8

Elizabeth W. Patton and Magdy Milad

Advances in gynecologic minimally invasive surgical techniques coupled with basic and translational research have led to the development of multiple laparoscopic surgical applications for fertility preservation. Procedures discussed in this chapter include salpingolysis and fimbrioplasty for tubal occlusion, reversal of tubal ligation and tubal reanastomosis, treatment of hydrosalpinx or salpingectomy to improve in vitro fertility rates, and removal of hysteroscopic sterilization devices. In addition, laparoscopic approaches for oophoropexy and ovarian transposition to prevent recurrent torsion or to avoid damage secondary to radiation treatment are reviewed.

Each procedure is described and includes patient selection and preparation as well as surgical approach and technique. Narrative descriptions are supplemented by multiple intraoperative images as well as figure drawings to illustrate the various techniques.

E.W. Patton, MD, MPhil (✉)
Department of Obstetrics and Gynecology,
University of Michigan,
2800 Plymouth Road Building 10, Room G016,
Ann Arbor, MI 48109-2800, USA
e-mail: pattone@umich.edu

M. Milad, MD, MS
Department of Obstetrics and Gynecology,
Northwestern University Feinberg School of Medicine,
250 East Superior, Suite 05-2177,
Chicago, IL 60611, USA
e-mail: mmilad@nmh.org

8.1 Introduction

As the field of gynecologic laparoscopy has become increasingly sophisticated, techniques and procedures related to fertility preservation, treatment, and enhancement have likewise been refined. Basic and translational research has also shaped the practice of gynecologic minimally invasive surgery. For example, as techniques of in vitro fertilization have become progressively successful, the role of tubal surgery for tubal repair or reanastomosis has become more limited, although it retains a role for select patients if performed by skilled providers. Robotic access may also improve the availability of these procedures by providers that previously did not have the requisite psychomotor skills. Additionally, ovarian preservation surgery remains an important area of gynecologic laparoscopy, particularly for younger patients facing radiation treatment for malignancy or those with recurrent ovarian torsion requiring repeated urgent surgeries. Surgical procedures such as oophoropexy to prevent recurrent torsion or transposition to attempt to preserve fertility by moving the ovaries outside of a proposed radiation field for treatment of malignancy are often relatively simple and within the scope of many gynecologists. These should be offered to appropriate patients during physician-patient counseling on surgical management.

In this chapter, the techniques of tubal repair and reanastomosis, oophoropexy and ovarian transposition, and removal of previously

P.F. Escobar, T. Falcone (eds.), *Atlas of Single-Port, Laparoscopic, and Robotic Surgery*,
DOI 10.1007/978-1-4614-6840-0_8, © Springer Science+Business Media New York 2014

hysteroscopically placed sterilization devices will be reviewed, along with illustrative intra-operative images and figure drawings. Each section in the chapter will review the technique, the patients for whom it is appropriate, and any particular preoperative and perioperative considerations accompanied by the images. In some cases, such as tubal repair and reanastomosis, the procedure requires highly specialized laparoscopic skills, which may necessitate referral to a specialist trained in these techniques.

8.2 Laparoscopic Tubal Surgery for Fertility Indications

8.2.1 Laparoscopic Tubal Repair and Reanastomosis and Removal of Previously Placed Tubal Occlusion Devices

Tubal disease plays a significant role in female-factor infertility, with rates ranging from 25 % to 35 % [1]. Besides the significant role of salpingitis and other contributors to tubal factor infertility, 20–30 % of women regret having pursued a tubal ligation [2]. Thus, there are many potential patients for whom a tubal repair or tubal reanastomosis surgery might be appropriate. However, in an era in which in vitro fertilization (IVF) treatments are becoming ubiquitous and effective, careful consideration must be given to patient counseling and selection. Bypassing the fallopian tubes entirely with IVF has further advantages for those affected by infertility. It is less surgically invasive, enables treatment of other infertility factors, and allows for frozen embryos that can be used years later when diminished ovarian reserve may have ensued. Additionally, tubal repair or reanastomosis requires a laparoscopic surgeon of sophisticated skill; such a surgeon may be unavailable to many patients.

On the other hand, tubal repair/reanastomosis is a minimally invasive outpatient surgery, and if successful, saves a patient from serial injections, the increased risk of multifetal gestations, and ovarian hyperstimulation syndrome, which can be seen with IVF. For patients whose location, socioeconomic status, or insurance does not afford them access to IVF treatment, tubal repair may be their only option for treatment of tubal factor infertility or to reverse the effects of a regretted prior tubal ligation. Finally, with severely diminished ovarian reserve, IVF may be associated with a dismal cycle specific pregnancy rate, in which case tubal repair with its associated cumulative success may be warranted.

Tubal repair surgery or reanastomosis surgery is therefore most appropriate for young healthy patients who do not have other known contributing factors to infertility except for the identified tubal factor or a prior tubal ligation. However, patients must be willing to accept the surgical risks of infection, bleeding, damage to adjacent structures, and the possibility that even a technically successful surgery may not result in pregnancy.

Once a patient has been thoroughly advised regarding her options and has, through collaborative discussion with her physician, opted for laparoscopic tubal repair surgery, the location of the tubal blockage of disease will determine the surgical approach and technique.

8.2.2 Proximal Tubal Occlusion

Appropriate candidates for tubal repair surgery to correct proximal tubal blockage are those who are young, without other obvious causes of female or male factor infertility, and those whose preoperative hysterosalpingogram (HSG) demonstrates inability to cannulate the tube only, without evidence of salpingitis isthmica nodosa or predisposing risk factors for concomitant distal disease.

Diagnosis of proximal tubal blockage can occur via fluoroscopy or by hysteroscopy with laparoscopic confirmation. An outer catheter is inserted in the ostia and a hysterosalpingogram is performed (Fig. 8.1). If blockage is confirmed, an inner catheter is advanced gently through the proximal tube, under fluoroscopic or hysteroscopic/laparoscopic guidance. If the catheter cannot be threaded with gentle pressure, an occlusion is considered confirmed. Meta-analysis review of patients with bilateral proximal tubal occlusion revealed an approximate 85 % success rate of unblocking with tubal cannulation and about 50 % patient conception thereafter [3].

Fig. 8.1 Transcervical tubal cannulation to assess for tubal patency

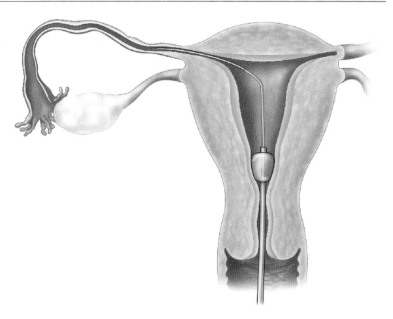

8.2.3   Distal Tubal Occlusion

If preoperative HSG has confirmed a more distal tubal occlusion, a diagnostic laparoscopy can be the next step for those patients not proceeding directly to IVF. Prior to these procedures patients should be counseled on both salpingostomy and tubal repair as well as salpingectomy, since large hydrosalpinges have been demonstrated to negatively affect IVF success [4]. Patients with the best chance of success for tubal repair are those with small amounts of filmy adhesions and mild dilation of the fallopian tubes (Fig. 8.2).

Salpingolysis and Fimbrioplasty. Once laparoscopic access is established, the fallopian tube is identified. The mesosalpinx can be injected with dilute vasopressin (5 international units per 20 mL of normal saline) to reduce bleeding. The tube is gently elevated with an atraumatic grasper, and adhesions are either lysed or excised using a harmonic scalpel or endoscopic scissors. Avoiding lateral damage may help improve long-term tubal function. Outcomes are best if distal tubal disease is limited to encapsulating adhesions.

A straight dissector can be used to resolve fimbrial agglutination or prefimbrial phimosis. If a small hydrosalpinx is present, an incision is made using a laparoscopic needle or scissors with harmonic, monopolar electrosurgery employed sparingly. This incision allows drainage of the hydrosalpinx fluid.

If the hydrosalpinx is large or the adhesions are extensive, salpingectomy should be undertaken and followed by IVF because a large hydrosalpinx (greater than 3 cm) has a poor response to neosalpingostomy. A blunt probe can be very useful in truly gauging the severity of a hydrosalpinx (Fig. 8.3).

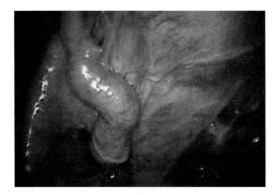

Fig. 8.2 Peritubal adhesions. Intraoperative laparoscopic image of peritubal adhesions (Courtesy of M. Milad)

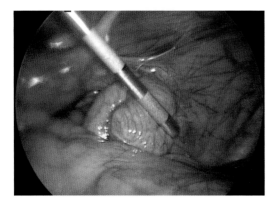

Fig. 8.3 Utilizing a blunt probe to assess the size of a hydrosalpinx (Courtesy of M. Milad)

Salpingectomy is performed by dividing the proximal tube at the cornua using an electrosurgical coagulation and cutting device. The same device is then used to coagulate and cut the mesosalpinx close to the tube along its length serially. Electrosurgery should be used sparingly, given the concern for thermal injury to the ovarian vessels and the potential for fewer oocytes retrieved at egg aspiration. To avoid any electrosurgery at the infundibulopelvic ligaments, sutures or an endoloop may be employed (Fig. 8.4).

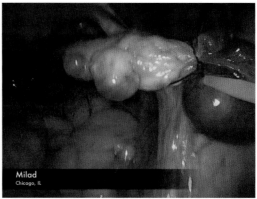

Fig. 8.4 Use of an endoloop to ligate the infundibulopelvic ligament as part of a salpingectomy, enabling minimal use of the electrocautery and maximal sparing of the ovarian blood supply (Courtesy of M. Milad)

Neosalpingostomy. If the fimbria have become severely adhered in such a way that the tubal opening is obliterated and no retention of normal fimbria is seen, a more complex tubal repair may be warranted. After placement of dilute vasopressin and salpingolysis, a stellate or cruciate incision is made at the distal end of the hydrosalpinx using a needle, harmonic shears, or scissors. Electrosurgery should be used sparingly to avoid tubal damage. The distal end "fimbriae" are then everted, and interrupted sutures are placed to maintain the increased size of the opening (see Fig. 8.5a, b). Owing to the technically difficult nature of placing these sutures in friable and delicate tubal tissue, this procedure should only be undertaken by laparoscopic surgeons who are very comfortable with the laparoscopic microsuturing technique and the use of 6–0 suture or finer. Alternatively, desiccation using electrosurgery or laser immediately behind the distal end may help facilitate retention of patency after the stellate or cruciate incision has been made (see Fig. 8.6).

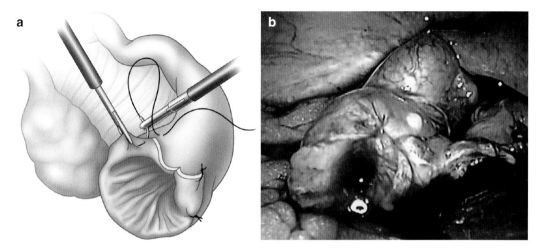

Fig. 8.5 Neosalpingostomy. (**a**) Line drawing of neosalpingostomy technique illustrating suturing of divided tubal edge to proximal tube to create a new tubal opening. (**b**) Intraoperative photograph demonstrating the resulting tubal opening after completion of the neosalpingostomy

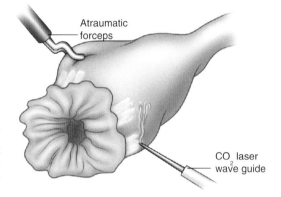

Fig. 8.6 Bruhat technique using carbon dioxide laser just behind the distal tubal edge to attempt to maintain tubal patency after lysis of adhesions of a blocked tubal opening

Success rates for these procedures range widely. Patients with only mild hydrosalpinx have had intrauterine pregnancy rates ranging from 58 to 77 % after the procedure, with an ectopic pregnancy rate of 2–8 % [5].

8.2.4 Reversal of Prior Tubal Ligation

Patients undergoing reversal of prior tubal ligation should be counseled about the alternate option of IVF. Most patients with tubal ligation have excellent IVF cycle specific success rates. If tubal reversal is warranted, it should be undertaken by an expert reproductive surgeon experienced with handling of fine suture and delicate tissue.

The laparoscopic approach is preferred because outcomes are the same as with laparotomy. New advances in robotic technology also make this an option for those with access to this technology and with a facility with the robotic suturing technique.

The previously ligated tubes are identified, and the two occluded ends of the distal and proximal ends are located. Vasopressin is again injected into the mesosalpinx prior to operating on the tube. If a clip or ring was used, the affected tubal segment is resected typically in a perpendicular fashion to the lumen. Each end is opened. A stent may be placed hysteroscopically and inserted through the proximal end into the distal end to ensure patency throughout the length of the tube. A retention suture can be placed in the mesosalpinx under the distal and proximal ends to ensure that the ends remain in close proximity while the approximating sutures are placed. The proximal and distal ends are reanastomosed using interrupted nonreactive sutures placed circumferentially at the cardinal angles. A single suture along the antimesosalpingeal corner has been suggested as an alternative but has not been well studied. The stent is withdrawn. Reanastomosis requires surgeons skilled in microsurgical laparoscopic technique.

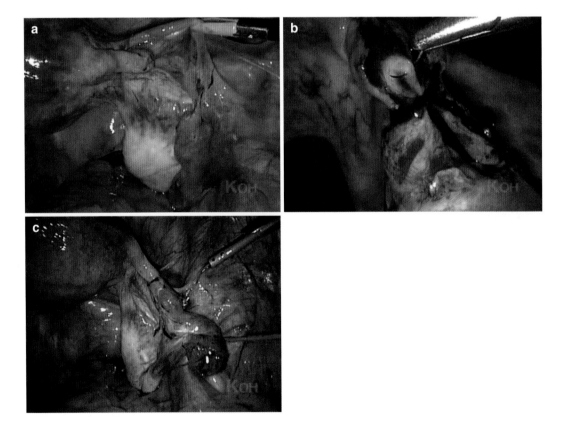

Fig. 8.7 (**a**) Intraoperative image demonstrating the appearance of a fallopian tube in a patient with a history of prior tubal ligation; (**b**) laparoscopically suturing the uterine tubal stump to the tubal stump at the fimbriated end of the fallopian tube; (**c**) appearance after suturing is complete; chromopertubation with spillage of blue dye at fimbriated end confirming patency of the fallopian tube after reanastamosis (Courtesy of Charles Koh, MD, Co-Director, Milwaukee Institute of Minimally Invasive Surgery.)

8.2.5 Removal of Previously Placed Hysteroscopic Sterilization Device

The advent of hysteroscopic sterilization with coil devices has resulted in a new group of patients pursuing surgery for fertility indications—those with such previously placed devices who desire their removal for pursuit of fertility or owing to chronic post-placement pain. Like patients with second thoughts regarding a previous tubal ligation, patients with prior hysteroscopic sterilization should also be counseled about the option of IVF if fertility is their goal.

Once laparoscopic access to the abdomen has been achieved, the location of the microinsert within the tube is identified. Needlepoint monopolar electrosurgery is used to incise over the end portion of the microinsert, and then graspers are used to gently remove the microinsert from the tube and withdraw it through the port [6]. If fertility is desired, the procedure is terminated. If the goal of the procedure was to reduce pain and the patient does not desire fertility, a laparoscopic tubal ligation is performed at this time.

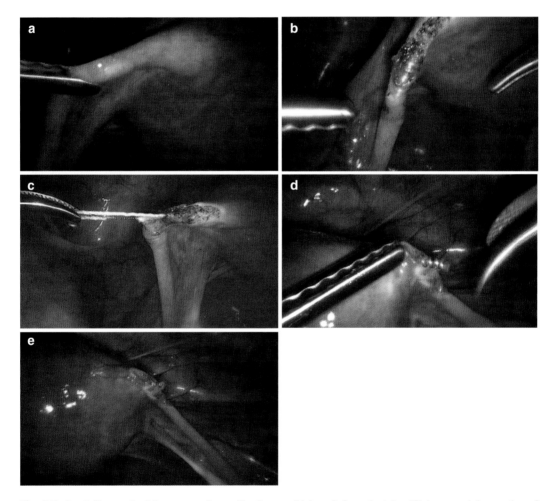

Fig. 8.8 (**a–e**) Removal of hysteroscopic sterilization device. (**a**) Elevation of tube with laparoscopic grasper to locate the end of the hysteroscopic sterilization device within the tube. (**b**) Incision using monopolar needle electrosurgery along the length of the tube parallel to the hysteroscopic sterilization device to expose the end of the device. (**c**) Laparoscopic graspers such as a Maryland grasper are used to grasp the end of the device and withdraw it from the tube. (**d**) Any remaining portion of the coil that did not emerge with the initial portion of the device may be grasped similarly and withdrawn from the tube. (**e**) Excellent hemostasis noted after removal of the device. If the procedure was pursued to relieve pain symptoms and the patient desires tubal ligation, it may be done at this time (Courtesy of Dr. Amanda Yunker, DO, MSCR, Assistant Professor, Vanderbilt Medical Center.)

8.3 Laparoscopic Ovarian Surgery for Fertility Indications

While most gynecologic surgeons are familiar with ovarian surgery for removal of ovarian masses and cysts, ovarian surgery for fertility indications is less widely performed. However, for the appropriate patient, these procedures may provide significant benefit. This section will review the reasons for and the techniques of oophoropexy.

Oophoropexy can principally benefit two groups of patients: those younger women undergoing radiation for various malignancies before completing childbearing and desiring ovarian preservation and those women with recurrent ovarian torsion of normal- sized adnexa. Although data are limited regarding these techniques and outcomes, it seems that the best approach to oophoropexy in the setting of planned radiation treatment is fixation of the ovary to the anterolateral pelvic side wall at or above the level of the pelvic brim [7]. In the setting of recurrent torsion of the adnexa, an alternate technique involves plication of the utero-ovarian ligament rather than oophoropexy [8].

8.3.1 Oophoropexy

Once laparoscopic access to the abdomen has been achieved, the ovaries and the utero-ovarian ligament are identified. To facilitate transposition, the utero-ovarian ligament is divided close to the uterine cornua. The tube is left intact. The ovary is then transposed lateral and anterior, approximately at the level of the anterior superior iliac spine. It is securely sutured in place with permanent suture to the peritoneum. The lower border of the ovary can be marked with hemoclips for later identification. Prior to surgery, the field of planned radiation can be outlined to

ensure that the ovaries are placed lateral and superior to the field.

8.3.2 Plication of the Utero-Ovarian Ligament

The utero-ovarian ligament and ovary are identified. Suture is brought into the pelvis and inserted with the needle parallel to the ligament. The needle enters into the ligament from the lateral end, and several stitches are placed along the length of the ligament running toward the cornua to plicate the extra length of the ligament. The suture is tied once the ligament is felt to be sufficiently shortened. The process can be repeated on the opposite site. The ovary and fallopian tube are not disturbed by this technique nor is undue tension placed on the ligament.

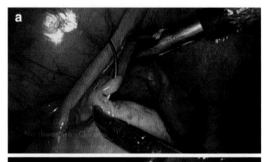
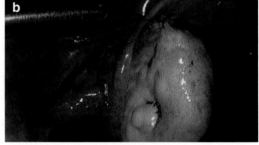

Fig. 8.9 (**a, b**) Intraoperative image demonstrating suture plication of the utero-ovarian ligament to prevent recurrent torsion (Courtesy of M. Milad)

Conclusion

The laparoscopic techniques in this chapter range from the relatively straightforward (plication of the utero-ovarian ligament, salpingectomy in the case of large hydrosalpinges to promote improved IVF success rates) to those requiring exquisite laparoscopic surgical skill (tubal reanastomosis). All illustrate the multiple applications of laparoscopic gynecologic surgery in the arena of fertility, a trend that is likely to continue with further developments in minimally invasive techniques and ever more sophisticated equipment.

References

1. The Practice Committee of the American Society for Reproductive Medicine. Committee opinion: role of tubal surgery in the era of assisted reproductive technology. Fertil Steril. 2012;97:539–45.

2. Borrero SB, Reeves MF, Schwarz EB, Bost JE, Creinin MD, Ibrahim SA. Race, insurance status, and desire for tubal sterilization reversal. Fertil Steril. 2008;90:272–7.

3. Honore GM, Holden AE, Schenken RS. Pathophysiology and management of proximal tubal blockage. Fertil Steril. 1999;5:785–95.

4. Kassabji M, Sims JA, Butler L, Muasher SJ. Reduced pregnancy outcome in patients with unilateral or bilateral hydrosalpinx after in vitro fertilization. Eur J Obstet Gynecol Reprod Biol. 1994;56:129–32.

5. Nackley AC, Muasher SJ. The significance of hydrosalpinx in in vitro fertilization. Fertil Steril. 1998;69:373–84.

6. Lennon BM, Lee SY. Techniques for the removal of the Essure* hysteroscopic tubal occlusion device. Fertil Steril. 2007;88:497.e13–4.

7. Bisharah M, Tulandi T. Laparoscopic preservation of ovarian function: an underused procedure. Am J Obstet Gynecol. 2003;188:367–70.

8. Fuchs N, Smorgick N, Tovbin Y, Ben Ami I, Maymon R, Halperin R, Panksy M. Oophoropexy to prevent adnesal torsion: how, when and for whom? J Minim Invasive Gynecol. 2010;17:205–8.

Part II

Single/Reduced Laparoscopy

Instrumentation for Single-Site Gynecologic Surgery

9

Jessica R. Woessner and Jason A. Knight

In minimally invasive surgery, the surgeon neither directly visualizes nor handles the tissue but rather gains access to the surgical field via cannulae through multiple incisions or a single incision. Access is provided by an optical system that allows visualization of the surgical field. Well-selected laparoscopic instrumentation provides traction and the capacity to seal and divide tissue pedicles to achieve the surgical goal. Access systems are categorized into single-site platforms and multi-incision platforms. The successful single-site surgeon should be thoroughly familiar with surgical instrumentation and should select a complement of instruments that satisfy his or her operative needs and experience. Laboratory experience in a simulated surgical environment allows surgeons to explore instrumentation and thereby provides the surgeon with a comprehensive understanding of an instrument. This chapter reviews the instrumentation for single-site gynecologic surgery.

9.1 Introduction

Traction, countertraction, and exposure are the familiar mantras of successful surgery. While these principles remain relevant in minimally invasive surgery, the surgical environment is one in which the surgeon neither directly visualizes nor handles tissue. Therefore, the mantras of traction, countertraction, and exposure may be better rephrased in minimally invasive surgery as access, dissector, and optics, since these three elements are necessary in minimally invasive surgery in order to successfully achieve traction, countertraction, and exposure.

The ability to provide traction, countertraction, and exposure is directly related to one's ability to gain access to the surgical field, which in minimally invasive surgery is through cannulae, entering through multiple incisions or a single incision. Access must be coupled with an optical system allowing visualization of the surgical field. A well-selected dissector in conjunction with laparoscopic instrumentation provides traction and the capacity to seal and divide tissue pedicles to achieve the surgical goal.

J.R. Woessner, MD
Women's Health Institute, Cleveland Clinic,
9500 Euclid Avenue, Cleveland,
OH 44195, USA

J.A. Knight, MD (✉)
Women's Health Institute, Section of Gynecologic Oncology, Cleveland Clinic, 9500 Euclid Avenue, Cleveland, OH 44195, USA
e-mail: knightj3@ccf.org

P.F. Escobar, T. Falcone (eds.), *Atlas of Single-Port, Laparoscopic, and Robotic Surgery*,
DOI 10.1007/978-1-4614-6840-0_9, © Springer Science+Business Media New York 2014

9.2   Access

The hallmark of minimally invasive surgery is a decrease in incision burden with a consequent reductions in postoperative pain, analgesic use, and hernia incidence compared to laparotomy [1, 2]. Minimally invasive surgery has itself evolved from multi-incision techniques to single-site techniques with a similar although smaller magnitude and reduction in postoperative pain and analgesic use [3].

Several access platforms for minimally invasive gynecologic surgery exist. The surgeon is encouraged to select the platform appropriate for the planned surgery and his or her experience.

Successful gynecologic and gynecologic oncology procedures are feasible with all of these platforms [4, 5]; however, each platform has its advantages and limitations.

9.2.1   Single-Site Platforms

9.2.1.1 SILS Port (Covidien; Mansfield, MA)

This port requires a 2.5-cm skin and fascial incision. The foam port is 5 cm long and can accom-

modate a body wall that is 3.5 cm thick (Fig. 9.1). In addition to the insufflation cannula, the port accommodates three instrument cannulae. The standard configuration is composed of three 5-mm cannulae; alternatively, one of the 5-mm cannulae can be replaced with a 12- or 15-mm cannula.

The SILS Port is most notable for its relative ease of use; however, it is sensitive to incision size. An incision <2.5 cm will make port placement difficult, whereas incisions >2.5 cm will result in gas leak. Furthermore, in cases where morcellation is contraindicated or not feasible, continuing single-site surgery after extension of the umbilical incision for specimen removal is not possible because the abdominal aperture will be too large for the SILS port. Finally, the SILS port is not well suited to patients with a thick abdominal wall greater than 3.5 cm. In such cases, the flanges at either side of the port will become buried within the wound instead of resting on the skin and peritoneal surfaces.

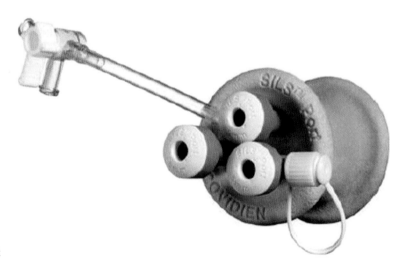

Fig. 9.1 Covidien SILS Port

9.2.1.2 The QuadPort+(Olympus America; Center Valley, PA)

This port accommodates a 2–6-cm skin and fascial incision. The adjustable sleeve accommodates an abdominal wall up to 10 cm thick. In addition to the insufflation cannula, the port has five trocars: two 5 mm, one 10 mm, one 15 mm, and one 12 mm (Fig. 9.2). The configuration of the trocars cannot be changed, except that the larger trocars can be stepped down to 5 mm with an adapter.

The QuadPort+is notable for its adjustable wound sleeve and feature of five trocars. The limitation is that surgeons rarely utilize more than three trocars at any moment and the other two can get in the way. More importantly, the drag force that the trocars impart upon entry and withdrawal of instruments is much more than other trocar systems. The added force required to introduce, adjust, and withdraw instruments has the potential to contribute to surgeon fatigue. Furthermore, the added force required to make fine instrument adjustments has the potential to negatively impact the precision of these fine movements.

9.2.1.3 GelPOINT Advanced Access Platform

The platform is composed of an Alexis Wound Retractor (Applied Medical; Rancho Santa Margarita, CA) and a GelPort cover (Applied Medical; Rancho Santa Margarita, CA). It accommodates a skin and fascial incision between 1.5 and 7 cm. The adjustable wound retractor accommodates an abdominal wall up to 10 cm thick. The platform comes with four trocars: three 10 mm and one 15 mm (Fig. 9.3). The trocars can be oriented in the GelPort cover in any configuration. They can be removed and repositioned as needed given the GelPort's self-healing capability.

Because the GelPOINT utilizes an Alexis Wound Retractor and a GelPort cover, it affords the surgeon the greatest degree of configuration flexibility among the single-site access platforms. The surgeon may utilize any of the four trocars in any desired configuration as he or she places the trocars into the GelPort according to the needs of the case. The trocars can be removed and replaced at any time. The self-healing property of the GelPort prevents gas leaks even after configuration changes. The incision can be extended to facilitate specimen removal. Single-site surgery can continue with the GelPOINT as long as the incision diameter does not exceed 7 cm. Portions of the procedure, such as an omentectomy, can be performed open using the Alexis Wound Retractor without the GelPort cover, followed by single-site pelvic laparoscopy (e.g., hysterectomy, bilateral salpingo-oophorectomy with lymphadenectomy).

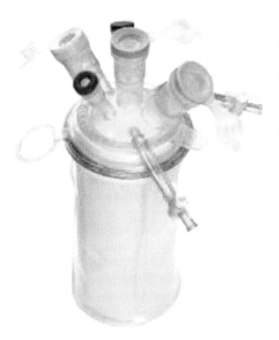

Fig. 9.2 Olympus QuadPort+

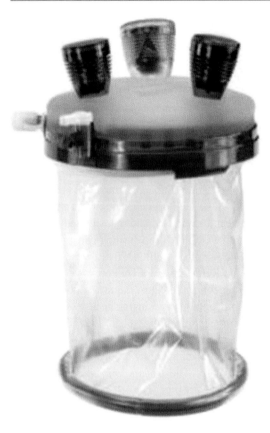

Fig. 9.3 Applied Medical GelPOINT Advanced Access Platform

9.3 Dissectors

Successful completion of single-site gynecologic surgery requires a dissector capable of sealing and dividing vascular pedicles. Although many energy sources are available, the most applicable to gynecologic surgery are bipolar and ultrasonic dissectors. Ionized noble gas dissectors and laser dissectors, while useful in specific circumstances, are not sufficient by themselves in completing common gynecologic procedures such as hysterectomy.

9.3.1 Bipolar Dissectors

The most basic bipolar dissector uses a bipolar waveform supplied by a generator such as the ForceTriad (Covidien; Mansfield, MA) or an older ValleyLab electrosurgical generator (Covidien; Mansfield, MA) connected to a bipolar grasper such as the Sovereign Bipolar Maryland forcep (Aesculap, Inc.; Center Valley, PA). While effective, this configuration lacks the security afforded by dynamic tissue impedance detection. Thus, the surgeon has no objective measure of therapeutic effect and no objective means to determine treatment length. Undertreatment risks pedicle bleeding; overtreatment increases thermal spread and risk of occult injury to nearby tissues.

Several vendors provide bipolar dissectors that incorporate tissue impedance detection during the treatment cycle. Some systems automatically end treatment cycles once a threshold impedance is achieved, e.g., LigaSure (Covidien; Mansfield, MA; Fig. 9.4), while others provide dynamic audible cues regarding tissue impedance, allowing the surgeon to titrate the energy dosage to the desired impedance: Plasma Kinetic Dissecting Maryland Forceps, Fig. 9.5 (Gyrus Medical; Maple Grove, MN). The Caiman Dissector (Aesculap; Center Valley, PA; Fig. 9.6) combines impedance detection with pulse wave form modulation to achieve vessel sealing with less current and lower thermal spread. This dissector features an articulating jaw.

Fig. 9.4 Covidien LigaSure

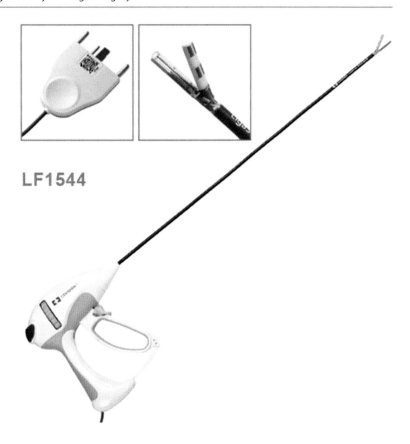

Fig. 9.5 Plasma Kinetic Dissecting forceps

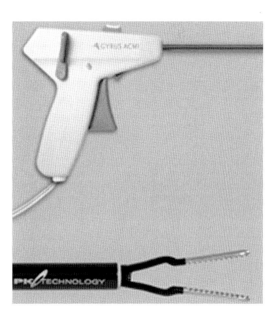

Fig. 9.6 The Aesculap
Caiman Dissector

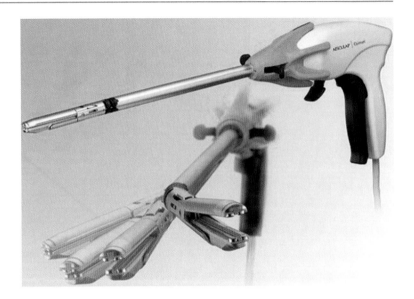

9.3.2 Ultrasonic Dissectors

Ultrasonic dissectors deliver mechanical energy
to tissues, resulting in vessel sealing via protein
denaturation. The primary limitation of ultrasonic dissectors is that vessel sealing cannot easily be performed without cutting tissue. Tissue
grasped by the jaw is divided during the process
of applying energy. This is of little consequence
when hemostasis is successfully achieved.
However, if a pedicle bleeds, each subsequent
attempt to secure the pedicle shortens it, which
in the case of the uterine artery pedicle decreases

the distance between the area of dissection and
the ureter.

Two ultrasonic dissectors that are currently
available are the Harmonic Ace by Ethicon
(Ethicon; Somerville, NJ; Fig. 9.7) and the
Sonocision (Covidien, Mansfield, MA), the only
cordless dissector commercially available. The
Sonocision (Covidien; Mansfield, MA) is powered
by a rechargeable battery pack and is entirely self-
contained, not requiring a bedside generator.

Table 9.1 compares the thermal spread and
vessel size limits associated with bipolar and
ultrasonic dissectors [6].

Fig. 9.7 The Harmonic Ace
by Ethicon

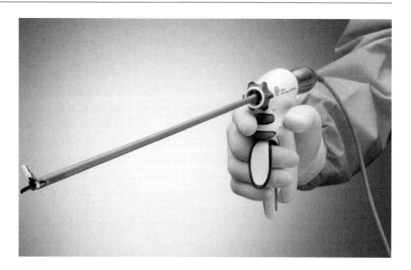

Table 9.1 Thermal spread and vessel size of bipolar and ultrasonic dissectors

Dissector	Thermal spread, mm[a]	Maximum vessel size, mm[a]
Plasma kinetic dissecting forcep (Gyrus Medical; Maple Grove, MN)	3.6[b]	5[b]
Aesculap Caiman (Aesculap, Center Valley, PA)	1	7
Ligasure (Covidien; Mansfield MA)	3	7
Sonicision (Covidien; Mansfield MA)	1.6	5
Harmonic Ace (Ethicon; Somerville, NJ)	1.5	5

[a]As reported by manufacturer
[b]Pietrow et al. [6]

9.4 Optics

Visualization of the surgical field is a necessary element of single-site surgery. Selecting an optical platform that meets the needs of the surgical approach is essential to successful completion of the planned surgery. Two classes of optical systems are available for minimally invasive surgery: rigid telescopes and flexible-tipped endoscopes.

Single-site surgery presents a unique surgical environment compared to traditional laparoscopy. Whereas traditional laparoscopy maintains triangulation of the surgical field via strategic positioning of trocars, single-site laparosocopy presents a challenge in that all instruments enter in parallel through a single incision, with a coincident loss of triangulation. Successful single-site surgery requires the intracorporeal reproduction of triangulation. As three points define a plane, the surgical plane is defined by the target organ and the two operating instruments. In traditional laparoscopy, the camera is typically outside of the plane of surgery by virtue of entering through a separate trocar site. Maintaining the camera outside of the surgical plane allows visualization of the surgical plane and prevents the camera from physically interfering with the surgical plane. In single-site laparoscopy, maintaining the camera outside of the surgical plane is important because failure to do so risks extracorporeal and intracorporeal conflict or clashing between the camera and operating instruments. In this circumstance, a flexible-tipped endoscope is preferred over a traditional rigid telescope. The flexible tip allows the camera to look down on the surgical field, thereby keeping the camera tip out of the field intracorporeally and the camera head out of conflict of the operating instruments extracorporeally. Examples of flexible tipped endoscopes are the Olympus EndoEYE (Center Valley, PA; Fig. 9.8) and the Stryker IDEAL EYES (Kalamazoo, MI).

Fig. 9.8 The Olympus EndoEYE

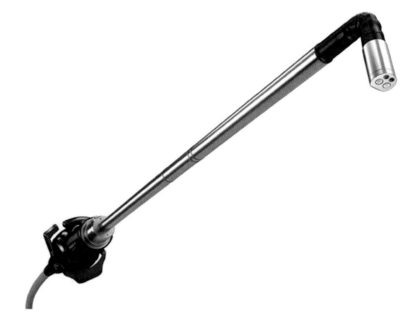

Conclusion

The successful single-site surgeon should be thoroughly familiar with surgical instrumentation. Laboratory experience in a simulated surgical environment is useful in allowing surgeons to explore instrumentation up to and beyond their designed limits, which in our opinion, provides understanding of an instrument's safety envelope during patient care.

Each surgeon should find instruments that satisfy his or her operative needs and experience. We routinely use the GelPOINT system for single-site surgery because of its versatility coupled with a Ligasure blunt-tipped dissector (Covidien; Mansfield, MA) and a flexible-tipped endoscope. We prefer the single-site approach over traditional laparoscopy for most patients because it reduces the number of incisions and is more cosmetically acceptable. Benign and oncologic staging procedures are feasible with the single-site approach with adequate surgical experience.

References

1. Falcone T, Paraiso MF, Mascha E. Prospective randomized clinical trial of laparoscopically assisted vaginal hysterectomy versus total abdominal hysterectomy. Am J Obstet Gynecol. 1999;180:955–62.
2. Walker JL, Piedmonte MR, Spirtos NM, Eisenkop SM, Schlaerth JB, Mannel RS, et al. Laparoscopy compared with laparotomy for comprehensive surgical staging of uterine cancer: Gynecologic Oncology Group Study LAP2. J Clin Oncol. 2009;27:5331–6.
3. Chen YJ, Wang PH, Ocampo EJ, Twu NF, Yen MS, Chao KC. Single-port compared with conventional laparoscopic-assisted vaginal hysterectomy: a randomized controlled trial. Obstet Gynecol. 2011;117: 906–12.
4. Escobar PF, Fader AN, Paraiso MF, Kaouk JH, Falcone T. Robotic-assisted laparoendoscopic single-site surgery in gynecology: initial report and technique. J Minim Invasive Gynecol. 2009;16:589–91.
5. Escobar PF, Nickles Fader A, Rasool N, Rojas-Espaillat L. Single-port laparoscopic pelvic and para-aortic lymph node sampling or lymphadenectomy: development of a technique and instrumentation. Int J Gynecol Cancer. 2010;20:1268–73.
6. Pietrow PK, Weizer AZ, L'Esperance JO, Auge BK, Silverstein A, Cummings T, et al. Plasma kinetic bipolar vessel sealing: burst pressures and thermal spread in an animal model. J Endourol. 2005;19: 107–10.

Single-Port Laparoscopic Adnexal Surgery

10

Chad M. Michener

Laparoscopic management of the adnexa in gynecology dates back to the initial descriptions of diagnostic laparoscopy and laparoscopic tubal surgery in the early 1900s. In 1910, a Swedish physician named Jacobeus was credited with coining the term *laparoscopy* when he performed the first intraperitoneal "scope" using a cystoscope. Despite the discovery of this novel technique to see inside the abdomen with only a small incision, laparoscopy got off to a slow start in the United States. In the late 1940s, TeLinde and colleagues [1] described the use of a rigid scope placed though the vagina for evaluation of the adnexa. TeLinde termed this *culdoscopy* and used it in the work-up of fertility patients, as well as to assess for ectopic pregnancy before laparotomy. The visualization of the pelvic abdominal cavities via a transvaginal approach was one of the foundations for natural orifice surgery [2]. Transabdominal laparoscopic visualization of the peritoneal cavity took a little longer to catch on in the United States. It was not until the late 1960s, when descriptions of laparoscopic tubal cauterization using a single-channel operative laparoscope with a mirrored lens began to surface, that operative laparoscopy gained more interest [3].

Since that time, innovations in technology have greatly improved the optics and the safety of laparoscopic equipment, while technical innovations and forward-thinking surgeons have identified new potential applications for operative laparoscopy. The result has been a recent surge in publications on standard laparoscopic, robotic-assisted laparoscopic, and, more recently, single-port laparoscopic management of benign and malignant adnexal conditions. This chapter focuses on single-port laparoscopic management of the adnexa in gynecologic surgery.

10.1 Patient Selection and Indications

Indications for single-port laparoscopic adnexal surgery do not differ from indications for standard laparoscopic procedures. The choice of which patients should be offered laparoscopy for the management of pelvic pathology should be based on sound clinical judgment and the skills of the surgeon. A patient with a highly suspicious, malignant-appearing mass on ultrasound and a CA-125 of 300 may not be the best candidate for single-port (or even standard) laparoscopic management. On the other hand, a woman with a mostly simple but enlarging 8-cm ovarian cyst with a thin septation and a normal CA-125 would be a perfect candidate for a trial of single-port laparoscopy.

C.M. Michener, MD
Department of Obstetrics and Gynecology,
Women's Health Institute, Cleveland Clinic,
Cleveland, OH 44195, USA
e-mail: michenc@ccf.org

P.F. Escobar, T. Falcone (eds.), *Atlas of Single-Port, Laparoscopic, and Robotic Surgery*,
DOI 10.1007/978-1-4614-6840-0_10, © Springer Science+Business Media New York 2014

Mass size has been used in the past for patient selection for both surgery and laparoscopy. Ghezzi et al. [4] found that women with adnexal masses larger than 10 cm and no evidence of ascites or metastases had an 8.6 % risk of ovarian cancer, a 4.3 % risk of low malignant potential tumors, and a 0.5 % risk of metastatic tumors in the ovary. Thus more than 85 % of tumors larger than 10 cm were benign and could safely be managed by laparoscopy.

10.2 Potential Benefits and Risks

One of the most important benefits of single-port laparoscopy is the slightly larger size of the incision, approximately twice that of a standard 12-mm laparoscopic port but small enough to hide within the umbilicus in most patients. This extra length of the incision allows for more flexibility in surgery, with easier extraction of the mass. Nevertheless, the requirement persists that larger cystic masses must be drained and more solid masses must be morcellated; both of these procedures should be carried out within a laparoscopic specimen retrieval bag (Fig. 10.1). Use of the umbilical incision, which may be enlarged as needed, avoids the need to "stretch" or extend lateral 12-mm port incisions to help with specimen retrieval, which may increase postoperative pain and hernia formation. Smaller ovaries can often

be removed intact and sometimes do not require a specimen retrieval bag at all, especially if the single-port device has a transabdominal wall sleeve, such as seen with the Applied Medical Gel Point™ (Rancho Santa Margarita, CA) or Olympus TriPort/Quadport (Center Valley, PA).

That said, several challenges with single-port laparoscopic surgery in gynecology have been well documented (Table 10.1). The most

Table 10.1 Potential benefits and drawbacks of single-port laparoscopy for adnexal masses

Potential benefits
Easier specimen extraction
Easy conversion if cancer
Better cosmesis
Decreased pain
Better exposure for fascial closure
Potential drawbacks
Difficult learning curve
Instrument clashing
Possible increased rupture risk
Increased operative time (initial)

Table 10.2 Potential etiologies of adnexal masses

Benign etiologies
Ovarian cysts
Ovarian torsion
Hemorrhagic cyst
Theca lutein cyst
Benign ovarian neoplasms
Epithelial
Germ cell
Sex-cord/stromal
Infectious/inflammatory
Tubo-ovarian abscess
Appendiceal abscess
Diverticular abscess
Endometrioma
Fallopian tube lesions
Hydrosalpinx
Paratubal cyst
Ectopic pregnancy
Other masses
Peritoneal inclusion cyst
Leiomyomas
Malignant etiologies
Ovarian malignancy
Epithelial carcinoma
Germ cell tumors
Sex cord/stromal tumors
Sarcomas
Fallopian tube carcinoma
Low malignant potential tumors
Metastatic lesions of adnexa
Carcinomas
Gastrointestinal
Breast
Pancreatic
Pseudomyxoma/appendiceal tumors
Sarcomas

common themes listed are instrument collision (both inside and outside of the peritoneal cavity), lack of triangulation of instrumentation, and loss of depth perception when the instruments are in line with the laparoscope. Some of these limitations have been overcome by novel instrumentation including articulating laparoscopes, articulating instruments, and improved camera optics. Nevertheless, even advanced laparoscopic surgeons experience a short learning curve when switching to a single-port laparoscopic approach. This learning curve has been documented by several studies looking at operative time and proficiency in single-port procedures. Fader et al. [5] studied all laparoendoscopic single-site surgeries (LESS) by gynecologic oncologists with advanced laparoscopic skills at three institutions and showed that both port placement and operative times markedly decreased between the first 10 cases and the 11th and 20th cases. Moreover, operative times stabilized after the first 20 cases. Additionally, Lee et al. [6] reviewed a single surgeon's experience over 500 gynecologic cases in Korea and found that the majority of benign gynecologic procedures could be performed by single-port laparoscopy. In this study, there was progression in each quintile of cases from the use of multiple ports to a single port (use of 2 or

more ports in 48 % of the first 100 cases versus less than 10 % in the last group of 100 cases), and a continued decline in laparotomy (29 % in the first 100 cases to 4 % for the last 100 cases). The quintiles did not differ with regard to surgical indication, procedure, prior laparotomies, adnexal size, or uterine weight. These findings make an argument for attempting to increase any form of laparoscopic surgery versus laparotomy in gynecologic surgery.

The selection of surgical candidates for single-port laparoscopic surgery for adnexal masses is no different than selection for standard laparoscopy. Etiologies of adnexal masses vary and can sometimes be identified preoperatively (Table 10.2). Ovarian masses can be segregated into high-risk and low-risk based on patient age, family history, symptoms, ultrasound findings, and tumor markers. These criteria can also be used to identify which patients should be referred to a gynecologic oncologist (Table 10.3) [7]. There is no absolute contraindication for the use of single-port laparoscopy compared with standard laparoscopy. However, several studies on single-port adnexal mass management have used various exclusion criteria, including suspicion of malignant tumor, emergent surgery, coexistence of other surgeries [8], tumor larger than 7 cm, age older than 70 years, and previous abdominal surgery for malignancy [9]. We have found that most gynecologic procedures can be adapted to the single-port approach with relatively few true contraindications. Even patients with one or more prior abdominal surgeries may be considered for the single-port laparoscopic approach, given that this is an open laparoscopy placement with a slightly larger incision. We have found that we are able to take down adhesions around the entry site enough that the single-port system can be placed and additional adhesiolysis, ureterolysis, extensive sidewall dissection can be performed laparoscopically (Figs. 10.2, 10.3, and 10.4). Nonetheless, clinical judgment should dictate each individual surgeon's comfort in choosing laparoscopy over laparotomy.

Table 10.3 SGO/ACOG guidelines for referral to a gynecologic oncologist

Postmenopausal	Premenopausal
Elevated CA-125	CA-125 >200 U/mL[a]
Ascites	Ascites
Nodular or fixed pelvic mass	–
Evidence of metastasis	Evidence of metastasis
Family history of one or more first-degree relatives with ovarian or breast cancer	Family history of one or more first-degree relatives with ovarian or breast cancer

Adapted from Im et al. [7]
ACOG American College of Obstetricians and Gynecologists, *SGO* Society of Gynecologic Oncologists
[a]Sensitivity and positive predictive value for referral in premenopausal women was low and can be increased by using a lower cutoff for CA-125

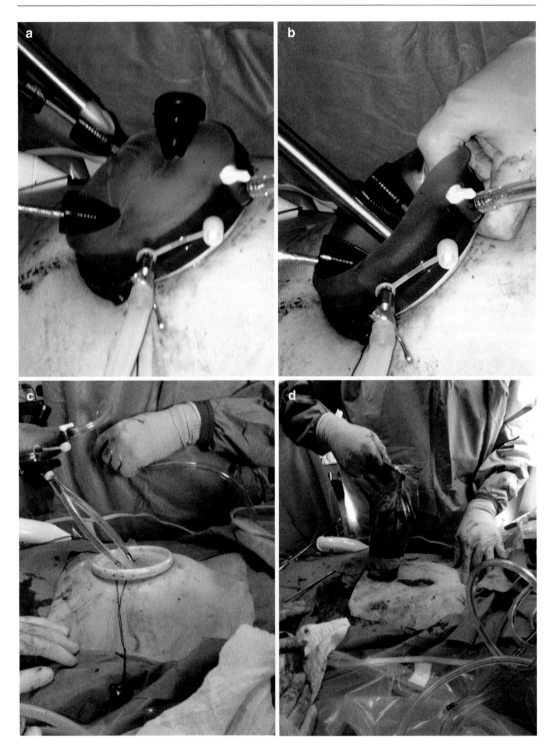

Fig. 10.1 Direct insertion of a large Endocatch bag through a Gel Point™ device (Applied Medical; Rancho Santa Margarita, CA). (**a**) The tip of the metal ring is advanced. (**b**) The bag is inserted directly through the gel. (**c**) Bag is cinched and metallic ring is withdrawn. (**d**) String is cut, gel cap removed, and specimen retrieved from the abdomen within the bag. Note that the incision in this case was extended to retrieve a very large, solid mass

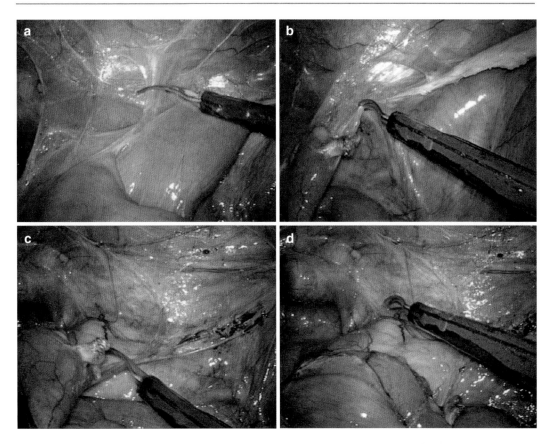

Fig. 10.2 Lysis of adhesions to expose adnexal mass using bowel grasper and endoscopic shears. (**a**) Lysis of filmy small bowel adhesions. (**b**) Cauterization of thick band and continued lysis of filmy adhesions. (**c**) Final lysis of small bowel adhesions. (**d**) Dissection of colon off of side wall to expose infundibulopelvic ligament

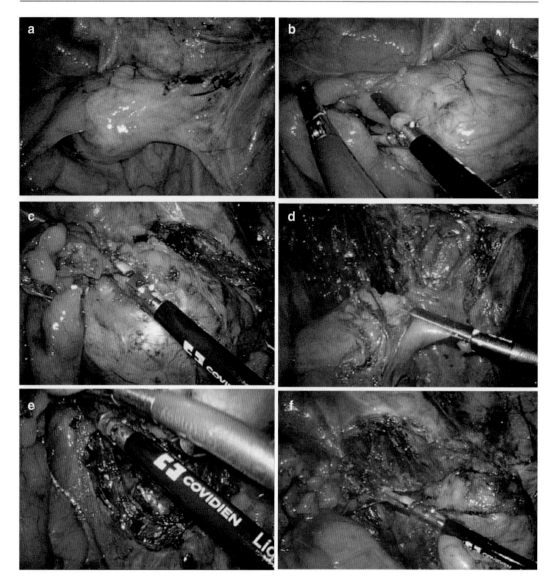

Fig. 10.3 Lysis of adhesions and excision of right ovarian fibroma. (**a**) Fibroma attached to sigmoid epiploica and side wall. Note ureter running posterior to anterior. (**b**) Lysis of epiploica adhesions. (**c**) Side wall open laterally and lower pole adhesions lysed. (**d**) Transection of infundibulopelvic ligament. (**e**) Mobilization away from the side wall. (**f**) Retrograde transection of inferior side wall attachments

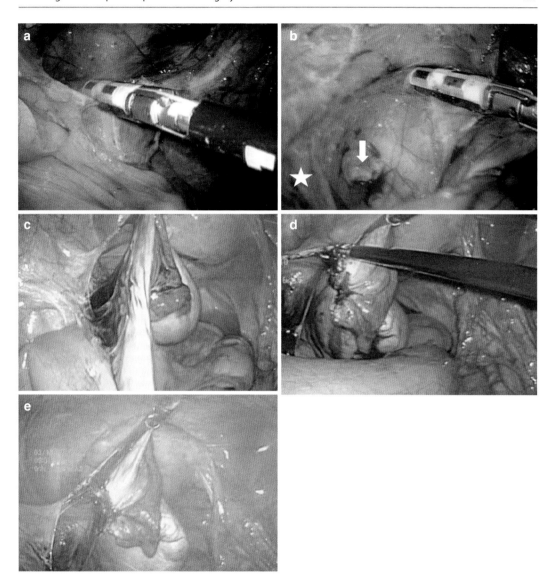

Fig. 10.4 Exposure of side wall and left salpingo-oopho-rectomy in patient with prior hysterectomy. (**a**) Opening of left pelvic side wall. (**b**) Exposure of iliac vessels (*star*) and ureter (*arrow*). (**c**) Traction on ovary to isolate infun-dibulopelvic ligament. (**d**) Transection of broad ligament. (**e**) Transection of distal side wall attachments

10.3   Procedure

The steps for single-port laparoscopic management of adnexal masses are listed in Table 10.4. Positioning is typically done as seen in Fig. 10.5. Most adnexal surgery is best performed via a transumbilical single-port approach. Entry into the peritoneal cavity should be carried out using the technique described by Hasson et al. [10]. Occasionally we have chosen an alternate site of entry, usually owing to a large uterus or a large adnexal mass, in which we make our incision in a supraumbilical location. Our preferred method of entry is to anesthetize the periumbilical region with bupivacaine. The edges of the umbilicus are grasped at 3 and 9 o'clock with Allis clamps, and we incise through the base of the umbilicus in the midline to make an incision measuring 1.5–2.5 cm. The fascial incision is extended, the peritoneum is grasped and entered, and a finger is swept into the peritoneal cavity to assess for adhesions. We then place an S-retractor into the peritoneal cavity at the inferior portion of the incision. The single-port system is then inserted into the peritoneal cavity and fixed in place, and the abdomen is insufflated. Once the camera is inserted into the peritoneal cavity, we use articulation of the flexible camera to evaluate the anterior abdominal wall around the port site and to evaluate the peritoneal cavity for ascites, carcinomatosis, and other pathology. The operative procedure itself can be carried out using standard, straight laparoscopic instruments (Fig. 10.6), but an increasing number of articulating instruments are available to decrease instrument clashing. The development of multifunctional instruments that enable us to dissect, seal vessels, and cut tissue without instrument exchanges has been a key to efficient single-port (and standard laparoscopic) procedures. Once the procedure is complete, we typically close the fascia with 0 delayed absorbable suture in a running fashion. If there was a previous umbilical hernia, we often use interrupted, figure-of-eight, nonabsorbable sutures. The skin is closed with a running subcuticular 4-0 absorbable suture.

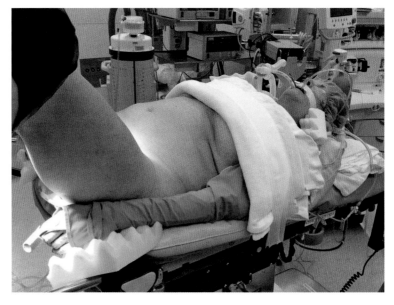

Fig. 10.5 Patient positioning. Typical positioning used with patient in lithotomy, both arms tucked and padded at sides, shoulders padded with a "beanbag" deflated to conform to the patient. The chest is taped/strapped with padding beneath. The beanbag can also be taped to the table if extra support is needed

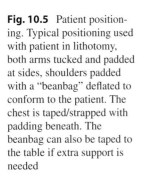

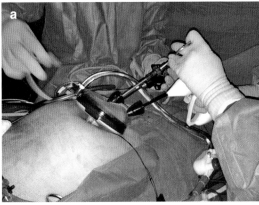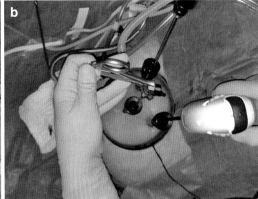

Fig. 10.6 Hand position in single-port laparoscopy with straight instruments. (**a**) Lateral view of hand positions. The nondominant hand (i.e., left) is toward the pelvis, with the handle of the instrument inverted. The dominant hand (i.e., right) is cephalad, with the instrument held in normal position. (**b**) Top view of hand positions. Note the port set-up of two ports cephalad and one caudad. The camera is in the right cephalad port

Table 10.4 Steps for single-port laparoscopic excision of an adnexal mass

Examination under anesthesia
Umbilical/abdominal entry via Hasson technique
Placement of single-port device and insufflation of abdomen
Inspection of mass and peritoneal surfaces, including diaphragm (easier with 30° or flexible-tip laparoscope)
Pelvic and abdominal washings
Biopsy of sites suspicious for metastasis; get frozen section
If malignant, convert to laparotomy for staging, if feasible; carry out laparoscopic staging, if it can be performed adequately; or discontinue laparoscopy and refer for staging
If benign/no evidence of malignancy, proceed with single-port laparoscopy
Cystectomy, oophorectomy, salpingectomy (excision of mass)
Identify ureter
Identify and ligate gonadal vessels for oophorectomy
If prophylactic bilateral salpingo-oophorectomy, ensure all ovarian tissue is removed, including adhesions—typically 2–3 cm up infundibulopelvic ligament from ovary
Place mass in laparoscopic specimen retrieval bag
Open bag at abdominal wall and remove specimen for frozen section
Inspect for hemostasis, irrigate, and close

10.4 Single-Port Laparoscopic Adnexal Surgery in Gynecology

10.4.1 Tubal Sterilization

One of the first reports on the use of single-port laparoscopy was for tubal sterilization. Wheeless and Thompson [3] reported on 2,600 women who underwent tubal sterilization at Johns Hopkins between 1968 and 1972, via a one-incision peri-umbilical technique utilizing either one burn or three burns using electrocautery through an operative laparoscope with an eyepiece. This technique was compared to a two-incision technique for sterilization in an additional 1,000 patients. Of the total of 3,600 patients, there were 24 pregnancies following the sterilization procedure. Injury of the intestinal tract from electrocautery occurred in 11 women. Miller [11] described single-puncture sterilization in an office setting using a single-puncture laparoscope with intravenous conscious sedation and local anesthesia in over 1,100 women. Ismail et al. [12] described a single-puncture tubal sterilization technique using Filshie clips in 42 women. More recently, Sewta [13] published a report on single-port laparoscopic sterilization using fallopian tube rings in 2011 patients in India. There were no sterilization failures and no major complications.

10.4.2 Management of Ectopic Pregnancy

Bedaiwy et al. [14] described the management of 11 hemodynamically stable women with isthmic and ampullary ectopic pregnancies using laparoendoscopic single-site salpingectomy using a commercially available single-port device. In this study, the tubal mass measured 1–6.5 cm and fetal cardiac activity was present in 6 of the 11 patients. The median operative time was 35 min and blood loss was 30 mL. They reported no conversions and no intraoperative or postoperative complications. Yoon et al. [15] described their experience with 20 women with ectopic pregnancy treated by single-port salpingectomy using a homemade "glove port." Outcomes in this series were similar, with no conversions in their series.

10.4.3 Management of Adnexal Masses

Increasing data have shown the utility of a variety of single-port laparoscopic techniques in the management of adnexal masses and other pathology (Table 10.5) [9, 16–25]. Risk-reducing salpingo-oophorectomy (RRSO) is an indication that appears favorable for laparoscopic management. Escobar et al. [16] described their initial experience with RRSO and found short operative times and no major complications in the RRSO group. Kim et al. [17] describe single-port access transumbilical laparoscopic-assisted adnexal surgery (SPATULAAS) for benign-appearing adnexal masses greater than 8 cm, using a homemade glove port. We have found that many adnexal masses up to 18 cm and some pedunculated leiomyomas with stalk width of ≤3 cm can be managed with a single port laparoscopic approach (Figs. 10.7 and 10.8).

Single-port access hand-assisted laparoscopic surgery (SPA-HALS) was developed for the management of large adnexal tumors Rho et al. [9] compared 43 patients with large adnexal tumors managed by SPA-HALS with 96 patients managed by standard single-port laparoscopic surgery (SPL). Despite a larger median mass size in the SPA-HALS group (10.9 vs. 6.3 cm), they noted a significant reduction in tumor spillage (10.3 % vs. 31.3 %) and more frequent adnexa-conserving procedures (76.7 % vs. 43.8 %) in the SPA-HALS group, compared with the standard SPL group.

Isobaric single-port laparoscopy has also been described using an abdominal wall elevator with a subcutaneous surgical wire or "rope" and steep Trendelenburg to visualize the pelvis without the use of pneumoperitoneum. This technique has been used for a variety of procedures on the ovaries and in the management of ectopic pregnancy

[26–28]. The number of applications for single-port laparoscopy in the management of adnexal pathology continues to grow and will only be limited by the gynecologist's imagination and skill set.

Although culdoscopy enjoyed popularity in the 1950s and 1960s, its use is more limited today. However, there are still papers published detailing transvaginal management of a variety of adnexal and uterine pathology. Tsin and colleagues [29] described a variety of surgical procedures performed via transvaginal laparoscopy, including ovarian cystectomy, oophorectomy, myomectomy, appendectomy, and cholecystectomy. There were no major complications in their series, but reported bowel injury rates for a transvaginal approach have ranged from 0.25 to 0.65 % [30]. In their retrospective review, 22 of 24 injuries resolved with conservative management consisting of hospital observation and antibiotics.

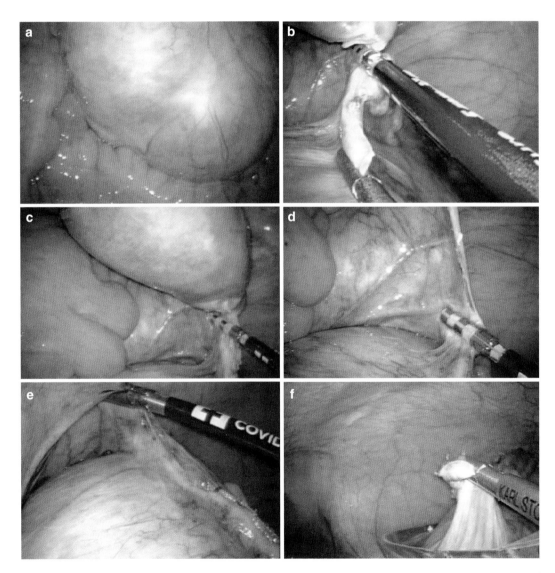

Fig. 10.7 Retrograde excision of 15-cm right ovarian mass. (**a**) 15-cm mass in situ. (**b**) Transection of proximal tube. (**c**) Transection of utero-ovarian ligament. (**d**) Transection of upper broad ligament. (**e**) Transection of infundibulopelvic ligament. (**f**) Placement of specimen into 15-mm specimen retrieval bag

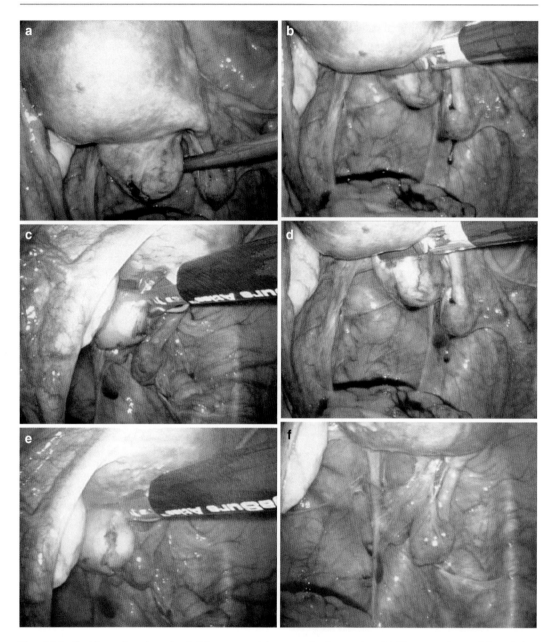

Fig. 10.8 Excision of pedunculated leiomyoma. (**a**) Pedunculated leiomyoma. (**b**) 10-mm Ligasure (Covidien, Mansfield, MA) used with slow closure of jaws on several cauterization cycles. (**c**) Energy active and jaws being closed slowly. (**d**) Complete closure of jaws. (**e**) Transection of last pedicle. (**f**) Leiomyoma completely excised

Table 10.5 Studies on single-port laparoscopy for adnexal mass

Study	Year	Cases, *n*	Mean tumor diameter, *cm*	Notes
Kim et al. [18]	2009	24	5.0	LESS successful in 92 %, 1 case added trocar for adhesions, 1 conversion for LMP tumor. Median operative time 70 min. No major complications
Escobar et al. [19]	2010	8	5.3	1 conversion, 1 additional 3-mm trocar for adhesions
Escobar et al. [16]	2010	58	n/a	LESS risk-reducing salpingo-oophorectomy, 13 cases also had hysterectomy. Wound cellulitis in 1.7 %. No umbilical hernias
Lee et al. [20]	2010	17	5.6	No differences in operative time, pain, or EBL compared with 34 patients undergoing laparoscopic procedures. Majority had cystectomy. No complications
Jung et al. [21]	2011	86	n/a	Majority of cases for endometriosis; 4 complications (3 pelvic infections, 1 postop hemorrhage); 2 converted to multiport laparoscopy. Safe and feasible
Kim et al. [17]	2011	94	6.3	Homemade glove port, single surgeon, 2 conversions for possible cancer, 2 cases with extra trocar for lysis of adhesions, No major complications
Bedaiwy et al. [22]	2012	28 (50 controls)	5.5	Compared with 50 control standard laparoscopies. Safe, feasible: similar EBL, operative time, hospital stay
Cho YJ et al. [23]	2012	33	6.6	Compared single-port and conventional laparoscopic cystectomy for adnexal mass. 1 postop ileus and 1 ovarian hematoma in single-port group. No conversion. No comment on cyst rupture rates
Gunderson et al. [24]	2012	70	n/a	70/211 cases for adnexal masses. Overall 2.4 % (3/70) umbilical hernia risk
Roh et al. [9]	2012	43	10.9	Single-port hand-assisted laparoscopy for large tumors; 10.3 % spill, 0 % hernia
Hoyer-Sorenson et al. [25]	2012	20	All <6 cm	Compared with 20 control standard laparoscopies. Higher rate of shoulder tip pain in SPL group at 6 and 24 h. Similar use of analgesics

EBL estimated blood loss, *LESS* laparoendoscopic single-site surgeries, *LMP* low malignant potential, *SPL* single-port laparoscopy

10.5 Complications

Expected complications are similar to those for standard laparoscopy, such as visceral injury, port-site hernia, and tumor rupture (Table 10.6) [8, 9, 17, 18, 20, 22, 31–35]. However, the risk of umbilical (port-site) hernia has been a major concern with increasing the size of the umbilical access site. Standard laparoscopic approaches have noted increasing umbilical hernias with increased size of the umbilical port size. Given that most standard laparoscopic procedures would use a port size of up to 10–12 mm with a typical umbilical hernia rate of 1–3 % [36, 37], concern has been that increasing the umbilical incision to 20–25 mm may increase the hernia risk. Most single-port laparoscopy studies in the gynecology literature have noted umbilical hernia risk up to 2.4 % [6, 24]. Based on early data, visceral injury and increased blood loss do not appear to be any more frequent with single-port laparoscopy. The rate of cyst rupture varies between studies and by definition of rupture, as some authors perceive only gross leakage of cyst fluid as a spill, whereas others feel that any breach in the cyst wall would count. Overall rates appear to be about 20 % with laparoscopy, but they do vary widely based on definitions. Moreover, it appears that rupture risk is increased with cystectomy versus oophorectomy, and it increases with the size of the mass [38].

Table 10.6 Complications of single-port laparoscopic management of adnexal masses

Year	Study	Cases, n	Mean size, cm	Mean operative Time, min	EBL, mL	Cyst rupture, %	Umbilical hernia	Cellulitis or abscess	Visceral injury	Comments
2009	Kim et al. [18]	24	5	70	10	NR	0	0	0	1 additional trocar for adhesiolysis, 1 conversion for LMP tumor
2010	Lee et al. [20]	17	5.6	64	80	NR	0	0	0	Compared with 34 CL cases, similar operative time, pain, EBL
2010	Mereu et al. [32]	16	–	42	<10	NR	0	1 (6.2 %)	0	Reusable port and curved graspers
2011	Im et al. [33]	18	8.3	62.8	100	NR	0	0	0	No conversions. 7 mild postop fever
2011	Kim et al. [8]	22	11.9	50	38	9.1	0	0	0	Extracorporeal cystectomy or cyst drainage. Fever 9 %. 1 extra trocar for adhesiolysis
2011	Kim et al. [17]	94	6.3	50	83	10.7	0	0	0	95 % successful SPL (2 conversion, 2 extra trocars)
2012	Bedaiwy et al. [22]	28	5.5	45	20	NR	0	0	0	Operative time, EBL similar to standard laparoscopy. Less postop narcotic use in SPL
2012	Fagotti et al. [34]	125	6.0	48	10	NR	0	1 (0.8 %)	0	3 additional ports used: 2 for control of bleeding, 1 to remove large specimen. Learning curve=15 procedures
2012	Kim et al. [35]	94	5.0	77.5	50	NR	0	NR	NR	Compared to CL. 49 % prior abdominal surgery. 6 cases had additional trocars placed. Less pain in SPL group at 24 h
2012	Roh et al. [9]	96 (SPL)	6.3	70	105	31.3	0	1 (1 %)	0	1 umbilical wound infection and 2 ileus in SPL group
		43 (hand-assist)	10.9	75	50	10.3	0	0	0	

CL conventional laparoscopy, *EBL* estimated blood loss, *LMP* low malignant potential, *NR* not recorded, *SPL* pure single-port laparoscopy

Conclusions

Single-port laparoscopic management of the adnexa in gynecology is safe and feasible. With continued advances in technology, the instrumentation will become easier to use, and increasing dissemination of this knowledge and equipment will allow single-port laparoscopy to become more readily available to a larger number of gynecologic surgeons. In benign gynecology, a large number of cases should be amenable to minimally invasive approaches, whether single-port or conventional laparoscopy, but increased availability of novel technologies should not replace sound clinical judgment and surgeon comfort in deciding which patients should undergo single-port laparoscopic procedures. A focused approach to increasing the number of minimally invasive cases in one's practice can lead to a successful decline in the number of open procedures performed and subsequently can decrease postoperative complications. Certainly many adnexal masses should be amenable to laparoscopic excision. Further data should help to clarify whether single-port laparoscopic cystectomy and oophorectomy have any higher risk of tumor rupture and whether the outcome is affected for women found to have ovarian cancer.

References

1. TeLinde RW, Rutledge F. Culdoscopy, a useful gynecologic procedure. Am J Obstet Gynecol. 1948;55: 102–16.
2. Christian J, Barrier BF, Schust D, et al. Culdoscopy: a foundation for natural orifice surgery–past, present, and future. J Am Coll Surg. 2008;207:417–22.
3. Wheeless Jr CR, Thompson BH. Laparoscopic sterilization. Review of 3600 cases. Obstet Gynecol. 1973; 42:751–8.
4. Ghezzi F, Cromi A, Bergamini V, et al. Should adnexal mass size influence surgical approach? A series of 186 laparoscopically managed large adnexal masses. BJOG. 2008;115:1020–7.
5. Fader AN, Rojas-Espaillat L, Ibeanu O, et al. Laparoendoscopic single-site surgery (LESS) in gynecology: a multi-institutional evaluation. Am J Obstet Gynecol. 2010;203:501.e1–6.
6. Lee M, Kim SW, Nam EJ, et al. Single-port laparoscopic surgery is applicable to most gynecologic surgery: a single surgeon's experience. Surg Endosc. 2012;26:1318–24.
7. Im SS, Gordon AN, Buttin BM, et al. Validation of referral guidelines for women with pelvic masses. Obstet Gynecol. 2005;105:35–41.
8. Kim WC, Im KS, Kwon YS. Single-port transumbilical laparoscopic-assisted adnexal surgery. JSLS. 2011;15:222–7.
9. Roh HJ, Lee SJ, Ahn JW, et al. Single-port-access, hand-assisted laparoscopic surgery for benign large adnexal tumors versus single-port pure laparoscopic surgery for adnexal tumors. Surg Endosc. 2012;26: 693–703.
10. Hasson HM, Rotman C, Rana N, Kumari NA. Open laparoscopy: 29-year experience. Obstet Gynecol. 2000;96:763–6.
11. Miller GH. Office single puncture laparoscopy sterilization with local anesthesia. JSLS. 1997;1:55–9.
12. Ismail MT, Arshat H, Halim AJ. Filshie clip sterilization – single puncture laparoscopic approach (a preliminary report). Malays J Reprod Health. 1988;6: 90–6.
13. Sewta RS. Laparoscopic female sterilisation by a single port through monitor – a better alternative. J Indian Med Assoc. 2011;109:262–3, 266.
14. Bedaiwy MA, Escobar PF, Pinkerton J, Hurd W. Laparoendoscopic single-site salpingectomy in isthmic and ampullary ectopic pregnancy: preliminary report and technique. J Minim Invasive Gynecol. 2011;18:230–3.
15. Yoon BS, Park H, Seong SJ, et al. Single-port laparoscopic salpingectomy for the surgical treatment of ectopic pregnancy. J Minim Invasive Gynecol. 2010; 17:26–9.
16. Escobar PF, Starks DC, Fader AN, et al. Single-port risk-reducing salpingo-oophorectomy with and without hysterectomy: surgical outcomes and learning curve analysis. Gynecol Oncol. 2010;119:43–7.
17. Kim WC, Lee JE, Kwon YS, et al. Laparoscopic single-site surgery (LESS) for adnexal tumors: one surgeon's initial experience over a one-year period. Eur J Obstet Gynecol Reprod Biol. 2011;158:265–8.
18. Kim TJ, Lee YY, Kim MJ, et al. Single port access laparoscopic adnexal surgery. J Minim Invasive Gynecol. 2009;16:612–5.
19. Escobar PF, Bedaiwy MA, Fader AN, et al. Laparoendoscopic single-site (LESS) surgery in patients with benign adnexal disease. Fertil Steril. 2074;2010(93):e7–10.
20. Lee YY, Kim TJ, Kim CJ, et al. Single port access laparoscopic adnexal surgery versus conventional laparoscopic adnexal surgery: a comparison of perioperative outcomes. Eur J Obstet Gynecol Reprod Biol. 2010;151:181–4.
21. Jung YW, Choi YM, Chung CK, et al. Single port transumbilical laparoscopic surgery for adnexal

lesions: a single center experience in Korea. Eur J Obstet Gynecol Reprod Biol. 2011;155:221–4.
22. Bedaiwy MA, Starks D, Hurd W, Escobar PF. Laparoendoscopic single-site surgery in patients with benign adnexal disease: a comparative study. Gynecol Obstet Invest. 2012;73:294–8.
23. Cho YJ, Kim ML, Lee SY, et al. Laparoendoscopic single-site surgery (LESS) versus conventional laparoscopic surgery for adnexal preservation: a randomized controlled study. Int J Womens Health. 2012;4:85–91.
24. Gunderson CC, Knight J, Ybanez-Morano J, et al. The risk of umbilical hernia and other complications with laparoendoscopic single-site surgery. J Minim Invasive Gynecol. 2012;19:40–5.
25. Hoyer-Sørensen C, Vistad I, Ballard K. Is single-port laparoscopy for benign adnexal disease less painful than conventional laparoscopy? A single-center randomized controlled trial. Fertil Steril. 2012;98:973–9.
26. Takeda A, Imoto S, Mori M, et al. Wound retraction system for isobaric laparoendoscopic single-site surgery to treat adnexal tumors: pilot study. J Minim Invasive Gynecol. 2010;17:626–30.
27. Takeda A, Imoto S, Mori M, et al. Isobaric laparoendoscopic single-site surgery with wound retractor for adnexal tumors: a single center experience with the initial 100 cases. Eur J Obstet Gynecol Reprod Biol. 2011;157:190–6.
28. Ülker K, Hüseyinoğlu Ü, Kılıç N. Management of benign ovarian cysts by a novel, gasless, single-incision laparoscopic technique: keyless abdominal rope-lifting surgery (KARS). Surg Endosc. 2013;27:189–98.
29. Tsin DA, Colombero LT, Lambeck J, Manolas P. Minilaparoscopy-assisted natural orifice surgery. JSLS. 2007;11:24–9.
30. Gordts S, Watrelot A, Campo R, Brosens I. Risk and outcome of bowel injury during transvaginal pelvic endoscopy. Fertil Steril. 2001;76:1238–41.
31. Jansen FW, Kolkman W, Bakkum EA, et al. Complications of laparoscopy: an inquiry about closed- versus open-entry technique. Am J Obstet Gynecol. 2004;190:634–8.
32. Mereu L, Angioni S, Melis GB, Mencaglia L. Single access laparoscopy for adnexal pathologies using a novel reusable port and curved instruments. Int J Gynaecol Obstet. 2010;109:78–80.
33. Im KS, Koo YJ, Kim JB, Kwon YS. Laparoendoscopic single-site surgery versus conventional laparoscopic surgery for adnexal tumors: a comparison of surgical outcomes and postoperative pain outcomes. Kaohsiung J Med Sci. 2011;27:91–5.
34. Fagotti A, Bottoni C, Vizzielli G, et al. Laparoendoscopic single-site surgery (LESS) for treatment of benign adnexal disease: single-center experience over 3-years. J Minim Invasive Gynecol. 2012;19:695–700.
35. Kim TJ, Lee YY, An JJ, et al. Does single-port access (SPA) laparoscopy mean reduced pain? A retrospective cohort analysis between SPA and conventional laparoscopy. Eur J Obstet Gynecol Reprod Biol. 2012;162:71–4.
36. Coda A, Bossotti M, Ferri F, et al. Incisional hernia and fascial defect following laparoscopic surgery. Surg Laparosc Endosc Percutan Tech. 2000;10:34–8.
37. Kadar N, Reich H, Liu CY, et al. Incisional hernias after major laparoscopic gynecologic procedures. Am J Obstet Gynecol. 1993;168:1493–5.
38. Smorgick N, Barel O, Halperin R, et al. Laparoscopic removal of adnexal cysts: is it possible to decrease inadvertent intraoperative rupture rate? Am J Obstet Gynecol. 2009;200:237.e1–3.

Single-Port Laparoscopic Hysterectomy

Kevin J.E. Stepp and Anjana R. Nair

For the last 10–15 years, access and instrumentation for laparoscopic hysterectomy have improved, but the techniques have remained relatively unchanged. Although they are still minimally invasive options, the conventional laparoscopic and robotic hysterectomy techniques typically require three to five small incisions in the abdominal wall. Surgeons are now able to complete laparoscopic surgeries through a single small incision that can be hidden in the base of the umbilicus for an excellent cosmetic result and reduced port site complications. This chapter illustrates a step-by-step approach for an effective, efficient, and reproducible technique to perform laparoendoscopic single-site surgery (LESS) for hysterectomy. The basic concepts illustrated here can be further utilized in any pelvic surgery. This technique is easily understood, replicated, and useful in learning the LESS technique while shortening the learning curve and minimizing frustration.

K.J.E. Stepp, MD (✉) • A.R. Nair, MD
Department of Obstetrics and Gynecology,
Carolinas HealthCare System,
2001 Vail Avenue, Suite 360, Charlotte,
NC 28277, USA
e-mail: kevin.stepp@carolinashealthcare.org;
anjana.nair@carolinashealthcare.org

P.F. Escobar, T. Falcone (eds.), *Atlas of Single-Port, Laparoscopic, and Robotic Surgery,*
DOI 10.1007/978-1-4614-6840-0_11, © Springer Science+Business Media New York 2014

11.1 Introduction

Since the late 1980s and early 1990s, surgeons have been vigorously exploring minimally invasive techniques to decrease the complication rates of traditional hysterectomy when vaginal hysterectomy is not an option. This has led to the development and advancement of conventional laparoscopic hysterectomy. For the last 10–15 years, access and instrumentation for laparoscopic hysterectomy have improved, but the techniques have remained relatively unchanged. Although they are still minimally invasive options, the conventional laparoscopic and robotic hysterectomy techniques typically require three to five small incisions in the abdominal wall. Each additional port contributes a small but not negligible risk for port site complications [1]. In an effort to minimize risks and improve cosmesis, alternatives to traditional laparoscopic surgery are being explored. Several centers are investigating techniques that gain access to the peritoneal cavity via natural orifices using a specialized endoscope and therefore do not require any abdominal wall incisions. Natural orifice transluminal endoscopic surgery (NOTES) has been described in animal models and in humans [2, 3]. A less dramatic and perhaps less risky approach is to perform laparoscopic surgery through a single port in the abdominal wall. The advent of multichannel ports for laparoscopy has enabled surgeons to complete laparoscopic surgeries through a single small incision that can be hidden in the base of the umbilicus. Several retrospective studies suggest the potential for decreased pain with single-port laparoscopy; however, two randomized controlled trials have conflicting results [4, 5]. Fagotti and coworkers [4] showed lower postoperative pain in patients undergoing single-port procedures, whereas Jung and colleagues [5] found no evidence of reduction in postoperative pain. Since its first description, several authors around the world have used multiple terms to describe laparoscopy carried out via a single incision. A recent multispecialty international consortium has recommended the name laparoendoscopic single-site surgery (LESS) [1, 6]. Nevertheless, a list of the multiple terms still being used is listed in Table 11.1.

The objective of this chapter is to illustrate an effective, efficient, and reproducible technique to perform LESS for hysterectomy. The basic concepts illustrated here can be further utilized in any pelvic surgery. This technique is easily understood, replicated, and useful in learning the LESS technique for hysterectomy. Escobar and coworkers examined the learning curve for LESS and found results similar to those in published conventional laparoscopy learning curves [7]. Although many of these techniques work well for complex surgical cases, we strongly recommend that surgeons first become familiar with the technique for benign indications and ovary preservation. Complex situations such as endometriosis, large fibroid uteri, malignancy, and significant adhesions are not covered here and are for advanced LESS surgeons. We describe a technique for surgeons who are interested in learning the LESS technique. Understanding the procedure and technique described here will help the surgeon proceed efficiently, resulting in minimal instrument exchanges and less external and internal clashing as well as avoiding a frustrating experience.

Table 11.1 Terms and abbreviations used to describe LESS

eNOTES	Embryonic natural orifice transluminal endoscopic surgery
LESS	Laparoendoscopic single-site surgery
NOTUS	Natural orifice transumbilical surgery
OPUS	One-port umbilical surgery
SAS	Single-access site laparoscopic surgery
SILS	Single-incision laparoscopic surgery
SPA	Single-port access laparoscopic surgery
SPLS	Singe-port laparoscopic surgery
SSA	Single-site access laparoscopic surgery
SSL	Single-site laparoscopy
TUES	Transumbilical endoscopic surgery
TULA	Transumbilical laparoscopic assisted surgery
U-LESS	Transumbilical laparoendoscopic single-site surgery

Adapted from Tracy et al. [1]

11.2   Instrumentation

There are specialized articulating instruments available. This may be helpful in certain situations, although there is an additional learning curve to using those instruments. When learning a new technique, we suggest minimizing the number of learning curves as much as possible. Using the technique described below, the majority of cases can be performed using only conventional straight instrumentation available in all operating rooms.

11.3   Camera Options

Most experts agree that an articulating camera is preferred and can sometimes facilitate an efficient procedure (*see* Fig. 11.1b). However, bariatric length or longer 30° or 45° laparoscopes can also be successful using the techniques and principles described here. If a non-articulating laparoscope is used, we recommend that a 90° adaptor be used to minimize interference with the light cord (*see* Fig. 11.1a and inset).

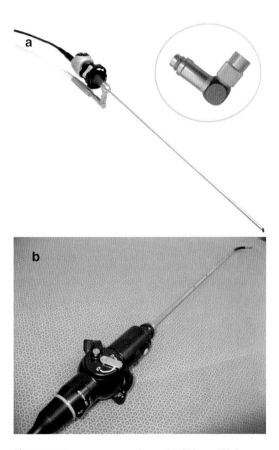

Fig. 11.1 Laparoscope options. (**a**) 30° or 45° laparoscopes work well for LESS. The longer and more angled the scope, the greater the minimization of external clashing. (*a Inset*), A 90° light cord adaptor will minimize interference with the light cord and other instruments. (**b**) An articulating scope provides excellent ability to position the camera away from other instruments (EndoEye [Olympus Surgical and Industrial America; Center Valley, PA, USA])

11.4 Technical Principles

1. Plan the procedure and choose instrumentation and techniques that minimize the need for
   instrument exchanges.
2. Always retract in such a way so that the handle of the instrument moves lateral, away from
   the camera and central area above the umbilicus. This prevents clashing of instruments
   externally.
3. Use a good uterine manipulator with a colpotomizer or ring to delineate the vaginal
   fornix.
4. If significant difficulty is encountered at any
   time during the procedure, an additional port
   can always be considered.

11.5 Ports and Gaining Access

Various access devices and techniques have been
described for peritoneal access. The skin incision
should be created to provide the most cosmetic
result possible. The umbilicus itself is a scar, and
each one has unique folds and shape. In some
patients, a vertical skin incision may be preferred.
In others, a circumferential or "omega" incision
may produce a better cosmetic result [8]. General
surgeons use this incision to provide additional
space to manipulate multiple laparoscopic instruments while providing ample space for specimen
removal and maintaining excellent cosmesis [9,
10]. Some have raised concerns regarding umbilical infections. A retrospective study of 120
patients did not find a difference in rate of infection when comparing vertical to circumferential
umbilical incision for LESS [8]. As with all laparoscopy, we advocate thorough attention to the
umbilicus during the surgical preparation prior to
surgery. Overlimiting the size of the incision may
place excess pressure on the incision edges that

may result in pressure necrosis at the edges.
Although this condition usually heals well, this
should be considered when making the skin incision and choosing ports for each patient.

There are a number of commercially available
ports designed to be placed through a single fascial incision (Fig. 11.2).

A. The X-CONE (Storz Endoscopy, Tuttlingen,
   Germany) (three 5-mm valves).
B. AnchorPort SIL Kit device (Surgiquest Inc.,
   Orange, CT) (allows three or more 5-mm tro-
   cars through a 1-in. skin incision).
C. SILS Port (Covidien, Norwalk, CT) (three
   5-mm cannulas, one of which can be upsized
   to 15 mm).
D. GelPoint (Applied Medical, Rancho Santa
   Margarita, CA) (includes four 5- to 12-mm
   universal cannulas. Additional instruments
   can be placed as needed).
E. TriPort Plus (Advanced Surgical Concepts,
   Wicklow, Ireland) (three 5-mm and one
   10-mm channel).
F. TriPort 15 (Advanced Surgical Concepts,
   Wicklow, Ireland) (two 5-mm and one 15-mm
   channel).

The majority of commercially available ports
have two attachments that can be used for insufflation, outflow, smoke evacuation, or an additional insufflation port as needed.

Ports that make use of a single open fascial
incision maximize space for additional instruments. However, ports that have multiple channels or cannulas minimize instrument friction
and unintended crossing at the level of the fascia
at the expense of needing a slightly larger fascial
incision.

When necessary, an additional port can be
placed at an alternate location to facilitate the
procedure. Conversion to two-port or multiport
conventional laparoscopy should not be considered a complication.

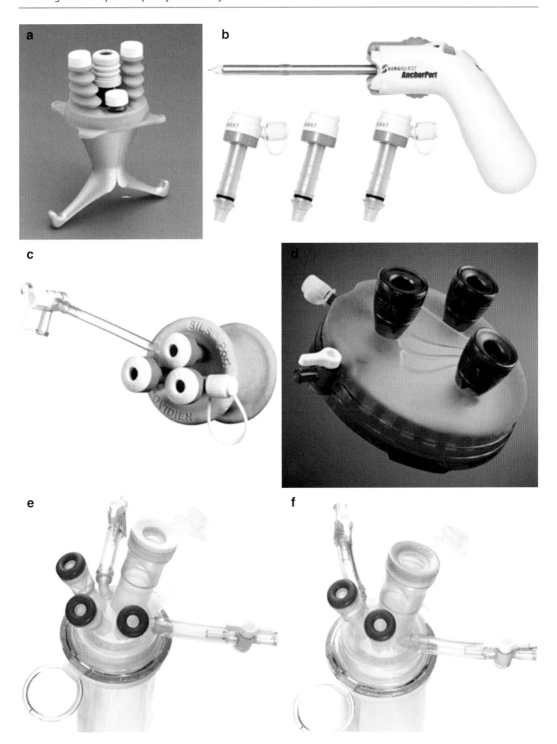

Fig. 11.2 (**a**) The X-CONE (Storz Endoscopy, Tuttlingen, Germany). (**b**) AnchorPort SIL Kit device (Surgiquest; Orange, CT, USA). (**c**) SILS Port (Covidien; Norwalk, CT, USA). (**d**) GelPoint (Applied Medical; Rancho Santa Margarita, CA, USA). (**e**) TriPort Plus (Advanced Surgical Concepts; Wicklow, Ireland). (**f**) TriPort 15 (Advanced Surgical Concepts; Wicklow, Ireland)

11.6   Technique

What follows is a step-by-step outline for an efficient procedure. The temptation is to skip steps or alter the order. We cannot stress enough the importance of completing the first step before moving on to the next. This will eliminate extraneous or duplicative movements. It also will ensure that instruments are positioned away from each other and avoid clashing, both internally and externally.

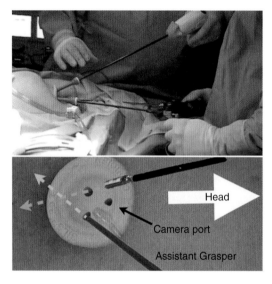

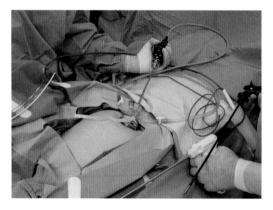

Fig. 11.3 Port orientation and camera placement. The port should be oriented so that the laparoscope may be placed through the most cephalad channel, valve, or cannula

11.6.1   Step 1. Initial Port Placement and Orientation

The surgeon should choose the port based on the individual characteristics of the patient, the case, his or her preference and experience, and the advantages and disadvantages of the specific ports. The ports should be placed in accordance with the manufacturer's instructions for use. Once securely placed in the peritoneal cavity, the port should be oriented as in Fig. 11.3. The channels or valves should be oriented so that the laparoscope can be placed through the most cephalad channel. The laparoscope should be positioned so that externally, the camera will be placed as close to the chest as possible. Then position the camera laterally as much as is practical (Fig. 11.4). This places the camera low and lateral, thereby maximizing space for other instruments and positioning the primary surgeon's hands directly above the port. With the hands and camera close to the chest, the internal end of the laparoscope is elevated toward the anterior abdominal wall. With the hands and camera close to the chest, the internal end of the laparoscope is elevated toward the anterior abdominal wall out of the way of the additional instruments within the pelvis. The greater the angle of the scope (30-degree, 45-degree, or flexible), the easier it is to get the laparoscope and camera away from the operative field and avoid clashing.

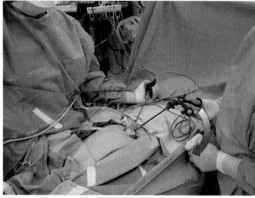

Fig. 11.4 Camera placement. The camera should be placed first prior to any additional instruments. It should be positioned close to the chest and deviated laterally to maximize space for additional instruments

Fig. 11.5 Insert the assistant grasper. Retraction should always be in the direction resulting in lateral movement of the handle, away from the midline

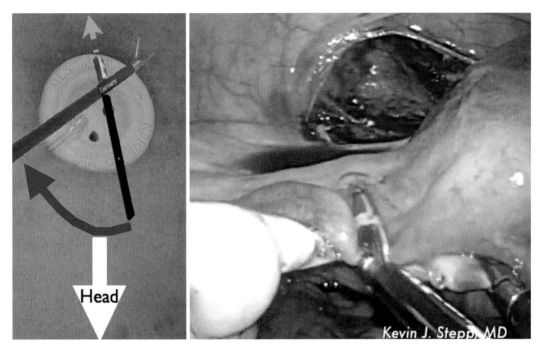

Fig. 11.6 Begin the left side of the hysterectomy. The assistant grasper and uterine manipulator deviate the uterus to the contralateral side, providing an excellent position for the bipolar device to begin the hysterectomy

11.6.2 Step 2. Insert the Assistant Instrument/Grasper

Here we assume that the primary surgeon is on the patient's left side and will begin the hysterectomy on the patient's left. (This process may be reversed if the surgeon is standing on the opposite side.) An assistant grasper instrument is inserted through the *left* channel and controlled with the surgeon's left hand (Fig. 11.5). The technical principle should be maintained: the direction of traction should always be to move the instrument handle away from the midline externally. Retract or manipulate the tissue internally so the handle falls lateral and away from the camera. This maximizes room for the laparo-scope and instrument handles externally. A good uterine manipulator will be able to adequately ele-vate and position the uterus toward the right shoul-der. The assistant grasper can be used to augment and maximize this positioning to present the left uterovarian and broad ligaments for the electrosur-gical device (Fig. 11.6).

11.6.3 Step 3. Insert the Operating Electrosurgical Instrument

The operating instrument is inserted through the *right* channel (Fig. 11.7). It enters the internal operative field through the center and usually is directed straight toward the utero-ovarian liga-ment. It is often easier to begin by sealing and transecting the utero-ovarian ligament, leaving the ovaries until after the hysterectomy is com-plete (Fig. 11.6). This allows the ovaries to remain on the pelvic side wall, away from the uterus and out of the way. After the hysterectomy is complete, the ovaries can be simply removed if desired. In the event that the instrument handles interfere with each other or with the camera, they should be positioned opposite each other (Fig. 11.8).

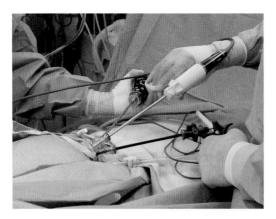

Fig. 11.7 External view showing set-up and instrument positions without clashing. Note that the handles of the bipolar device and assistant grasper are facing in opposite directions

11.6.4 Step 4. Performing the Left Side of the Hysterectomy

Grasp and seal the utero-ovarian ligament with the electrosurgical device. Continue to seal and transect the broad ligament until it is beyond the round ligament. Separate the broad ligament to begin to expose the uterine vessels (Fig. 11.9). Separating the anterior and posterior leafs of the broad ligament too soon will cause bleeding from the round ligament. Upward traction on the uterine manipulator exposes the uterine vasculature and increases the distance to the ureters. If the uterine vessels are clearly visible, they may be sealed at this time; inside the ring or cup of the uterine manipulator they will be at a safe distance from the ureters and thus be able to avoid lateral electrosurgery injury (Fig. 11.10).

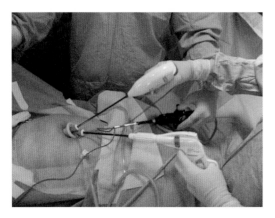

Fig. 11.8 External view showing the camera low and a comfortable surgical position with the handles of the instruments facing outward

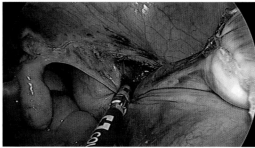

Fig. 11.10 The uterine vasculature is sealed while upward traction is placed on the uterine manipulator. The bipolar device should stay inside the colpotomizer ring or cup of the uterine manipulator to minimize the risk of injury to the ureter

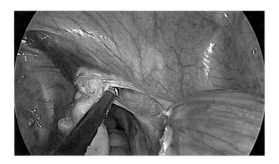

Fig. 11.9 Once the round ligament is completely sealed, begin to separate the anterior and posterior broad ligaments to expose the uterine vasculature and begin the bladder flap

11.6.5 Step 5. Create the Bladder Flap

The assistant grasper now can be moved inferiorly on the uterus if necessary. Alternatively, it may elevate the bladder peritoneum cephalad and upward toward the anterior wall. Ideally, the assistant grasper will also be used to elevate the bladder peritoneum, thus minimizing instrument exchanges. If necessary, rotation of the open jaws of the energy device will provide an additional few millimeters toward the right side (Fig. 11.11).

Variation: If necessary, the operative instrument/energy device can be exchanged with a monopolar or bipolar hook or spatula to create the bladder flap (Fig. 11.12). Remove the hook or spatula when the bladder flap is complete.

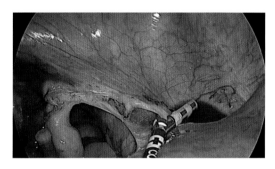

Fig. 11.11 Creating the bladder flap. Often the bladder flap is created with the bipolar instrument. Opening the jaws and rotating will help get around the front of the uterus

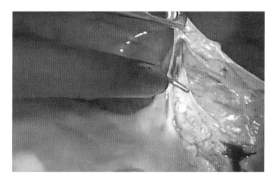

Fig. 11.12 Creating the bladder flap. An alternate method involves elevation of the anterior bladder peritoneum in the midline while incising the peritoneum to expose the vaginal cuff and fornix

11.6.6 Step 6. Perform the Right Side of the Hysterectomy

Early during the learning curve, we believe that the simplest option for the right side is to remove both the assistant grasper and the operative instrument/energy device. The primary surgeon can move to the patient's contralateral side (Figs. 11.13 and 11.14) or remain on the patient's left side (Fig. 11.15). The uterus should be repositioned toward the left with the manipulator. Then Steps 2 through 5 should be performed from the right side or from opposite directions.

Reinsert the assistant grasper from the *right* channel and retract laterally (Fig. 11.13) while deviating the uterus toward the left shoulder. Insert the electrosurgical instrument through the *left* channel (Figs. 11.14 and 11.15). Seal and transect the utero-ovarian ligament, round ligament, and broad ligament. Complete the bladder flap from the right side. Expose and seal the right uterine vessels (Fig. 11.16).

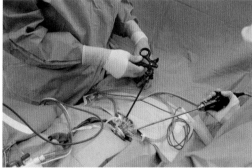

Fig. 11.13 Performing the right side of the hysterectomy. In this view, the primary surgeon has switched sides and is now on the patient's right side. The camera is positioned on the contralateral side. All instruments are removed to set up the operative technique again. The assistant grasper is placed through the right channel, and the handle is retracted laterally

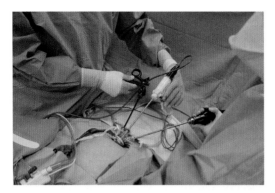

Fig. 11.14 Insert the bipolar device to perform the right side of the hysterectomy. Note that the handles are not clashing with each other or the camera

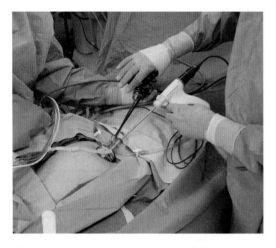

Fig. 11.15 Performing the right side of the hysterectomy without switching sides. The instruments are still switched as in Fig. 11.14. However, the primary surgeon remains on the patient's left side. To maintain a comfortable position requires that the surgeon place the bipolar device in his or her left hand

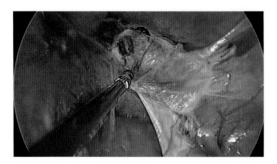

Fig. 11.16 Sealing the right uterine vasculature with upward traction on the uterine manipulator. The bladder flap is completed if necessary

11.6.7 Step 7 (Supracervical Hysterectomy) – Amputate the Fundus

Position the uterus toward the right shoulder with the uterine manipulator. Remove the assistant grasper and operative instrument. Move the assistant grasper to the contralateral channel on the *left* and insert. Grasp the uterine fundus or place it posteriorly behind the cervix to elevate the uterus toward the right shoulder and away from the bowel. The instrument handle will fall laterally to the left and down away from the camera. Insert a monopolar or bipolar hook or spatula through the contralateral (*right*) channel for amputation (Fig. 11.17). The instrument should appear at the midline as it approaches the lower uterus (Fig. 11.18).

Complete 50 % of the amputation from the left side (Fig. 11.19). Continued and increasing upward traction on the uterus with the assistant grasper will create a reverse cone ensuring maximal resection of the internal cervical os. To complete the amputation from the right side, reposition the uterus to the right with the uterine manipulator and repeat the steps from the contralateral side. Remove the assistant grasper and operative instrument. Now place the assistant grasper through the *right* channel and create the upward traction by grasping the uterine fundus or by placing the instrument posteriorly behind the cervix. Elevate the uterus toward the left shoulder and away from the bowel by placing the handle laterally to the right and down away from the camera. Reinsert the monopolar/bipolar hook or spatula via the *left* channel to complete the amputation. Coagulate the endocervix.

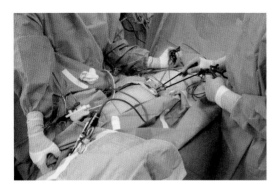

Fig. 11.17 Set-up for supracervical amputation or colpotomy. The assistant grasper handle is retracted laterally, providing space for the hook or spatula without clashing or touching the other instruments. The assistant can comfortably manipulate the uterus and the camera for exposure

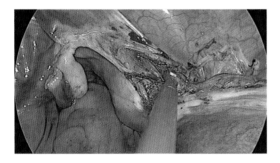

Fig. 11.18 Internal view of a monopolar hook beginning the supracervical amputation on the left

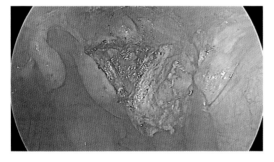

Fig. 11.19 Internal view of amputation. The left side is completely amputated before proceeding to the contralateral side in order to minimize going back and forth

11.6.8 Step 8 (Total Laparoscopic Hysterectomy) – Perform the Colpotomy

This procedure is very similar to the supracervical amputation technique. Careful positioning of the uterus to expose the cervicovaginal junction will allow efficient creation of the colpotomy with limited instrument exchanges.

The external position of the instruments and hands are similar to that in supracervical amputation (Fig. 11.17).

With the uterus positioned to the right with the uterine manipulator, place the assistant grasper now through the *left* lateral channel and grasp the uterine fundus or place it posteriorly behind the cervix to elevate the uterus toward the right shoulder and away from the bowel. Insert a monopolar or bipolar hook or spatula through the contralateral channel to start the colpotomy (Fig. 11.20). Complete 50 % of the amputation from the left side.

To complete the amputation from the right side, reposition the uterus to the left with the uterine manipulator and repeat the process from the contralateral side (Fig. 11.21). Occasionally it may be necessary to reposition the uterus anteriorly to complete the colpotomy in the posterior midline.

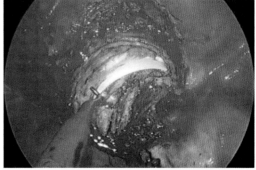

Fig. 11.20 Internal view of the colpotomy. Upward traction will increase the distance from the ureters laterally and help identify the colpotomizer ring or cup of the uterine manipulator. Begin the colpotomy anteriorly and proceed laterally and posteriorly as much as possible before moving to the contralateral side

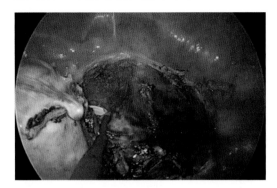

Fig. 11.21 The colpotomy is then completed on the right side, staying medial to the sealed uterine vessels

11.6.9 Step 9 (Total Laparoscopic Hysterectomy) – Vaginal Cuff Closure

In the case of total hysterectomy, the authors suggest closing the vaginal cuff from a vaginal approach. Laparoscopic suturing is the most complicated task to perform with LESS. We recommend that traditional suturing be considered only by those well experienced with LESS. If laparoscopic closure is attempted, we strongly suggest utilizing suturing assist devices such as Endostitch (Covidien, Norwalk, CT), barbed-suture, or Laparo-Ty (Ethicon Endo Surgery, Inc., Cincinnati, OH).

11.7 Risks Specific to LESS

As with any laparoscopy, it is imperative that surgeons have a thorough knowledge of electro-surgery to avoid electrosurgical complications. Surgeons should be aware of the different types of electrosurgical complications. There may be a theoretical increased risk of capacitive coupling when performing LESS. Working with instruments in close quarters may predispose them to insulation damage. Therefore, we recommend meticulous inspection of the instruments. Disposable electrosurgical instruments may have

a decreased risk of insulation damage and thus a lower risk of direct coupling. We believe that good technique should mitigate these risks.

Acknowledgement The authors would like to acknowledge Dr. K Anthony Shibley for assistance in creating some of the surgical photos.

References

1. Tracy CR, Raman JD, Cadeddu JA, Rane A. Laparoendoscopic single-site surgery in urology: where have we been and where are we heading? Nat Clin Pract Urol. 2008;5:561–8.
2. Marescaux J, Dallemagne D, Perretta S, Wattiez A, Mutter D, Coumaros D. Surgery without scars: report of transluminal cholecystectomy in a human being. Arch Surg. 2007;142:823–6.
3. Wagh MS, Thompson CC. Surgery insight: natural orifice transluminal endoscopic surgery – an analysis of work to date. Nat Clin Pract Gastroenterol Hepatol. 2007;4:386–92.
4. Fagotti A, Bottoni C, Vizzielli G, Alletti SG, Scambia G, Marana E, Fanfani F. Postoperative pain after conventional laparoscopy and laparoendoscopic single site surgery (LESS) for benign adnexal disease: a randomized trial. Fertil Steril. 2011;96:255–9.
5. Jung YK, Lee M, Yim GW. A randomized prospective study of single-port and four-port approaches for hysterectomy in terms of postoperative pain. Surg Endosc. 2011;25:2462–9.
6. Gill IS, Advincula AP, Aron M, Caddedu J, Canes D, Curcillo PG, et al. Consensus statement of the consortium for laparoendoscopic single-site surgery. Surg Endosc. 2010;24:762–8.
7. Escobar PF, Starks DC, Fader AN, Barber M, Rojas-Espalliat L. Single-port risk-reducing salpingo-oophorectomy with and without hysterectomy: surgical outcomes and learning curve analysis. Gynecol Oncol. 2010;119:43–7.
8. Kane S, Stepp KJ. Circumumbilical (Omega) incision for laparoendoscopic single-site surgery. Oral Presentation: Society Gynecologic Surgeons Annual Clinical Meeting, San Antonio, April 2011.
9. Huang CK, Houng JY, Chiang CJ, Chen YS, Lee PH. Single incision transumbilical laparoscopic Roux-en-Y gastric bypass: a first case report. Obes Surg. 2009;19:1711–5.
10. Hong SH, Seo SI, Kim JC, Hwang TK. Cosmetic circumumbilical incision for extraction of specimen after laparoscopic radical prostatectomy. J Endourol. 2006;20:519–21.

Single-Port Laparoscopic Management of Endometriosis

12

Mohamed A. Bedaiwy and Leticia Cox

Endometriosis is a chronic gynecologic condition that often presents in patients during the reproductive years with complaints of pelvic pain or infertility or both. Diagnosis has been made easier as a result of the growing use of laparoscopy. The exact pathogenesis is not known. Surgical management is indicated in women who suffer severe disease and do not do well on medical therapy, the objective being to ablate all visible disease. There are currently four primary surgical options: laparotomy, laparoscopy, robotic-assisted laparoscopy, and laparoendoscopic single-port surgery (LESS). Laparoendoscopic single-port surgery is associated with better cosmetic results, shorter hospital stay, and less postoperative pain. This technique is reviewed here.

M.A. Bedaiwy, MD, PhD (✉)
Department of Obstetrics and Gynaecology,
The University of British Columbia,
D415A, 4500 Oak Street,
Vancouver, BC V6H 3V4, Canada
e-mail: bedaiwymmm@yahoo.com,
mohamed.bedaiwy@cw.bc.ca

L. Cox, MD
Department of Obstetrics and Gynecology,
University Hospitals Case Medical Center,
Case Western Reserve University,
Cleveland, OH 44106, USA
e-mail: leticia.cox@uhhospitals.org

P.F. Escobar, T. Falcone (eds.), *Atlas of Single-Port, Laparoscopic, and Robotic Surgery*,
DOI 10.1007/978-1-4614-6840-0_12, © Springer Science+Business Media New York 2014

12.1 Introduction

Endometriosis is a chronic gynecologic condition defined by heterotopic implantation of endometrial glands and stroma [1]. Patients often present during the reproductive years with complaints of pelvic pain and infertility or both. The diagnosis requires direct visualization of endometriotic spots, and therefore laparoscopy or laparotomy is indicated for definitive diagnosis. Although the incidence appears to have increased in recent years, this is likely a reflection of the diagnosis having been made easier by the growing use of laparoscopy. Currently, the incidence is estimated to be 5–15 % of laparotomies and laparoscopies, 30 % in women with longstanding pelvic pain and 40 % in women with infertility [1]. The exact pathogenic mechanisms leading to this condition are not entirely clear. Proposed mechanisms include retrograde menstruation, lymphatic and vascular spread, mesothelial metaplasia, genetic predisposition, immunologic factors, and hormonal influences.

Endometriosis is usually pelvic in location, involving the left hemipelvis and ovary more commonly than the right. Endometriosis sites are summarized in Table 12.1. This is thought to be a result of the restriction of peritoneal fluid movement by the left-sided sigmoid colon. A cystic collection of endometriosis in the ovary is referred to as an endometrioma or chocolate cyst. Other commonly affected pelvic sites include the posterior cul-de-sac, the peritoneum, the uterovesical pouch, and the uterosacral round and broad ligaments. Less commonly the cervix, vagina, and vulva are involved. The rectosigmoid is involved in up to 15 % of cases, while the urinary tract is involved in 10 % of cases with small superficial bladder involvement being the most common. The topographic distribution of endometriosis is best assessed by the American Society for Reproductive Medicine (ASRM) classification despite its limitations (Fig. 12.1). To felicitate a standardized approach to examine the pelvis in endometriosis patients, it was recently proposed that the pelvis could be topographically divided into two midline zones (Zone I & II) and two paired (right and left) lateral zones (Zone III & IV). Zone I is the area between the two round ligaments from their origin at the uterine cornua to their insertion in the deep inguinal rings. Zone II is the area between the two uterosacral ligaments from their origin from the back of the uterus to their insertions in the sacrum posteriorly. Zone III is the area between the uterosacral ligament inferiorly and the entire length of the fallopian tube and the infundibulopelvic ligament superiorly. Zone IV is the triangular area lateral to the fallopian tube and the infundibulopelvic ligament and medial to the external iliac vessels up to the round ligament (Fig. 12.2) [2].

Table 12.1 Potential sites of endometriosis

Genital pelvic sites	Extragenital pelvic sites	Rare locations
Ovaries	Sigmoid colon	Umbilicus
Rectovaginal septum	Rectum	Small bowel
Anteroposterior cul-de-sac	Appendix	Lungs
Broad ligament	Bladder	Kidney
Cervix		Cesarean section/episiotomy scar
Vagina		Sciatic nerve
Fallopian tubes		Arms
		Nasal mucosa
		Spinal column
		Liver

Fig. 12.1 (**a, b**) American Society for Reproductive Medicine Endometriosis Classification assigned points according to the severity of endometriosis on the basis of size and depth of implants and severity of adhesions. Stage I (1–5 points): minimal disease; Stage II (6–15 points): mild disease; Stage III (16–40 points): moderate disease; Stage IV (>40 points): severe disease

a

THE AMERICAN FERTILITY SOCIETY
REVISED CLASSIFICATION OF ENDOMETRIOSIS

Patient's Name _____   Date _____

Stage I (Minimal) · 1-5
Stage II (Mild) · 6-15   Laparoscopy _____ Laparotomy _____ Photography _____
Stage III (Moderate) · 16-40   Recommended Treatment _____
Stage IV (Severe) · >40
Total _____   Prognosis _____

	ENDOMETRIOSIS		<1cm	1-3cm	>3cm
PERITONEUM		Superficial	1	2	4
		Deep	2	4	6
OVARY	R	Superficial	1	2	4
		Deep	4	16	20
	L	Superficial	1	2	4
		Deep	4	16	20

	POSTERIOR CULDESAC OBLITERATION	Partial		Complete
		4		40

	ADHESIONS		<1/3 Enclosure	1/3-2/3 Enclosure	>2/3 Enclosure
OVARY	R	Filmy	1	2	4
		Dense	4	8	16
	L	Filmy	1	2	4
		Dense	4	8	16
TUBE	R	Filmy	1	2	4
		Dense	4*	8*	16
	L	Filmy	1	2	4
		Dense	4*	8*	16

*If the fimbriated end of the fallopian tube is completely enclosed, change the point assignment to 16.

Additional Endometriosis: _____ | Associated Pathology: _____
_____ | _____
_____ | _____
_____ | _____

To Be Used with Normal   To Be Used with Abnormal
Tubes and Ovaries   Tubes and/or Ovaries

L   R | L   R

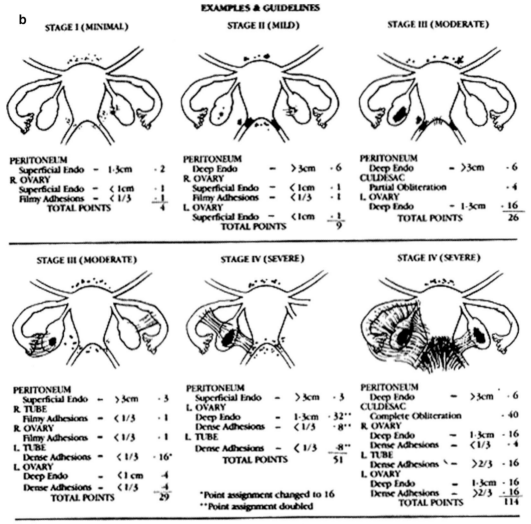

Fig. 12.1 (continued)

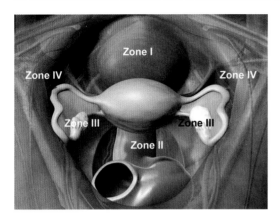

Fig. 12.2 **A color-coded illustration of the anatomical boundaries and the contents of all pelvic zones.** Zone I: Midline anterior abdominal cavity limited by the round ligaments bilaterally. Zone II: Midline posterior zone of the abdominal cavity limited by the uterosacral ligaments bilaterally. Zone III: Lateral pelvic side walls limited by the uterosacral ligament and the adnexae and infundibulo-pelvic ligamentsone IV: Pelvic side wall limited by the round ligament, adnexae and infundibular ligament, and external iliac vessels

12.2   Surgical Management of Endometriosis

Surgery may be indicated in women who suffer severe disease, do not respond to medical therapy, or desire fertility. The indications for surgical intervention are summarized in Table 12.2. Endometriosis can be challenging to manage surgically because of the peculiarities of the disease. Because it is adhesive, widespread, infiltrative, and recurrent, the objective of surgical management is to safely resect or ablate all visible disease. To date there are four primary surgical options. Traditional laparotomy is associated with longer recovery and hospital stay but may be necessary for advanced disease with extensive adhesions or involvement of the ureter, bladder, uterine arteries, and/or bowel. Laparoscopy is an alternative minimally invasive approach that has been shown to be equally effective in resecting endometriomas. Robotic-assisted laparoscopy is another new modality that has been reported.

Most recently, laparoendoscopic single-port surgery (LESS) has emerged as a minimally invasive approach. Compared to traditional laparoscopy, it is associated with better cosmetic results, a shorter hospital stay, and less postoperative pain. It has been used extensively for a wide variety of gynecologic indications. More recently, LESS was used in an attempt to treat endometriosis requiring a single incision [3–6].

Table 12.2 Indications for surgical management of endometriosis

Severe incapacitating symptoms with significant functional impairment
Advanced disease with distortion of pelvic organs
Failure of expectant or medical management
Noncompliance with or intolerance to medical treatment
Endometriosis emergencies
Ruptured or torsed endometrioma
Obstructive uropathy
Bowel obstruction

12.3 LESS Technique for Endometriosis Resection

The LESS technique for the surgical resection of endometriosis was described by Bedaiwy and coworkers [7]. Briefly, after induction of general anesthesia and endotracheal intubation, the patient is placed in Allen stirrups, a Foley catheter and an orogastric tube are inserted, and abdominal access is attained using a modified open Hasson technique with a vertical 1.8–2.0 cm infraumbilical incision. The rectus fascia is sharply incised, and a single access multichannel SILS port (Covidien, Mansfield, MA) is inserted in the peritoneal cavity. Pneumoperitoneum was attained with the pressure set at 15–20 mmHg. A 5-mm, 0° lens laparoscope with a flexible tip—the Endoeye (Olympus Surgical, Orangeburg, NY)—or a 30° bariatric length rigid scope is used. Articulating graspers (Covidien, Mansfield, MA) are helpful in providing efficient retraction to optimize surgical exposure.

Pelvic side wall adhesions are released from the lateral pelvic wall using laparoscopic endoshears. Lysis of periovarian adhesions is performed in a similar fashion when needed. The ureters are identified at the pelvic brim and followed toward the true pelvis. The pelvic side wall peritoneum is opened, and the ureter is identified and isolated along the medial leaflet of the peritoneum. Subsequently, the deep infiltrating lesions are dissected and excised. Similarly, the deep infiltrating lesions in the cul-de-sac are dissected and excised.

If the cul-de-sac is obliterated, its sharp dissection with scissors while a sponge stick is distending the rectum creates the pouch of Douglas. The rectum is confirmed to be intact by performing an underwater leak test. Endometriosis implanted on the bladder surface is also removed in a similar fashion.

Endometriomas, whether unilateral or bilateral, are managed following the principle of excision of the cyst wall in its entirety. Ovarian cystectomy is started by grasping the utero-ovarian ligament to stabilize the ovary. The antimesenteric border of the ovary is then incised using endoshears (Fig. 12.3). Subsequently, the cyst wall is identified and bidirectional dissection of the surrounding ovarian cortex is completed using a combination of blunt and sharp technique, traction and countertraction, and electro-coagulation. Endometriomas usually rupture during dissection in virtually all patients. Once the endometrioma is excised, the bed is then carefully inspected, and bleeding areas are secured with a cautery. The cyst bed is left open for spontaneous healing.

The excised peritoneal tissue/endometrioma is placed in 5–12 mm Endo Catch (Covidien) bags and removed through the multichannel port after detaching all the trocars from the abdomen. At the end of all procedures, the fascia of the umbilical incision is closed with 0 Vicryl absorbable sutures (polyglactin 910; Ethicon Inc., Somerville, NJ) in a running fashion and then the skin of the umbilicus is closed with 4–0 Vicryl absorbable sutures in a subcuticular fashion. All incisions are injected with 0.5 % bupivacaine hydrochloride at the end of the procedure.

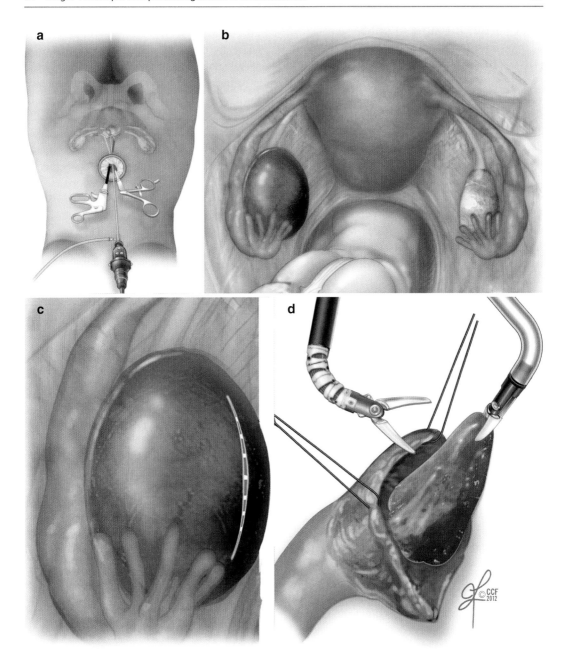

Fig. 12.3 Laparoendoscopic single-site resection of endometriomas. (**a**) An outside view showing the orientation of the instruments. (**b**) Left-sided ovarian endometrioma. (**c**) The initial incision on the mesenteric border of the ovary. (**d**) The combined blunt and sharp dissection of the cyst wall

12.4 The Outcome of LESS Technique for Endometriosis Resection

Data about the use of LESS for the management of endometriosis are limited. In a retrospective study Bedaiwy and colleagues demonstrated that LESS is a feasible initial surgical approach to treating unilateral endometriomas [7]. This study, however, did highlight a need to use an additional side port in 41 % of patients, particularly those with cul-de-sac disease, lateral pelvic side wall disease, or bilateral endometriomas. This could be explained by the adhesive and the deep infiltrating nature of the disease. In addition, surgical dissection of endometriosis and dissection of ovarian cysts require ergonomically challenging movements of surgical instruments. This is not offered by the currently available instruments for LESS.

When compared to conventional laparoscopy, this study [7] showed that the operative time and blood loss for this single-port series was similar to those of a matched series treated laparoscopically.

Overall, minimally invasive approaches have been shown to be safe and associated with shorter hospital stays, reduced postoperative pain, speedy recovery, and reduced surgical wound morbidity compared to open surgery [8–10]. The LESS technology is a recent modification of laparoscopic surgery that has several potential merits. One of the benefits that has been shown in several studies, including one randomized, controlled trial, is significantly less postoperative pain compared to conventional laparoscopy. This is particularly important in endometrioma patients, whose most common presentation is chronic pelvic pain [5, 6], However, in a recent randomized trial comparing LESS with conventional laparoscopy, Hoyer-Sorensen and colleagues reported similar postoperative pain perception in both groups, with more shoulder pain in the LESS group [11]. This was also shown in a retrospective control study [12]. A potential benefit of the LESS approach is the ability to retrieve specimens after cystectomy via the umbilical incision even without the use of Endo Catch.

Conclusion

Currently, the LESS technique for surgical management of endometriosis should be considered experimental. It is a reasonable initial approach for the treatment of endometriomas. In our experience, an additional side port is usually needed to treat pelvic side wall and cul-de-sac endometriosis that often accompanies endometriomas. Therefore, reduced port laparoscopy may be more feasible for the performance of ovarian cystectomy and resection of endometriosis, particularly when gonadal preservation is attempted or deeply infiltrating endometriosis is evident. The benefit of LESS surgery in endometriosis should be substantiated in a prospective randomized controlled trial.

References

1. Giudice LC. Clinical practice. Endometriosis. N Engl J Med. 2010;362:2389–98.
2. Bedaiwy MA, Pope R, Henry D, Zanotti K, Mahajan S, Hurd W, Falcone T, Liu J. Standardization of laparoscopic pelvic examination: a proposal of a novel system. Minim Invasive Surg. 2013:153235. doi:10.1155/2013/153235.
3. Escobar PF, Bedaiwy MA, Fader AN, Falcone T. Laparoendoscopic single-site (LESS) surgery in patients with benign adnexal disease. Fertil Steril. 2010;93:2074 e7–e10.
4. Bedaiwy MA, Starks D, Hurd W, Escobar PF. Laparoendoscopic single-site surgery in patients with benign adnexal disease: a comparative study. Gynecol Obstet Invest. 2012;73:294–8.
5. Bucher P, Ostermann S, Pugin F, Morel P. Female population perception of conventional laparoscopy, transumbilical LESS, and transvaginal NOTES for cholecystectomy. Surg Endosc. 2011;25:2308–15.
6. Georgiou AN, Rassweiler J, Herrmann TR, Georgiou AN, Rassweiler J, Herrmann TR, et al. Evolution and simplified terminology of natural orifice transluminal endoscopic surgery (NOTES), laparoendoscopic single-site surgery (LESS), and mini-laparoscopy (ML). World J Urol. 2012;30:573–80.
7. Bedaiwy MA, Farghaly T, Hurd WW, Liu J, Mansour G, Nickles-Fader A, Escobar P. Laparoendoscopic single site surgery (LESS) for management of ovarian endometriomas. JSLS (in press).
8. Kuhry E, Schwenk W, Gaupset R, Romild U, Bonjer J. Long-term outcome of laparoscopic surgery for colorectal cancer: a cochrane systematic review of randomised controlled trials. Cancer Treat Rev. 2008;34:498–504.

9. Keus F, de Jong JA, Gooszen HG, van Laarhoven CJ. Laparoscopic versus open cholecystectomy for patients with symptomatic cholecystolithiasis. Cochrane Database Syst Rev. 2006;(4):CD006231.

10. American College of Obstetricians and Gynecologists. ACOG practice bulletin. Management of adnexal masses. Obstet Gynecol. 2007;110:201–14.

11. Hoyer-Sorensen C, Vistad I, Ballard K. Is single-port laparoscopy for benign adnexal disease less painful than conventional laparoscopy? A single-center randomized controlled trial. Fertil Steril. 2012;98:973–9.

12. Yim GW, Lee M, Nam EJ, Kim S, Kim YT, Kim SW. Is single-port access laparoscopy less painful than conventional laparoscopy for adnexal surgery? A comparison of postoperative pain and surgical outcomes. Surg Innov. 2013;20:46–54.

Techniques for Single-Port Gynecologic Oncology

13

Anna Fagotti, Francesco Fanfani, Cristiano Rossitto, and Giovanni Scambia

Single-port or laparoendoscopic single-site surgery (LESS) is an advanced minimally invasive procedure that utilizes a single, small incision within the umbilicus. The feasibility and advantages of this type of surgery in benign gynecologic conditions indicate a promising surgical innovation for gynecologic or gynecologic-oncologic patients.

13.1 Introduction

Single-port surgery or laparoendoscopic single-site surgery (LESS) is an advanced minimally invasive procedure in which the surgeon operates exclusively through a single, small skin incision concealed within the umbilicus. Considering the feasibility and advantages related to this type of surgery in benign gynecologic conditions, its application in gynecologic oncology has been a

natural evolution. Our research group and others have described techniques, feasibility, safety, and outcomes associated with the performance of various gynecologic-oncologic procedures via the LESS approach (Table 13.1) [1–7]. These experiences indicate that LESS is a promising surgical innovation that demonstrates several practical applications in oncologic surgery and potential clinical benefits for the patients. This chapter describes LESS techniques in the treatment of various gynecologic oncology conditions.

Table 13.1 Gynecologic oncology indications to single port surgery

Adnexa
Retrieval of ovarian tissue for freezing before any type of RT and/or CT in young cancer patients
Ovarian suspension before pelvic radiation for cervical cancer
RRSO
Conservative and not conservative treatment and (re)staging of borderline ovarian tumors
Potential conservative and demolitive treatment and (re)staging of apparently stage 1 ovarian cancer (both epithelial and others)
Uterus
Treatment and staging of early endometrial cancer
Treatment and staging of IB1 small tumor cervical cancer
Staging for conservative treatment in early stage cervical cancer
Retroperitoneal staging in LACC
RT radiotherapy, *CT* chemotherapy, *RRSO* risk reducing salpingo oophorectomy, *LACC* local advanced cervical cancer

A. Fagotti, MD (✉)
Division of Minimally Invasive Gynecologic Surgery,
St. Maria Hospital, University of Perugia,
Via Tristano di Joannuccio 1, 05100 Terni, Italy
e-mail: annafagotti@libero.it

F. Fanfani • C. Rossitto • G. Scambia
Department of Obstetrics and Gynecology,
Catholic University of the Sacred Heart,
Largo Agostino Gemelli 8, 100168 Rome, Italy
e-mail: francesco.fanfani@rm.unicatt.it;
cristiano.rossitto@rm.unicatt.it;
giovanni.scambia@rm.unicatt.it

P.F. Escobar, T. Falcone (eds.), *Atlas of Single-Port, Laparoscopic, and Robotic Surgery*,
DOI 10.1007/978-1-4614-6840-0_13, © Springer Science+Business Media New York 2014

13.2 Operating Room Organization

A well-organized operating room is a prerequisite not only for the success of the intervention but also to optimize the timing of surgery and to lower related costs. Surgical team position radically changes during LESS surgery compared with standard laparoscopy, because single-site incisions force surgeons to change their position to maximize mobility of the instruments. In this case, the first surgeon, after inserting the port, stands behind the shoulders of the patient, at the level of the head, the place usually occupied by the anesthesia team. The assistant is positioned at the right shoulder of the patient. An appropriate Trendelenburg position is required to decrease the distance between the surgeon and the patient, which is more extreme than in standard laparoscopy. A third surgeon may be placed between the legs of the patient to manipulate the uterus.

13.3 Surgical Technique

Surgical procedures are performed through a single multiport reusable or disposable trocar (LESS) inserted into the umbilicus. We generally use an Olympus multiport trocar (Olympus Winter & IBE GMBH; Hamburg, Germany). This device consists of three components: the introducer, the fixing valve, and the trocar itself. The trocar, made of a doubled-over cylindrical sleeve of pliable film material fixed to the proximal ring, flows down around the distal ring and then back up and out. To introduce the trocar, the distal ring is passed through an open access into the abdominal cavity using the introducer. A 1.5–2-cm longitudinal transumbilical skin incision is made. The subcutaneous fat is opened, with exposure and incision of the abdominal fasciae for approximately 2 cm. The parietal peritoneum is smoothly dissected with blunt scissors, achieving access into the peritoneal cavity. After the skin incision is made, the distal ring is mounted on an introducer, an instrument used to insert and push the distal ring through the abdominal wall. Then the introducer is removed, the retractable sleeve is gripped to the proximal end, and the outer ring is pushed down to create a perfect seal with the abdominal wall. The excess sleeve is finally cut off. Through the adjustable length of the sheath, the outer part of the trocar can be positioned in contact with the skin regardless of the thickness of the abdominal wall or body mass index of the patient, making it comfortable even in obese patients. Triport (Olympus Winter & IBE GMBH; Hamburg, Germany) has two channels for the transit of gas and three ports for surgical instruments: two measuring 5 mm and one measuring 12 mm. Although a model with four ports is available, three ports seem sufficient to perform any gynecologic-oncologic procedure. The cannula positions are adjustable within the flexible port, and a separate channel allows for carbon dioxide insufflation. In order to maintain the pneumoperitoneum, the ports are sealed with a gelatinous plastic material, which prevents the escape of gas during surgical maneuvers; this does make it necessary to lubricate the instruments to avoid excessive friction. Once pneumoperitoneum (12 mmHg) is achieved, intra-abdominal visualization is obtained with a 5-mm 30° telescope or, alternatively, a 5-mm 0° laparoscope with a flexible tip (EndoEYE; Olympus Winter & IBE GMBH; Hamburg, Germany) (Fig. 13.1). Straight conventional 5-mm instruments are inserted into the remaining two ports, namely, the surgeon's choice of graspers, scissors, suction/irrigation, bipolar coagulator, and a multifunctional versatile laparoscopic device that grasps, coagulates, and transects simultaneously. The combination of one standard 33-cm long instrument with a 43-cm

long instrument is preferred to prevent excessive contact between the surgeon's instruments outside the abdominal cavity and to facilitate stripping and traction maneuvers (Fig. 13.2). Changes in the positions of the instruments and camera are performed according to the needs of the surgeon. A steep Trendelenburg position is usually needed to complete the surgery (about 30°). At the end of the procedure, each layer of the access port is separately sutured to prevent subsequent umbilical hernia occurrence. In particular, the abdominal fascia is closed by separate delayed reabsorbable sutures, and the skin is repaired with rapid absorbable suture.

The following table describes some of the most common surgical procedures performed in gynecologic oncology (Table 13.2).

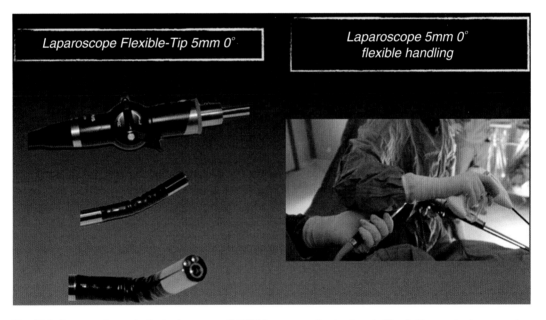

Fig. 13.1 Laparoendoscopic single-site surgery (LESS) for conservative treatment of borderline ovarian tumors: external view (**a**); internal view (**b**)

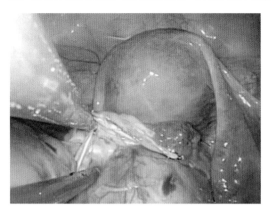

Fig. 13.2 The position of instruments during stripping of an ovarian cyst

Table 13.2 Single port surgical procedures in gynecologic oncology

Intraperitoneal
Abdominal inspection and washing
Peritoneal biopsies
Infra-colic omentectomy
Appendectomy
Extrafascial and radical hysterectomy
Adnexectomy, cystectomy, salpingectomy
Retroperitoneal
Pelvic and para-aortic lymphadenectomy

13.3.1 Risk-Reducing Salpingo-Oophorectomy, Bilateral Salpingo-Oophorectomy for Adnexal Masses, and Ovarian Cancer Staging

An intrauterine device (intrauterine manipulator-Olympus Winter & IBE; Hamburg, Germany) may be used to make surgery easier (i.e., pelvic endometriosis or large adnexal masses). Once pneumoperitoneum is achieved (12 mmHg), intra-abdominal visualization is obtained, and one grasper and one multifunctional versatile laparoscopic device that grasps, coagulates, and transects simultaneously are inserted to perform surgery. However, the use of different surgical instruments does not change the surgical technique. Pelvic washing is performed in all cases. The broad ligament is transected between the ovarian pedicle and the iliac vessels,

and the retroperitoneal structures and the ureter are identified. The infundibulopelvic ligament is skeletonized and transected using the 5-mm multifunctional device. The fallopian tube and mesosalpinx are dissected, and the utero-ovarian ligament is transected. The same procedure is repeated on the opposite side. The adnexa are inserted into a 10-mm Endocatch bag (Covidien; Mansfield, MA) and removed through the umbilicus after taking out the single-port device. In the case of large adnexal cysts, they may be emptied within an endobag to avoid spillage.

13.3.2 Simple Extrafascial Hysterectomy and Bilateral Salpingo-Oophorectomy

The patient is placed in the dorsal lithotomy position, and both arms are gently tucked and padded at the patient's sides. A high-quality uterine manipulator with a colpotomy valve is utilized in order to achieve the necessary counter-traction for LESS hysterectomy cases. It is positioned only after bilateral coagulation of the tubes in order to prevent tumor from spreading into the peritoneal cavity. In our experience, the use of a manipulator is not detrimental to any procedures in terms of increased bleeding or difficulty with pathologic evaluation. This was corroborated by Rakowski and colleagues and Fanfani and colleagues, who demonstrated that minimally invasive radical hysterectomy cases performed with a uterine manipulator did not show any clinical-pathologic differences in depth of invasion, lymphovascular space invasion, or parametrial involvement compared to open cases [8, 9].

A combination of one straight 33-cm long, 5-mm instrument with one 43-cm long, 5-mm instrument (such as graspers, cold scissors, suction/irrigator) and a 5-mm multifunctional device (that grasps, coagulates, and transects simultaneously) plus a 5-mm flexible-tipped laparoscope are used. After coagulation and section of the round ligament, entry into the retroperitoneal space is performed, and the ureter is visualized. Hemostatic clips or direct coagulation is performed at the origin of the uterine artery

(Fig. 13.3a, b) [10]. The infundibulopelvic ligaments are skeletonized and transected. A bladder flap is developed using the multifunctional instrument. An adequate margin of the vagina is ensured before colpotomy, which is performed using a monopolar hook. The uterus, cervix, and bilateral fallopian tubes and ovaries are removed through the vagina, and the vaginal vault may be closed either via the vagina with single stich technique or by a laparoscopic extracorporeal knotting technique. Vascular or visceral injuries, loss of pneumoperitoneum, or intraoperative port-site bleeding are in line with literature data such as wound hematoma, wound infection, or delayed bleeding postoperatively [1–6]. Median operative time reported in the literature is about 100 min (range, 45–155 min) with a median estimated blood loss of 30 mL (range, 10–500 mL) [10]. Most patients report complete satisfaction with cosmetic appearance and postoperative pain control. They are discharged home one day postoperatively with only optional analgesic therapy.

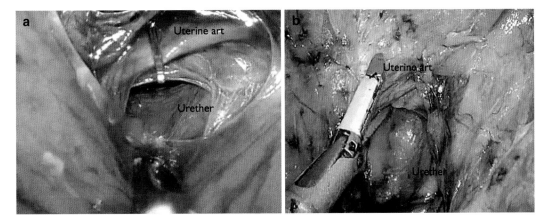

Fig. 13.3   (**a, b**) Hemostatic clip (**a**) or coagulation (**b**) at the origin of the uterine artery (*UA*) crossing over the ureter (*U*)

13.3.3 Radical Hysterectomy

Few cases of LESS radical hysterectomy have been reported in the literature [7, 11]. This may be considered one of the most advanced procedures performed by LESS currently. The first steps of preparation for radical hysterectomy are the same as those for simple extrafascial hysterectomy. After placing the patient in a steep Trendelenburg position (Fig. 13.4) and folding the small bowel out of the pelvis, a methodical survey of the abdomen, pelvis, and peritoneum as well as identification of bilateral ureters is performed.

It is our preference to perform bilateral pelvic lymphadenectomy prior to radical hysterectomy (see below for a technical description) to allow for frozen section assessment of pelvic nodes to tailor the extent of radical hysterectomy.

We usually work in an opposite way, which means having the active multifunctional instrument at the opposite side of the operating field (i.e., working on the right side of the pelvis and using the multifunctional device with the left hand). The laparoscopic grasper is usually positioned to obtain the right traction, but only the working device moves inside the surgical field. In fact, with LESS, instrument exchanges should be limited, and only one hand should be positioned at a time to limit intracorporeal instrument "sword fighting." It is important to utilize a multifunctional instrument that ligates, cauterizes, divides, and dissects the tissue. We will describe consecutive steps to perform LESS radical hysterectomy. Median operative time is about 260 min (including bilateral pelvic lymphadenectomy) comparable to those of published [6, 7] early experiences with multiport laparoscopic radical hysterectomy. A 10 % conversion rate from LESS to an alternate surgical approach has been reported for this type of surgery [6, 7]

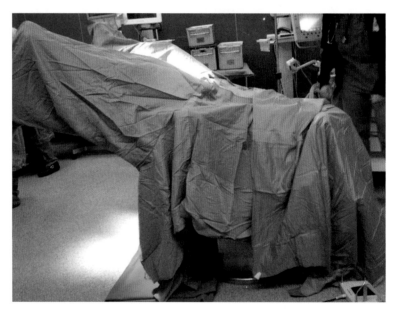

Fig. 13.4 Patient position for LESS surgery

13.3.3.1 Approach to the Retroperitoneum and Exposure of Pararectal and Paravesical Spaces

While moving the uterus to the opposite side with the uterine manipulator, a multifunctional instrument is used to coagulate and cut the round ligament at the lateral pelvic side wall. The broad ligament is opened, and the dissection is carried above the level of the pelvic brim in order to identify and expose the ureter. The ureter is mobilized medially and can be seen crossing the common iliac artery at the pelvic brim. Next, the pararectal and paravesical spaces are developed. Keeping the umbilical artery medially and the external iliac vessels laterally, the paravesical space is developed. Then, the surgeon can easily enter the pararectal fossa by displacing the ureter medially and dissecting bluntly toward the pelvic floor between the ureter and the internal iliac artery with either a suction irrigator instrument or a Maryland grasper (Medline Industries, Mundelein, IL). Development of these avascular spaces allows the surgeon to define the paracervix, which lies between the pararectal and paravesical spaces. The uterine artery and vein will easily come into view at the most caudal aspect of the spaces. Next, we move back to the left side of the uterine Dissection.

13.3.3.2 Isolation and Ligation of the Paracervix

The anterior division of the umbilical artery is identified, and the uterine artery and vein are isolated. One of the defining features of a class III radical hysterectomy is that the uterine vessels are ligated laterally to the ureters, near their origin. It is critical to isolate the artery from the vein and ligate them separately to ensure blood flow is halted and to optimize the radicality of the parametrial Dissection. A Maryland dissector and suction irrigator are used to perform the ureterolysis and dissect the ureter medially and away from the uterine vessels. Then the suction-irrigator, together with the bipolar grasper of monopolar scissors, are used to atraumatically continue taking down the bladder off the proximal vagina. If the ovaries are being removed, you can keep the infundibulopelvic ligament intact until the uterine vessels are ligated in order to maximize the degree of counter-traction applied to the medial leaf of the broad ligament. The same multifunctional instrument is used to ligate the infundibulopelvic ligament. Once one side is complete, the uterus is deviated to the opposite side, and the other uterine dissection is begun.

13.3.3.3 Anterior Paracervix

The ureter is further dissected from the medial peritoneum at the level of the uterosacral ligament. The ureter is dissected laterally with either a Maryland dissector or a suction-irrigator. The parametrial vasculature, once isolated and ligated with a multifunctional instrument, is flipped on the ureter that is rolled laterally out of the tunnel. The vesicouterine peritoneum is reflected caudally below the manipulator valve, exposing the proximal vagina. The ureter is dissected free from the surrounding tissue up to the level of the bladder. The procedure on the ureter is repeated on the opposite side until its insertion into the trigonal region of the bladder. Finally, the remaining attachments of the bladder and ureter to the anterior vagina are sharply dissected at the level of the inferior colpotomy valve.

13.3.3.4 Posterior Paracervix

The uterus is positioned upward and caudad using the uterine manipulator. The incision made in the posterior leaf of the broad ligament is extended across the cul-de-sac peritoneum between the cervicovaginal junction and rectum to develop the rectovaginal space. At this point, the ureters are mobilized laterally away from the point of dissection. The uterosacral ligaments are developed during this portion of the procedure. The multifunctional instrument, the suction irrigator, and the Maryland dissector serve as excellent dissecting tools to safely isolate the rectum from the cervix and the vagina. The posterior wall of the vagina is gently dissected off the anterior wall of the rectum. The uterosacral ligaments are coagulated and cut at this point, halfway down to the insertion point at the sacrum. The upper half of the uterosacral ligament is incised, and the lower half, containing the sympathetic nerves to the bladder, is spared. The surgeon can tailor the radicality of the procedure, and more of the uterosacral ligament may be ligated if necessary.

13.3.3.5 Colpotomy

The monopolar hook is used to perform a colpotomy. This results in the removal of the proximal 2–3 cm of vagina en bloc with the parametria, uterus, and cervix. It is our preference to perform cuff closure vaginally to decrease the risk of dehiscence compared with the laparoscopic approach.

13.3.3.6 Closure

Once hemostasis is obtained and no bladder injury has been identified, complete insufflation of carbon dioxide should be obtained to avoid significant postoperative pain. A well-positioned umbilical incision should be relatively concealed at the base of the navel once healing is complete, resulting in a scarless appearance. In order to minimize the risk of umbilical hernia at the incision site, we recommend a tight running closure of the umbilicus fasciae with a zero, delayed absorbable suture. Optimal cosmesis is achieved when the skin incision is closed with 3–4 single stitch using 2-0 absorbable suture, preferably Monocryl. The first stitch should bisect the incision and anchor the skin to the underlying umbilical tissue. This maneuver essentially results in reinverting the navel and restoring the native umbilical anatomy. The patient can be potentially discharged home on postoperative day 1 with a urinary catheter, which is removed 2 days later.

13.3.4 Pelvic and Low Para-Aortic Lymphadenectomy

With the patient in a steep Trendelenburg position, folding the small bowel and rectosigmoid colon gently out of the pelvis with atraumatic graspers optimizes pelvic exposure. It is our preference to perform bilateral pelvic lymphadenectomy prior to radical hysterectomy. While displacing the uterus to the opposite side with the uterine manipulator, the broad ligament is opened and the dissection is carried above the level of the pelvic brim in order to identify and expose the ureter and all the retroperitoneal lymph and vascular spaces. The pararectal and paravesical spaces are created by gentle blunt dissection using the Maryland grasper.

Some surgeons prefer to position the laparoscope so that the external iliac vessels are viewed

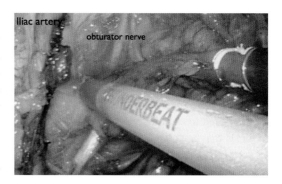

Fig. 13.5 Left pelvic lymphadenectomy

horizontally, similar to the view seen during open pelvic lymphadenectomy by the contralateral surgeon. The bifurcation of the common iliac, the right external iliac arteries and the hypogastric arteries, veins, and the right ureter are identified. Using a soft-tissue grasper and a multifunctional 5-mm laparoscopic instrument (which allows tissue fusion and/or vessel sealing, spot coagulation, and in some cases, endoscissor functions in one instrument), the dissection is initiated lateral to the external iliac artery. The peritoneum between the external iliac artery and the psoas muscle is elevated and incised parallel to the artery (Fig. 13.5).

The external iliac vessels are then skeletonized anteromedially and laterally, away from the psoas muscle, taking care to avoid injury to the genitofemoral nerve, which runs anteriorly along the muscle. All nodal tissue is then removed from the midportion of the common iliac artery superiorly to the circumflex iliac vein inferiorly and from the midportion of the psoas muscles laterally to the ureters and the hypogastric artery and vein medially. Furthermore, the nodal tissue within the obturator fossa is also carefully dissected and excised, anterior to the obturator nerve and vessels. The dissection is performed with a combination of gentle blunt dissection with either the reticulating Maryland soft-tissue grasper or the tip of a suction aspirator. The excised nodal tissue is placed in a sterile endoscopic bag, which is extracted through the umbilicus after removal of the single-port device and sent for frozen section analysis. The same procedure is performed on the opposite side in a similar fashion and within the same anatomic boundaries as the right pelvic lymph nodes. Notably, on the left side, it is often necessary to first divide physiologic adhesions from the sigmoid colon to the left pelvic side wall (with endoscissors or the tip of the multifunctional instrument) to optimize exposure of the left pelvic vasculature and node-bearing tissues.

The device is then reinserted into the umbilical incision, the abdomen is reinsufflated with carbon dioxide gas, and the pelvis is irrigated and inspected to ensure hemostasis. Endoclips are used generously to prevent blood loss and to close the lymphatic vessels [12].

Low para-aortic dissection is carried out to the level of the inferior mesenteric artery in a similar fashion. The peritoneum on top of the lower aorta is elevated and incised parallel to the artery starting cephalad to the bifurcation of the common iliac arteries. The ureter is dissected laterally using the graspers and the nodal tissue is then gently removed. The dissection is then carried out distally, exposing the bifurcation of the common iliacs and left common iliac vein. Of note, on the left side, the sigmoid colon has to be mobilized, depending on the approach to the dissection of lymph nodes around the left common iliac artery.

13.3.5 High Para-Aortic Lymphadenectomy

Single-port laparoscopic aortic lymphadenectomy to the level of the renal veins is a very complex procedure, which may be performed transperitoneally and extraperitoneally.

13.3.5.1 Transperitoneal

A 5-mm rotatable deflecting-tip laparoscope is inserted through the most inferior port on the single-port device (EndoEYE; Olympus Winter & IBE GMBH, Hamburg, Germany), and the first surgeon takes a place at the level of the right leg of the patient. The patient is then placed in the steep Trendelenburg and semiflank position (tilt to patient's right); folding the small bowel to the patient's right flank optimizes exposure of the aorta. The descending colon is either dissected and mobilized medially through the white line of Toldt or left in situ for a transmesenteric approach to the aorta, depending on patient characteristics (e.g., obesity, short intestinal mesentery, intestinal

adhesions, and/or distended bowel). The peritoneum and nodal tissue are grasped and dissected away from the aorta and vena cava from the aortic bifurcation to the left renal vein in caudal to cranial direction. The inferior mesenteric artery is preserved in all cases [13].

13.3.5.2 Extraperitoneal

A single 2–3-cm left iliac incision is made perpendicular to a point situated two thirds of the way along a line drawn from the umbilicus to the anterosuperior iliac spine or a point situated one third of the way along the line from the anterosuperior iliac spine toward the umbilicus. First, the fascia in front of the left rectus abdominis muscle is incised, and the muscles are divided in the direction of their fibers, plane by plane, up to the peritoneum, which is opened to introduce the single device used to perform a transperitoneal inspection. In the absence of peritoneal or ovarian spread, after peritoneal cytologic examination, the single-port device is removed, and a para-aortic lymphadenectomy is performed through the same incision via a left-sided extraperitoneal approach.

For this second step, through the same incision, the fascia in front of the anterolateral abdominal muscles is incised, and a large finger dissection of muscle fibers is performed to introduce the single port into the extraperitoneal space. Although the transperitoneal incision of the peritoneum is performed very close to the extraperitoneal approach, there is no gas transfer from the extraperitoneal to the intraperitoneal cavity.

The surgeon is positioned to the left of the patient during the procedure. The assistant stands on the left of the patient and to the left of the surgeon. For ergonomic reasons, the assistant can be placed between the legs of the patient during the dissection of the left renal vein.

The nodal tissues are grasped and dissected away from the aortic bifurcation to the left renal vein. The inferior mesenteric artery is preserved in all cases. Lymph nodes are extracted through the single-port device.

Conclusion

Laparoendoscopic single-site surgery oncologic surgery is feasible and safe in select patients. Future innovations that may allow greater diffusion of this surgical approach include refinement of single-port tools and techniques to merge robotics and single-site technology [14]. Further investigation is needed to determine the long-term outcomes of the LESS approach with oncologic patients.

References

1. Fader AN, Escobar PF. Laparoendoscopic single-site surgery (LESS) in gynecologic oncology: technique and initial report. Gynecol Oncol. 2009;114:157–61.
2. Fagotti A, Bottoni C, Vizzielli G, Alletti SG, Scambia G, Marana E, Fanfani F. Postoperative pain after conventional laparoscopy and laparoendoscopic single site surgery (LESS) for benign adnexal disease: a randomized trial. Fertil Steril. 2011;96:255.e2–9.e2.
3. Fagotti A, Gagliardi ML, Fanfani F, Salerno MG, Ercoli A, D'Asta M, et al. Perioperative outcomes of total laparoendoscopic single-site hysterectomy versus total robotic hysterectomy in endometrial cancer patients: a multicentre study. Gynecol Oncol. 2012; 125:552–5.
4. Marocco F, Fanfani F, Rossitto C, Gallotta V, Scambia G, Fagotti A. Laparoendoscopic single-site surgery for fertility-sparing staging of border line ovarian tumors: initial experience. Surg Laparosc Endosc Percutan Tech. 2010;20:e172–5.
5. Fanfani F, Fagotti A, Scambia G. Laparoendoscopic single-site surgery for total hysterectomy. Int J Gynaecol Obstet. 2010;109:76–7.
6. Garrett LA, Boruta 2nd DM. Laparoendoscopic single-site radical hysterectomy: the first report of LESS type III hysterectomy involves a woman with cervical cancer. Am J Obstet Gynecol. 2012;207:518.e1–e2.
7. Tergas AI, Fader AN. Laparoendoscopic single-site surgery (LESS) radical hysterectomy for the treatment of early stage cervical cancer. Gynecol Oncol. 2013;129:241–3.
8. Rakowski J, Tran TA, Ahmad S, James JA, Brudie LA, Pernicone PJ, et al. Does a uterine manipulator affect cervical cancer pathology or identification of lymphovascular space involvement? Gynecol Oncol. 2012; 127:98–101.
9. Fanfani F, Gagliardi ML, Zannoni GF, Gallotta V, Vizzielli G, Lecca A, et al. Total laparoscopic hysterectomy in early-stage endometrial cancer using an intrauterine manipulator: is it a bias for frozen section analysis? Case–control study. J Minim Invasive Gynecol. 2011;18:184–8.
10. Fagotti A, Boruta 2nd DM, Scambia G, Fanfani F, Paglia A, Escobar PF. First 100 early endometrial cancer cases treated with laparoendoscopic single-site surgery: a multicentric retrospective study. Am J Obstet Gynecol. 2012;206:353.e1–e6.
11. Desai R, Puntambekar SP, Lawande A, Kenawadekar R, Joshi S, Joshi GA, Kulkarni S. More with LESS: a novel report of nerve sparing radical hysterectomy performed using LESS. J Minim Invasive Gynecol. 2013;20:886–90.
12. Gallotta V, Fanfani F, Rossitto C, Vizzielli G, Testa A, Scambia G, Fagotti A. A randomized study comparing the use of the Ligaclip with bipolar energy to prevent lymphocele during laparoscopic pelvic lymphadenectomy for gynecologic cancer. Am J Obstet Gynecol. 2010;203:483.e1–e6.
13. Gouy S, Uzan C, Kane A, Scherier S, Gauthier T, Bentivegna E, Morice P. A new single-port approach to perform a transperitoneal step and an extraperitoneal para-aortic lymphadenectomy with a single incision. J Am Coll Surg. 2012;214:e25–30.
14. Fagotti A, Corrado G, Fanfani F, Mancini M, Paglia A, Vizzielli G, et al. Robotic single-site hysterectomy (RSS-H) vs. laparoendoscopic single-site hysterectomy (LESS-H) in early endometrial cancer: a double-institution case–control study. Gynecol Oncol. 2013; 130:219–23.

Techniques for Single-Port Urogynecology and Pelvic Reconstructive Surgery

14

Fariba Behnia-Willison and Anirudha Garg

This chapter introduces the use of single-port laparoscopy for surgical management of female pelvic floor repair. Degrees and types of pelvic organ prolapse are quantified. Patient care is covered, including preoperative and postoperative care and consent. The instruments, ergonomics, and learning curve are then discussed. Finally, descriptions of minimally invasive solutions to prolapse are described. Specifically, the use of sutures and mesh in apical vaginal vault repair with or without a previous hysterectomy are described.

F. Behnia-Willison (✉) • A. Garg, MD
Department of Obstetrics, Gynecology,
and Reproductive Medicine, Flinders Medical Centre,
Flinders University, Bedford Park,
Adelaide, SA 5042, Australia
e-mail: faribawillison@yahoo.com.au,
fariba.willison@gmail.com; anirgarg@gmail.com

P.F. Escobar, T. Falcone (eds.), *Atlas of Single-Port, Laparoscopic, and Robotic Surgery*,
DOI 10.1007/978-1-4614-6840-0_14, © Springer Science+Business Media New York 2014

14.1   Introduction

Historically, the treatment of genital prolapse dates back to 1500 B.C. to the Ebers Papyrus, which described the treatment of prolapse via the smearing of a mixture of honey and other sticky substances on the prolapsed organ [1]. Hippocrates subsequently described the treatment of uterine prolapse by securing the woman upside-down and shaking her. Management involved the insertion of a half pomegranate soaked in wine into the vagina. Suffice it to say, the treatment of prolapse has significantly improved since then. In the middle to late nineteenth century, surgical intervention to treat uterine prolapse consisted of narrowing the vaginal vault via astringents, colporrhaphy, or cautery. By the end of the nineteenth century, there were several surgical approaches to the treatment of uterine prolapse; however, achieving long-lasting repairs remained elusive [1].

An improved understanding of pelvic floor anatomy as well as aseptic surgical techniques brought about the concept of a vaginal/abdominal surgical approach to treat vaginal prolapse. Finally, the repair of vaginal prolapse was described in its current form in 1957 by Arthure and Savage, whose original description of abdominal sacrohysteropexy continues to be utilized today [2]. Although the surgical procedure largely remains the same, the approach toward pelvic floor repair has continually moved toward minimally invasive surgical techniques. In 2008, the present author performed one of the first mesh sacrohysteropexies as a laparoendoscopic single-site (LESS) surgery, thus helping to further minimize the invasiveness of prolapse repair.

The primary goals in surgical management of prolapse are not only to correct the prolapse but to correct the symptoms associated with this condition. This includes the reversal of urinary or fecal incontinence, urgency, and improvement of sexual dysfunction if present. There also are significant psychological consequences to prolapse, which may be improved with surgical correction [3].

Fig. 14.1 A sagittal view of the female pelvic floor. All measurements are taken with the vaginal orifice (hymen) as the midpoint with a value of 0. Points within the vaginal cavity are negative and points outside the vaginal cavity are positive (From Bump et al. [4]; with permission)

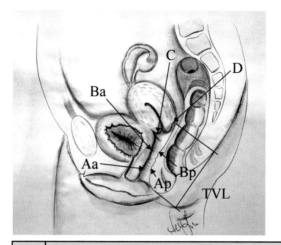

Point	Description	Range of Values
Aa	Anterior vaginal wall 3 cm proximal to the hymen	-3 cm to +3 cm
Ba	Most distal position of the remaining upper anterior vaginal wall	-3 cm to + tvl
C	Most distal edge of cervix or vaginal cuff scar	
D	Posterior fornix (N/A if post-hysterectomy)	
Ap	Posterior vaginal wall 3 cm proximal to the hymen	-3 cm to +3 cm
Bp	Most distal position of remaining upper posterior vaginal wall	-3 cm to + tvl

Genital higtus (pb) - Measured from middle of external urethral meatus to posterior midlline hymen

Perineal body (pb) - Measured from posterior margin of to gh middle of anal opening

Total vaginal length (tvl) - Depth of vagina when point D or C is reduced to normal position

Table 14.1 Staging criteria for POP-Q

POP-Q staging criteria	
Stage 0	Aa, Ap, Ba, Bp=−3 and C or D ≤ − (tvl − 2) cm
Stage I	Stage 0 criteria not met and leading <−1 cm
Stage II	Leading edge ≥ −1 cm but ≤+1 cm
Stage III	Leading edge >+1 cm but <+ (tvl − 2) cm
Stage IV	Leading edge ≥ +(tvl − 2) cm

From Bump et al. [4]

14.2 Prolapse Quantification

In order to describe pelvic floor dysfunction as it relates to gynecology, an objective system to quantify prolapse has been developed [4]. As described in Fig. 14.1, the Pelvic Organ Prolapse Quantification (POP-Q) system allows for a quick, one-line dissemination of the severity of pelvic organ prolapse, allowing the reader to understand the degree and type of prolapse (anterior versus posterior). Given this quantification system, a staging protocol, as described in Table 14.1, was concurrently developed.

14.3 Patient Care for Single-Port Pelvic Floor Repair

14.3.1 Preoperative

Women typically appear at the clinic with prolapse symptoms, which may include vaginal bulge, pelvic pain, sexual dysfunction (including dyspareunia), and urinary or fecal dysfunction. A standardized, comprehensive history that addresses prolapse, urinary, bowel, and sexual symptoms is completed. A physical examination, including assessment of the pelvic floor utilizing the POP-Q system, a cough test, and a Q-tip test are also performed. Perineal ultrasound analyzing detrusor and bladder neck caliber is carried out. The patient is further investigated with cystometric urodynamic studies, if indicated.

All patients are offered a vaginal support device to reduce vaginal bulge in the form of a ring pessary if they are sexually active or a mushroom pessary if they are not active. Conservative management is recommended initially for a minimum of 3–6 months and includes pelvic floor exercises, the use of estrogen cream if it is not contraindicated, lifestyle changes (including a reduction in caffeine intake and addressing constipation), reducing weight, reducing intra-abdominal pressure by decreasing heavy lifting (modifying gym activities such as lying down when lifting weights and increasing repetition with decreased load when lifting), and managing asthma or smoking (decreased coughing). Patients are advised to prolong the conservative management period until their family is complete. All patients are given bowel preparation the day before any laparoscopic pelvic floor surgery.

14.3.2 Consent Visit

If the patient's symptoms persist and she desires surgical management, she is asked to speak with the surgeon and her partner or support person about the postoperative period. They are informed about intraoperative prolapse staging, where 29 % of prolapses are upgraded and 9 % are downgraded, and subsequent modifications to the surgery that may be made owing to intraoperative findings [5]. Patients are reminded that pelvic floor repair is a major operation requiring strict and lifelong lifestyle management postoperatively. They are told about the risks of mesh repair as well as the limited data on the use of mesh in gynecology. This is an important aspect of the treatment because women with active lifestyles are prone to organ prolapse and, because the procedure is relatively pain-free postoperatively, they may relapse and compromise successful outcomes. Hence, strict follow-up visits at 1 week for detection of early complications, then 6 weeks, 3, 6, and 12 months, and annually thereafter are required.

14.3.3 Postoperative

An indwelling catheter (IDC) and vaginal pack are inserted immediately after the operation and removed the next day. A deep vein thrombosis prevention protocol is followed, and laxative medication in the form of a bulking agent is administered. It is recommended that patients stay in the hospital until there is no significant postvoid residual (<20 %) and the bowels are active.

Good patient selection, sound surgical skills, and postoperative patient lifestyle changes are cornerstones of a successful pelvic floor repair surgery.

14.4   Instruments, Ergonomics, and Learning Curve

14.4.1 Instruments (Commonly Used in LESS Pelvic Floor Repair)

- 30-degree, 5-mm bariatric scopes or 5-mm flexible scopes (Olympus; Center Valley, PA)
- Ligosure roticulating instruments (Covidien; Mansfield, MA)
- Endostitch (Covidien; Mansfield, MA) with Ethibond sutures (Ethicon; Somerville, NJ) or a straight needle-holder utilizing V-loc (Covidien; Mansfield, MA)
- Straight tooth and bowel graspers
- Roticulating graspers
- Smoke evacuator
- Suction irrigation
- Covidien (Mansfield, MA) or GelPOINT single-port surgical device (Applied Medical; Rancho Santa Margarita, CA)

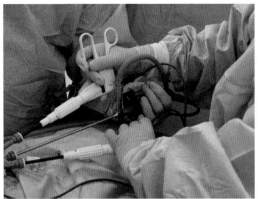

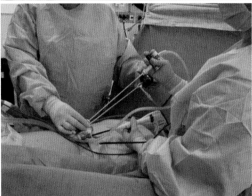

Fig. 14.2 Proper ergonomics are vitally important in a LESS procedure. Because of the single port access to the intra-abdominal cavity, the degrees of freedom are limited compared to those in conventional multiport laparoscopy. A surgical plan taking into account these limitations is important in producing successful outcomes for LESS pelvic floor repair. Note how the surgeons are standing as midline as possible with their arms in neutral positions and bodies facing away from the patient's head

14.4.2 Ergonomics

When using single-site ports of any kind, the ergonomics of the instruments will become crucial in performing the surgery. There are two important points regarding ergonomics in LESS pelvic floor repair. First, the operation can be cumbersome if a proper approach has not been thought through owing to the single fulcrum point at the abdomen as well as crowding of the instruments (Fig. 14.2). Second, there are issues regarding the body positioning of the surgeon and the assistant.

Unlike conventional laparoscopy in which crossing of instruments is discouraged, such a maneuver becomes necessary at times in LESS.

Crossing instruments is safe because of the insulating properties of roticulating graspers. This requires retraining for many conventional laparoscopic surgeons. Furthermore, the surgeon needs to be aware of possible instrument crowding issues. Thus, in order to minimize surgery time as well as reduce frustration, the surgeon needs to plan out the order and positioning of the instruments, taking into account the patient's anatomy, body mass index (BMI), and any surgical procedures performed previously on this patient prior to making an incision.

The operation is easier if a 5-mm bariatric 30° scope is used with a highly experienced assistant who will need to have both hands constantly on the camera and light lead to provide the best possible view. It is advisable to commence with the scope on the right side or most cephalic channel to enable the assistant to push the camera down toward the patient and away from the midline. The surgeon should place the instruments in a way that is physically most comfortable. As the operation proceeds, changing the channels of the instruments or changing the operating side may be required; therefore the surgeon should stand as close as possible to the head of the patient and in the midline. This provides the most accessible plane for operating on the pelvic floor. This is a particularly important point in LESS gynecology because of the limited degrees of freedom with a single-port approach and subsequent problems with needing to lean over patients (Fig. 14.2).

14.4.3 Learning Curve

A short learning curve for LESS requires sound anatomic knowledge, conventional laparoscopic surgical experience, and proficiency with laparoscopic suturing. Furthermore, an understanding of current surgical procedures for pelvic floor

repair is highly valued, since the approaches to these do not change significantly with the transabdominal approach (LESS versus multiport laparoscopy).

With regard to LESS versus conventional laparoscopic transabdominal pelvic floor repair surgeries, it has been noted that LESS takes more time (which decreases with experience) and is more strenuous if the ergonomics of the patient or operator have not been properly thought through. Current data are only available as case reports; however, the data from these reports appear encouraging both for patients and for surgeons [6]. This is probably because the surgeries themselves are the same, but the approach to them is simply being modified (single-port) in order to improve cosmesis and minimize invasiveness. Thus, the learning curve for a surgeon when training in LESS mainly deals with port insertion and ergonomics.

Prior to utilizing a LESS approach, as occurred with this chapter's first author, it is beneficial to have advanced skills in conventional laparoscopic pelvic floor repair surgeries utilizing Verress needles to establish the pneumoperitoneum. When switching to LESS, the author required approximately ten port insertions with the Covidien device (Mansfield, MA) in order to demonstrate efficiency and accuracy in the port insertion technique. This was achieved in dry laboratories, animal laboratories, and in the operating theater under supervision. Subsequently, the insertion of the GelPOINT port (Applied Medical; Rancho Santa Margarita, CA) required only one practice insertion with instruction in order to achieve proficiency. This was achieved following approximately 200 LESS procedures utilizing Covidien ports. Initially, port insertion took 7–10 min, but with practice (~25 procedures), this decreased to approximately 3–4 min per insertion.

14.5 Establishing the Pneumoperitoneum and Inserting the Port

14.5.1 Covidien SILS Port

All pelvic floor repair LESS procedures are performed under general anesthesia with the patient in the lithotomy position. Once the patient is prepared and draped, a periumbilical nerve block is performed by injecting 5 mL of 0.5 % bupivicaine and adrenaline at each of the 3, 6, 9, and 12 o'clock positions. A 15–20-mm vertical transumbilical skin incision is made. The rectus sheath is grasped with two graspers and a sharp incision made through the fascia with the tip of a scalpel, allowing intraperitoneal access. The incision is stretched with an artery clip and opened to its maximum opening width, which should accommodate the insertion of two S-retractors. A scalpel is used to extend the sheath incision to 2.5 cm under the skin without extending the skin incision.

The Covidien SILS port is inserted through the incision by grasping the base of the port with two Blake forceps. The Blake forceps are arranged so that the first forceps is positioned from the midsection of the port to the leading edge, and the second is arranged from the trailing edge to the midsection, such that the tip of the second clamp meets the heel of the first. The port is lubricated with paraffin, and the first clamp is inserted through the incision directed toward the right lateral abdominal wall. When the heel of the first clamp enters the sheath, it is removed while continued pressure is exerted on the second clamp in an arc-like motion until the lower lip of the port enters completely through the sheath. The trocars are then inserted. The present author has modified the Covidien SILS port by cutting it vertically between the channels at 120° angles so that a larger degree of freedom is attained for each trocar insertion port. Figure 14.3 briefly illustrates the process of incising the abdomen and inserting the port.

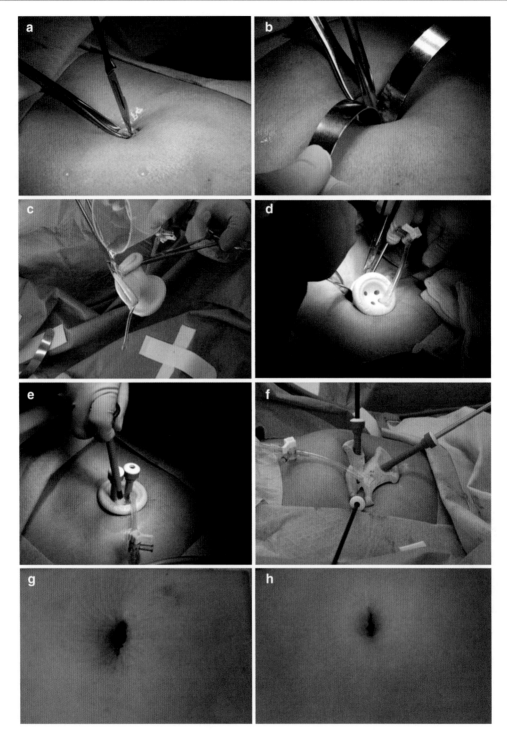

Fig. 14.3 An overview of the insertion, modification of the Covidien port, and postoperative cosmesis. (**a**) Incising and gaining access to the peritoneal cavity via the umbilicus. (**b**) Using S retractors to establish the pneumoperitoneum. (**c**) Lubricating the SILS port with paraffin wax. (**d**) Grasping the SILS port using two Blake forceps and inserting these into the umbilicus with the forceps as a guide. (**e**) Insertion of the trocars and insufflation of the abdomen. (**f**) Trocars are then inserted and the port is cut every 120° between the channels of the SILS port to allow for greater maneuverability. (**g**) The umbilicus is visualized immediately postoperatively. (**h**) Six weeks postoperative

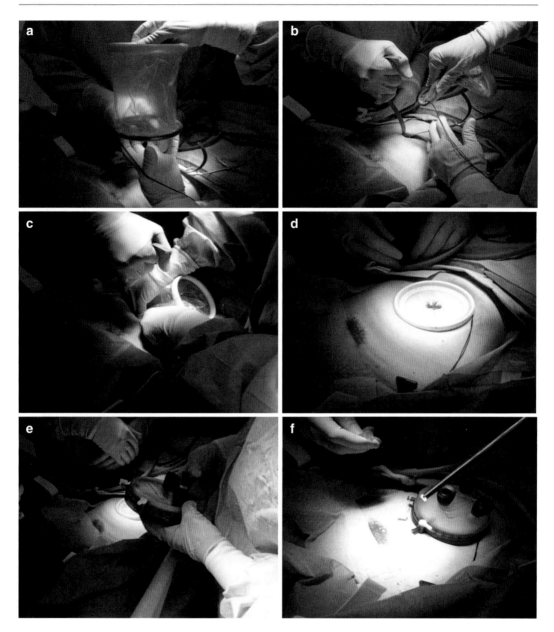

Fig. 14.4 Insertion of the GelPOINT port. (**a**) The purple ring is the intraperitoneal portion of the port, and the white ring remains outside the patient. (**b**) Using S retractors to keep the umbilicus open, the ring is squeezed tightly to allow entry through the umbilicus. (**c**) Fingers are used to move the port intra-abdominally. (**d**) The inserted port is visualized. (**e**) Trocar guides are inserted through the gel head of the port. (**f**) The gel head is attached to the port, and the surgery may now commence

14.5.2 Applied Medical GelPOINT Port

The GelPOINT port is inserted by squeezing one of the purple rings of the Alexis portion of the port system using an S-retractor and inserting it into the transumbilical incision with the force of the surgeon's hands directed toward the pelvis of the patient. A digital examination is then performed to ensure no bowel or omentum is caught between the purple ring and the abdominal wall. The outer ring is twisted inward to achieve more tension; this stretches the incision site and increases the diameter of the opening. The GelPOINT gel cap is pierced with three trocars whose locations are defined by the vertices of a triangle placed horizontally over the gel cap. This is placed over the Alexis part of the port and locked. The insertion of the GelPOINT device is illustrated in Fig. 14.4.

With the GelPOINT device it is easier to use straight instruments than with the Covidien port. In the case of suturing and utilizing conventional needle holders, one needs to learn and practice one-handed suturing technique because it makes the operation and suturing with LESS simpler.

14.6 Apical Compartment Repair Utilizing Nonabsorbable Sutures

Laparoscopic suture colpopexy (also known as vaginal vault suspension or McCall colposuspension) and laparoscopic hysteropexy using nonabsorbable suture material are valuable techniques in providing apical vaginal support dating back to 1957 [7]. Prophylactically,

they can be performed after vaginal or laparoscopic hysterectomy or in conjunction with anterior and posterior vaginal wall prolapse repair for further support and reinforcement of the apical compartment with or without uterine preservation. In the urogynecology unit at Flinders University, the preferred sutures are Ethibond (Ethicon; Somerville, NJ; nonabsorbable) or PDS (Ethicon; Somerville, NJ) or V-loc (Covidien; Mansfield, MA; absorbable after 6 months) sutures, that promote inflammation and scarring. A 15-cm barbed suture with a small loop at the end of the thread for locking is especially useful in LESS procedures because it eliminates the need for knot tying. These biologic processes act together to reinforce the uterosacral ligament supporting the vaginal vault or uterus in its correct anatomic position. This approach is sometimes preferable to laparoscopic mesh sacrohysteropexy because it may have fewer postoperative complications, such as new-onset urinary incontinence, pelvic pain and dyspareunia, damage to the surrounding pelvic floor organs, or subsequent surgical reintervention because of mesh exposure [8].

14.6.1 Typical Patient Presentation

A 65-year-old woman with a BMI of 25 and two prior vaginal deliveries presented with symptomatic global prolapse unresponsive to conservative management such as pelvic floor exercises, vaginal pessary, and estrogen cream. Her intraoperative POP-Q was GH 6 cm, Aa 0, Ba +0.5, Cx +1.5, Ap −1, Bp −0.5, total vaginal length (TVL) 10, resulting in a global prolapse, POP-Q Stage III.

Fig. 14.5 An outline of the use of sutures in apical vaginal prolapse repair using nonabsorbable sutures. (**a**) The utero-sacral ligament and ureters are identified on the left and right side. (**b**) 5–6 cm incisions (fenestrations) are made horizontally in the lateral portions of the left and right uterosacral ligaments. These are medial to the ureters and give subperi-toneal access for the insertion of the sutures. (**c**) A V-loc suture is placed through the right uterosacral ligament and locked at the proximal end. This method in LESS suturing requires one-handed suturing using the straight needle holder. The surgeon starts at the initial lateral incision site as proximal as possible and continues medially across the pos-terior vault/posterior cervix. (**d**) Bites of the right uterosac-ral ligament are continuously taken until the left uterosacral ligament is also incorporated. (**e**) The suture is tensioned once the left-most incision has been reached, bringing the uterosacral ligament and uterus/vault together. (**f**) A second suture is incorporated in the same plane for extra reinforce-ment of the uterosacral ligament. NB: In the case of using Endostitch with Ethibond sutures, the same incision is made medial to the ureter and over the uterosacral ligament. (**g**) The Endostitch is loaded and suturing starts from the proxi-molateral portion of the uterosacral ligaments, moving medially and ending at the level of posterior cervix/vault. (**h**) An extracorporeal suturing technique is then utilized. The sutures should then be tensioned such that there is a gap of 3–4 cm in the pouch of Douglas. This is done in order to prevent bowel entrapment and possible obstruction

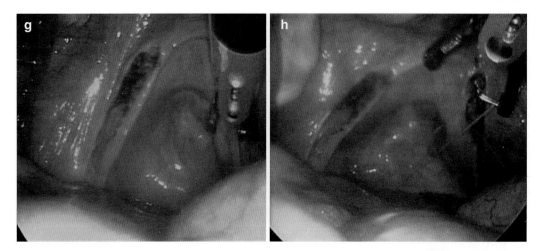

Fig. 14.5 (continued)

14.6.2 Procedure

Of particular importance in the apical repair of a vaginal vault or uterine prolapse is the integrity of the uterosacral ligament close to the uterus/vaginal vault. This important ligament is particularly prone to weakening and lengthening with age and multiparity. The relevant anatomy is shown in Fig. 14.3. Nonabsorbable sutures are used to strengthen and shorten the ligament by continuously suturing it from the lateral ends to the posterior cervix medially. The use of nonabsorbable sutures is important because it causes a local inflammatory reaction as well as providing support to the prolapsed organ. The inflammation causes scarring and fibrosis of the uterosacral ligament and subsequent elevation and correction of the prolapse. The steps to this procedure are outlined in Fig. 14.5.

14.7 Single-Incision Laparoscopic Mesh Sacrohysteropexy

The use of mesh in prolapse repair has been described successfully by Leron and coworkers [9] in 13 women who wished to retain their uteri and had significant prolapse. Mesh provides an alternative to suture-based prolapse repair in that it gives greater support to the apical portion of the vagina in the long term and is especially beneficial for women in whom child-bearing is incomplete [10]. Thus, mesh is sometimes preferred to suture-based prolapse repair, especially in younger, nulliparous women [11].

14.7.1 Typical Patient Presentation

A 70-year-old woman with a BMI of 26, Parity 3, who had always delivered vaginally, presented with symptomatic global prolapse, which was not improved with conservative management such as pelvic floor exercises, vaginal pessary, and estrogen cream. Her POP-Q was GH 4 cm, Aa −1, Ba +1.5, Cx +2, Ap −1, Bp +1, TVL 10, and right levator avulsion, resulting in a global POP-Q Stage III.

14.7.2 Procedure

Once pneumoperitoneum is established, the operation commences with the insertion of a bariatric 5 mm, 30° laparoscope and two instruments. The patient is tilted to the left, and the sigmoid colon pushed to the left side of the patient. In case of difficulty with bowel or ovarian mobilization, a straight needle can be passed through the abdominal wall and through the bowel mesentery or ovarian tissue and again through the abdominal wall outside of the body to assist with retraction. The right ureter and vessels as well as the sacral promontory are identified and a small incision is made in the peritoneum, on the top of the sacral promontory. There are now two possible approaches to mesh insertion: transperitoneal or retroperitoneal.

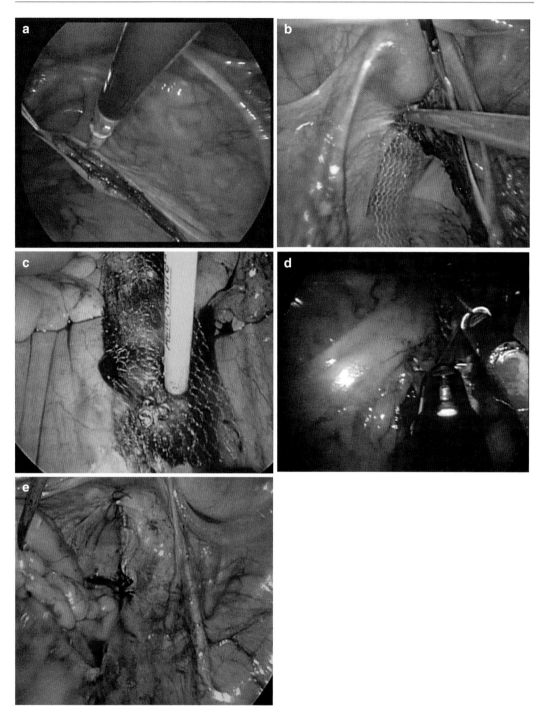

Fig. 14.6 Transperitoneal LESS mesh sacrohysteropexy. (**a**) The peritoneum over the sacral promontory is lifted and incised with Ligosure devices (Covidien; Mansfield, MA), and the incision is extended to the posterior cervix in the right pararectal space, just below the uterosacral ligament. (**b**) The mesh is attached to the posterior cervix using Absorbatack (Covidien; Mansfield, MA). Alternatively, one can attach the mesh utilizing one-handed suturing techniques or Endostitch. (**c**) The mesh is then secured to the sacral promontory using Protack fasteners. (**d**) The peritoneum is sutured over the mesh starting from the sacral promontory and moving caudally until the posterior cervix is reached. (**e**) The end product of enclosing the attached mesh in the peritoneum. Note that no mesh should be exposed because it can potentially cause bowel adhesions

14.7.3 Transperitoneal Mesh Sacrohysteropexy

The right ureter is identified, and a peritoneal incision is made from the sacral promontory in the right pararectal space inferior to the utero-sacral ligament to the posterior part of the cervix. Next, a polypropylene type-1 monofilament macroporous, nonabsorbable mesh is used to suspend the cervix from the sacral promontory. The length of mesh is measured and tailored to the anatomy of the patient, ensuring that the mesh is long enough to avoid tension and thus postoperative pain. The mesh is introduced through the transumbilical port. The distal end of the mesh is anchored to the posterior cervix with five absorbable 5-mm nonabsorbable helical Protack fasteners (Covidien; Mansfield, MA) or V-loc sutures. The mesh is then tacked to the sacral promontory with Protack fasteners. The aim is to lift the cervix at least 6–8 cm above the level of the introitus. The entire length of the mesh is closed and covered with peritoneum using Endostitch and Vicryl absorbable sutures. The use of mesh allows further shortening of the ligament via inflammation-induced fibrosis over time. A description of this procedure is given in Fig. 14.6.

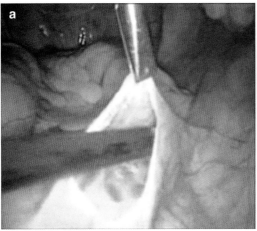 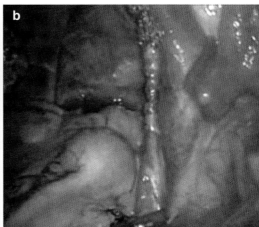

Fig. 14.7 Retroperitoneal LESS mesh sacrohystero-pexy. (**a**) An incision is made at the sacral promontory and at the posterior cervix. (**b**) A retroperitoneal tunnel is created from the initial incision in the sacral promontory to the posterior cervix with the assistance of two additional small incisions in the right pararectal space. An Elevate mesh kit wing (American Medical Systems, Inc.; Minnetonka, MN) is then passed through the mesh. (**c**) The portion of mesh protruding from the incision site at the sacral promontory is secured using Protack fasteners. (**d**) Sutures have been used to attach the caudal portion of the mesh to the posterior cervix. (**e**) The peritoneum at the sacral and posterior cervix incision sites is sutured over the mesh. The vaginal vault/uterus is lifted with tightening and subsequent fibrosis of the tissue surrounding the mesh

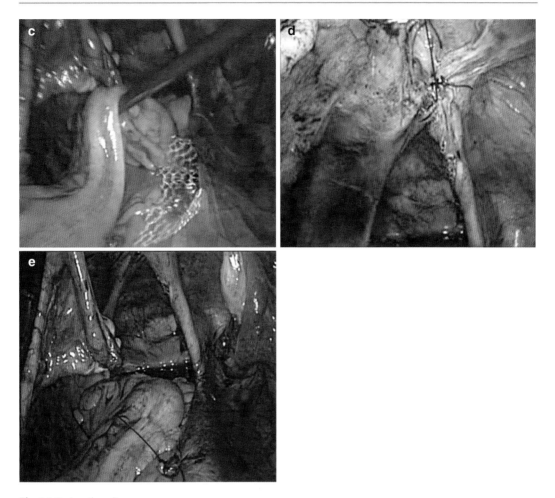

Fig. 14.7 (continued)

14.7.4 Retroperitoneal Mesh Sacrohysteropexy

This approach has been described by Behnia-Willison and colleagues [6] and is briefly covered here. Once the right ureter and vessels as well as the sacral promontory are identified, a small incision in the peritoneum on the top of the sacral promontory is made. Three small incisions into the peritoneum are made at intervals of 5 cm (avoiding complete incision of the peritoneum), and a tunnel is made in the retroperitoneum from the sacrum to the posterior cervix. Elevate mesh kit wings (American Medical Systems, Inc.; Minnetonka, MN) are used to anchor the mesh and feed it bluntly underneath the peritoneal membrane while maintaining patency of the membrane. There are three incisions (5 mm) made in the right pararectal space, and they are used to grasp the rigid portion of the wing and reinsert it again underneath the peritoneum in a linear fashion so that the mesh is fed underneath the peritoneum from the sacral promontory to the posterior cervix. The mesh is then anchored to the cervix and the sacral promontory utilizing Protack and/or V-loc. This particular methodology ensures the patency of the peritoneal membrane and avoids the need to fully dissect the peritoneum via sharp dissection. It is described in Fig. 14.7. The use of a subperitoneal tunneling technique for mesh insertion significantly shortens operation time.

Patients undergo cystoscopy at the end of these procedures to ensure ureteric patency. It is important to note that, following either of the procedures, anterior or posterior transvaginal repair with or without mesh is often undertaken in order to further strengthen the pelvic floor.

Acknowledgments The authors of this chapter would like to thank Dr. Marc Keirse for his valuable comments and Ms. Annie Yu for her illustration of Fig. 14.1.

References

1. Downing KT. Uterine prolapse: from antiquity to today. Obstet Gynecol Int. 2012;2012:1–9.
2. Arthure HG, Savage D. Uterine prolapse and prolapse of the vaginal vault treated by sacral hysteropexy. J Obstet Gynaecol Br Emp. 1957;64:355–60.
3. Azar M, Noohi S, Radfar S, Radfar MH. Sexual function in women after surgery for pelvic organ prolapse. Int Urogynecol J Pelvic Floor Dysfunct. 2008; 19:53–7.
4. Bump RC, Mattiasson A, Bo K, Brubaker LP, DeLancey JO, Klarskov P, et al. The standardization of terminology of female pelvic organ prolapse and pelvic floor dysfunction. Am J Obstet Gynecol. 1996;175:10–7.
5. Barber MD, Cundiff GW, Weidner AC, Coates KW, Bump RC, Addison WA. Accuracy of clinical assessment of paravaginal defects in women with anterior vaginal wall prolapse. Am J Obstet Gynecol. 1999;181:87–90.
6. Behnia-Willison F, Garg A, Keirse MA. Laparoendoscopic single-site surgery approach to mesh sacro-hysteropexy. Case Rep Med. 2013;2013:641675. doi:10.1155/2013/641675. Epub 2013 Feb 25.
7. McCall M. Posterior culdeplasty; surgical correction of enterocele during vaginal hysterectomy; a preliminary report. Obstet Gynecol. 1957;10:595–602.
8. Altman D, Väyrynen T, Engh ME, Axelsen S, Falconer C, Nordic Transvaginal Mesh Group. Anterior colporrhaphy versus transvaginal mesh for pelvic-organ prolapse. N Engl J Med. 2011;364: 1826–36.
9. Leron E, Stanton SL. Sacrohysteropexy with synthetic mesh for the management of uterovaginal prolapse. BJOG. 2001;108:629–33.
10. Busby G, Broome J. Successful pregnancy outcome following laparoscopic sacrohysteropexy for second degree uterine prolapse. Gynecol Surg. 2010;7:271–3.
11. Barranger E, Fritel X, Pigne A. Abdominal sacrohysteropexy in young women with uterovaginal prolapse: long-term follow-up. Am J Obstet Gynecol. 2003;189: 1245–50.

Instrumentation, Platforms, and Basic Principles of Robotics

15

Teresa P. Díaz-Montes, Edward J. Tanner, and Amanda Nickles Fader

Improvements in robotic surgical technology have refined the surgical devices and instrumentation, revolutionizing the approach to gynecologic surgery by overcoming the limitations of conventional laparoscopy. The advantages of robotic surgery over conventional laparoscopy have resulted in a more commonly adopted procedure by which gynecologic surgeons can treat patients. Advantages include three-dimensional optics, increased precision and dexterity, and ergonomic advantages for the surgeon that result in less muscle fatigue. The imitations of robotic surgery include the cost, training requirements, and lack of data supporting its efficacy. To increase the success of a robotic procedure, a variety of factors must be taken into account that include the platform being utilized, the appropriate selection and availability of instrumentation, and patient and procedural considerations. This chapter discusses these factors and the basic principles of robotic surgery.

T.P. Díaz-Montes, MD MPH
The Gynecology Oncology Center,
Mercy Medical Center,
227 St. Paul Place, Sixth Floor,
Baltimore, MD 21207, USA
e-mail: tdiazmo72@gmail.com

E.J. Tanner, MD
Department of Gynecology and Obstetrics,
The Kelly Gynecologic Oncology Service,
Johns Hopkins Hospital, 600 N. Wolfe Street,
Phipps 287, Baltimore, MD 21287, USA
e-mail: etanner4@jhmi.edu

A. Nickles Fader, MD (✉)
Department of Gynecology and Obstetrics,
Johns Hopkins Hospital, ,
600 N. Wolfe Street, Phipps 264,
Baltimore, MD 21287, USA
e-mail: afader1@jhmi.edu

P.F. Escobar, T. Falcone (eds.), *Atlas of Single-Port, Laparoscopic, and Robotic Surgery*,
DOI 10.1007/978-1-4614-6840-0_15, © Springer Science+Business Media New York 2014

15.1 Introduction

In recent years, robotic surgical technology has arguably revolutionized the approach to gynecologic surgery. It was largely developed to overcome the limitations of conventional laparoscopy, which include two-dimensional visualization, incomplete articulation of instruments, and limited ergonomics [1]. Since its approval for use in gynecologic surgery by the United States Food and Drug Administration in 2005, the da Vinci Surgical System platform (Intuitive Surgical, Inc.; Sunnyvale, CA) has been widely adopted by hospitals and gynecologic surgeons [2]. Gradual improvements in the robotic platform have further refined the device and instrumentation, which may result in even more widespread use. There are several purported advantages of robotic surgery over conventional laparoscopy. These include three-dimensional optics, increased precision and dexterity, and ergonomic advantages for the surgeon that result in less muscle fatigue. The limitations of robotic surgery include the cost, training requirements, and lack of Level I data supporting its efficacy and safety [3]. Additionally, the robotic platform is cumbersome to readjust once the robot has been docked and the surgeon is sitting at the console. For this reason, it is important to have a thoughtfully considered set-up for each case that is tailored to the operating room, the patient, and the procedure to be performed. To maximize the chance of a successful robotic procedure, a variety of factors must be considered: the platform being utilized, appropriate selection and availability of instrumentation, and patient and procedural factors. This chapter introduces how these factors influence robotic surgery.

15.2 Basic Set-Up and Instrumentation

The only current manufacturer of robotic surgical platforms for gynecologic surgery in the United States produces the da Vinci Surgical System. The most recent model (da Vinci Si System; Intuitive Surgical, Inc.; Sunnyvale, CA) includes support for high-definition video as well as the capacity to have dual surgeon consoles for training purposes. The platform consists of three major components: the surgeon console, the patient side cart, and the vision cart (Table 15.1, Fig. 15.1). At the surgeon console (Fig. 15.2), the surgeon operates while seated viewing a high definition, three-dimensional image of the pelvis. The surgeon grasps the master controls below the display (Fig. 15.3; this is the figure marked console surgeon and joysticks). The system translates the surgeon's hand and wrist movements into real-time movements of the robotic surgical instruments.

Table 15.1 da Vinci surgical system components

Component	Function
Surgeon console	3-D laparoscopic image projected from patient side cart camera
	Master controls to direct patient side cart instruments
	Foot pedal to adjust camera view
	Foot pedal ("clutch") to switch between first and third robotic arms
	Foot pedals to apply monopolar and bipolar cautery
	Master display to adjust video and audio properties of system
Patient side cart	Motorized cart to position robot
	Robotic camera arm
	Three robotic instrument arms
Vision cart	High-definition monitor of laparoscopic camera
	Image processing software

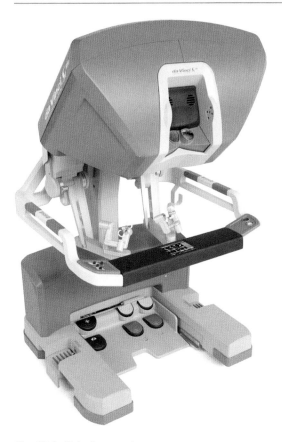

Fig. 15.1 Robotics console

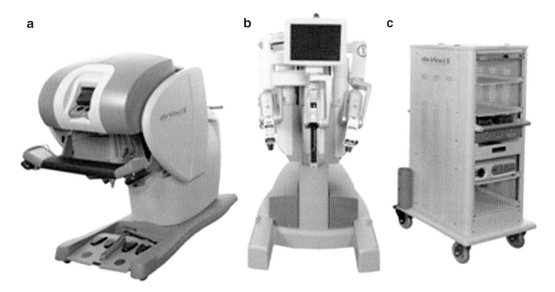

Fig. 15.2 (**a**) Robotic Console (**b**) Robot (**c**) Patient Cart

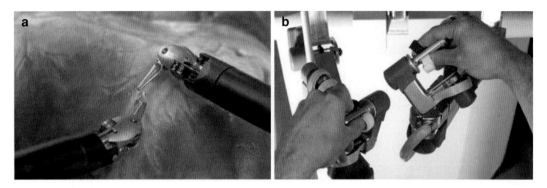

Fig. 15.3 (**a**) Robotic needle drivers (**b**) Robotics console joysticks

The operating room configuration depends on the procedure performed and the layout of the room. The patient side cart is positioned at the bedside during surgery. It includes either three or four robotic arms that respond to the commands of the surgeon at the surgeon console. The robotic arms move around fixed points at the level of the anterior abdominal wall, which may reduce trauma to patient incision sites. For pelvic surgery, at least three operating room configurations have been described: side docking, center docking (between the legs when the patient is in the dorsal lithotomy position), and parallel side docking (Figs. 15.4, 15.5, and 15.6) [4, 5]. If side docking is utilized, the location of monitors, surgical equipment, and the anesthesia staff should be organized to accommodate the patient side cart, which occupies one side of the bed. One possible operating room layout described below easily allows for side docking from the right side of the patient. In this scenario, it is recommended that the bedside surgeon and the accessory port are positioned on the patient's left side. One advantage of side docking versus center docking

is that it maximizes assistant access to the perineum/vagina. This allows for greater facility of uterine manipulation and facilitates vaginal delivery of the uterine specimen.

If center docking is preferred, the location of the equipment is flexible and may be organized so that the scrub nurse stands on the same side as the bedside assistant. An advantage of this set-up is that it allows placement of the fourth robotic arm on either side of the patient. In addition, this approach allows robotic trocars to be placed higher in the abdomen without instrument conflict, as may be required in cases with patients with large uteri, for para-aortic lymph node dissection, or for omentectomy in a gynecologic oncology procedure. To obtain better access to the upper abdomen, especially for oncologic procedures, the robot may also be docked from above the head of the patient. This set-up does not allow access to the pelvis and is frequently performed in conjunction with a docking position allowing pelvic access. This approach requires repositioning of both the patient bed and the bedside cart.

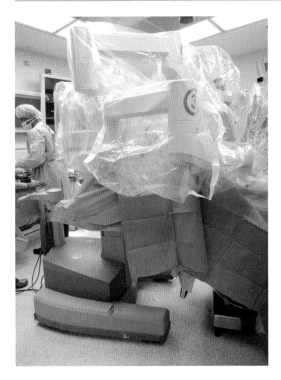

Fig. 15.4 Center docking position of the surgical robot

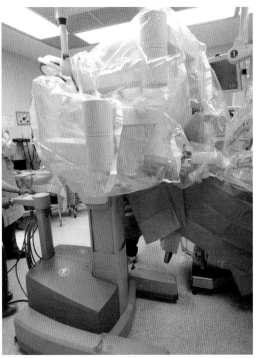

Fig. 15.6 Parallel docking position of the surgical robot

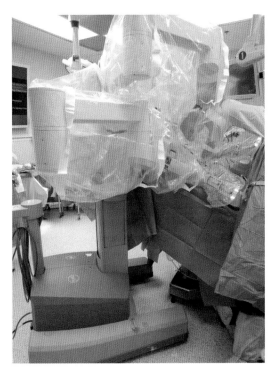

Fig. 15.5 Side docking position of the surgical robot

A variety of EndoWrist instruments (Intuitive Surgical, Inc.; Sunnyvale, CA) are available for robotic gynecologic surgery (Figs. 15.7 and 15.8). The surgeon should limit instrument exchange to improve efficiency and minimize cost. In most cases, the permanent cautery spatula or monopolar curved scissors is utilized in the medial right robotic arm, and fenestrated bipolar forceps or plasma kinetic (PK) dissecting forceps are placed in the left robotic arm. A grasper (ProGrasp forceps; Intuitive Surgical; Sunnyvale, CA, USA) instrument is inserted into the right lateral robotic arm whenever a fourth arm is used. When suturing is required, the medial robotic right instrument is switched for a Mega Suture Cut needle driver (Intuitive Surgical). The left robotic arm is switched to a Mega needle driver (Intuitive Surgical).

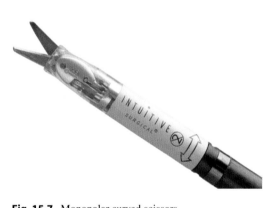

Fig. 15.7 Monopolar curved scissors

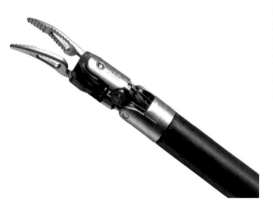

Fig. 15.8 Maryland bipolar forceps

15.3 Patient Selection

The selection of patients for robotic surgery is similar to the selection of patients for laparoscopic surgery. Most contraindications to robotic surgery are relative and depend on the skill set and experience of the surgeon (Table 15.2) [4]. Patients with decreased pulmonary reserve or poor cardiac function are at increased risk for complications. Patients with decreased pulmonary reserve may not tolerate prolonged ventilation or steep Trendelenburg positions that are required for pelvic robotic surgery. Patients with poor cardiac function may not tolerate prolonged pneumoperitoneum, as this may result in hypotension that may further compromise cardiac function.

The steep Trendelenburg position (30–40°) used during robotic gynecologic surgery plays a role in the tolerance of the procedure. A variety of medical comorbidities may limit patient tolerance of this position, and its judicious use is warranted. Patients are placed in a maximal Trendelenburg position to avoid undocking the robotic arms once the procedure has begun. In some cases, the degree of Trendelenburg positioning required to perform a complex gynecologic robotic-assisted procedure is more than the maximum amount possible on many beds. Surgeons should assess the positioning required at the beginning of the surgery rather than reflexively placing a patient in the maximum amount of Trendelenburg position tolerated. This may allow more patients to tolerate an extended period in this position. Insufflation pressures may also be decreased from the standard 15 mmHg to 10–12 mmHg after initial abdominal entry, as this may also allow more patients to tolerate robotic surgery.

Table 15.2 Relative contraindications to robotic surgery

Possible contraindications to robotic surgery
Contraindications related to patient inability to tolerate Trendelenburg positioning
Arteriovenous malformations (elevated intracranial pressures)
Closed-angle glaucoma (elevated intracranial pressure)
Severe cardiopulmonary disease
Contraindications related to inability to tolerate abdominal insufflation
Severe cardiopulmonary disease
Contraindications related to possible inferior clinical outcomes
Large solid abdominal mass (>15 cm in diameter) precluding laparoscopic removal with morcellation
Suspected metastatic cancer

15.4 Patient Positioning

Patient positioning during gynecologic surgery is an essential step to allow optimal surgical exposure and to prevent neuromuscular injuries. In addition to exposure, correct positioning will maximize range of motion of the robotic arms. The steep Trendelenburg position routinely used during robotic gynecologic surgery may cause the patient to slide in a cephalad direction (owing to gravity) and may result in serious injury. Patient slippage during the fixed portion of the peocedure places lateral tension on the laparoscopic incisions and can cause incisional tears, postoperative hernia formation, and increase postoperative pain owing to overstretching of the abdominal wall. The risk of these occurrences is potentially higher than in conventional laparoscopy because the primary surgeon is not operating at the bedside. Bedside assistants and anesthesia staff should monitor for changes in patient position throughout the procedure to ensure that no slipping has occurred.

To avoid patient slippage during the steep Trendelenburg position, a 3 by 5 foot surgical sheet is placed horizontally in the middle of the surgical table, corresponding to the position of the patient's arms and is later used to tuck the arms. A layer of egg crate foam is placed on top of the sheet and secured to the bed with tape. Upon arrival at the operating room, the patient's occiput should be padded with a gel donut to avoid ischemic necrosis. After the patient is in the supine position and anesthetized under general anesthesia, both arms should be gently tucked in the military position at the patient's side with generous corporeal padding. The legs of the patient should be placed in a dorsal lithotomy position in Allen stirrups (Allen Medical Systems; Acton, MA). Once positioning is complete, a Trendelenburg test may be performed in morbidly obese patients to ensure that they do not slide in a cephalad direction on the bed and are adequately ventilated in this position. Application of Velcro and a thin strip of egg crate foam as a band or cruciate pattern across the chest may also be considered to stabilize the patient and prevent slippage in cases in which the egg crate does not provide adequate support. Attention to patient ventilation should be emphasized if taping is required because the chest wall may become constricted.

Other alternatives to the egg crate include the use of surgical gel pads against the patient's bare skin or the Bean Bag Positioner (AliMed Inc.; Debham, MA). Both devices require disinfection after each case, and allergic reactions are possible. The Bean Bag Positioner is usually fastened to the surgical table and conforms to the shoulders and upper body of the patient. Potential drawbacks of this device include longer set-up time and the possibility of unrecognized deflation of the bean bag during the procedure, causing the patient to slide. The use of shoulder straps, braces, restraints, body straps, or head rests should be discouraged because of the potential risk of brachial plexus injuries.

The arms are tucked using sheets, or in morbidly obese patients with larger arms, sleds may be used. The arms should always be well padded. Overextension, flexion, or abduction of any extremity should be avoided. Adequate padding at all pressure points should be provided. Even though the face of the patient is outside the surgical field, it should be appropriately padded. The robotic camera system can come in close contact with the face and cause facial or ocular trauma. Instruments should not be placed on the face during the procedure.

15.5 Hysterectomy with or Without Salpingo-Oophorectomy

Hysterectomy is the most commonly performed major gynecologic surgical procedure in the United States (Fig. 15.9) [5]. Removal of tubes and ovaries may or may not be included as part of the surgery and should be individualized according to patient needs. The surgical principles and technique of robotic surgery are the same as those for open surgery. The main difference is equipment set-up (Table 15.3), instrumentation, and port placement. The operating room could be configured for side docking or docking between the legs, depending on the surgeon's preference and whether additional procedures are performed. For robotic hysterectomy, location of ports could vary, depending on the indication of the procedure. For benign cases, a 12-mm port is placed either at or above the umbilicus, depending on uterus size. The camera port should be placed at least 8–10 cm above the top of the elevated uterus to allow for adequate visualization and manipulation of the pelvis. In most cases, three robotic trocars are required to complete a hysterectomy. One 8-mm robotic trocar should be placed 2 cm superior to the anterosuperior iliac spine with care to avoid injuring the cecum during insertion. An additional 8-mm robotic trocar should be placed at least 10 cm lateral to the camera port and at least 10 cm away from the lateral trocar. In smaller patients, the robotic trocar may be placed 2 cm to the left of the midline to allow additional space for the two robotic trocars on the right side. One 8-mm robotic trocar should be placed 12 cm to the left of the camera trocar at a 15° downward angle toward the pelvis. An accessory trocar can then be placed in the left upper quadrant equidistant from the camera port and the left robotic trocar. This port is typically 10–12 mm in size to allow introduction of sutures as well as instruments used for retraction, irrigation, suction, or specimen retrieval. Based on surgeon preference, a variety of uterine manipulators can then be placed in order to facilitate the procedure.

Table 15.3 Instrument positioning by gynecologic procedure

Hysterectomy with/without bilateral salpingo-oophorectomy

    Arm 1 (right): Monopolar curved scissors or permanent cautery spatula

    Arm 2 (left): Fenestrated bipolar forceps or plasma kinetic dissecting forceps

    Arm 3 (right): Grasper forceps

    15-mm Accessory port in left abdomen: suction and irrigator

Suturing of vaginal cuff

    Arm 1 (right): Mega Suture Cut needle driver

    Arm 2 (left): Large needle driver

    Arm 3 (right): Grasper forceps

Myomectomy

    Arm 1 (right): Monopolar curved scissors

    Arm 2 (left): Fenestrated bipolar forceps

    Arm 3 (right): Grasper forceps

    15-mm incision: Morcellator

Suturing of myomectomy defect

    Arm 1 (right): Mega Suture Cut needle driver

    Arm 2 (left): Mega needle driver

    Arm 3 (right): Grasper forceps

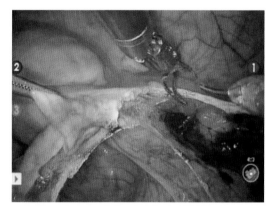

Fig. 15.9 Dissection of the anterior leaf of the broad ligament and vesicouterine peritoneum during a robotic-assisted hysterectomy procedure

15.6   Lymphadenectomy

To perform a lymphadenectomy as part of the gynecologic procedure, the operating room could be configured using any of the previously described docking approaches. For pelvic lymphadenectomy, side docking is preferred. For high para-aortic lymphadenectomy, docking between the legs or above the head of the patient may be considered (see Figs. 15.4, 15.5, and 15.6). Incisions should be placed higher in the abdomen. For example, the camera trocar should be placed approximately 25 cm above the pubic symphysis. The instrument trocars should similarly be placed higher in the abdomen to allow for improved access to the abdomen above the pelvic brim. For most cases, the monopolar curved scissors are placed in the medial right robotic arm, and fenestrated bipolar forceps or PK dissecting forceps are placed in the left robotic arm. A grasper instrument is placed in the robotic fourth arm.

15.7   Ovarian Cystectomy or Salpingo-Oophorectomy

Ovarian cystectomy or salpingo-oophorectomy should be performed laparoscopically in most cases, as these cases are often straightforward and will cost less to perform with conventional laparoscopy compared with robotic surgery [3]. However, indications for robotics-assistance may include anticipated case complexity, endometriosis, or an ovarian mass. Trocar placement is similar to that described for robotic hysterectomy. The trocar placement may vary, depending on the size of the ovarian cyst. Side docking or center docking may be utilized. For ovarian cystectomy, the following instruments are used: monopolar curved scissors in the medial right robotic arm, fenestrated bipolar forceps or Maryland bipolar forceps in the left robotic arm, and grasper forceps in the lateral right robotic arm. A suction and irrigation device can be used in the accessory port. For salpingo-oophorectomy, the following instruments are used: monopolar curved scissors in the medial right robotic arm, and fenestrated bipolar forceps or PK dissecting forceps in the left robotic arm. If a fourth robotic arm is required, grasper forceps can be used. A suction and irrigation device can be used in the accessory port.

15.8   Myomectomy

Robotic-assisted myomectomy should be organized to allow for the use of a laparoscopic morcellating instrument in the accessory port and at
least two robotic arms to facilitate laparoscopic
suturing. For large myomas extending outside the
pelvis, robotic trocars should be placed high
enough along the abdominal wall to allow for full
range of motion during excision and optimization
of the critical view of the uterus and pelvis.
During excision, monopolar curved scissors are
used in the right robotic arm and fenestrated
bipolar forceps in the left robotic arm. A grasper
or a robotic tenaculum may be used in the robotic
fourth arm if needed. If morcellation is required,
the morcellator device can be introduced through
one of the accessory trocar incisions after removing the respective trocar. During suturing, the
right robotic instrument should be switched to a
Mega Suture Cut needle driver and the left robotic
arm switched to a Mega needle driver. The use of
barbed suture may facilitate efficient closure of
the myomectomy defect (Fig. 15.10) [3].

15.9   Future Directions

Laparoendoscopic single-site surgery (LESS)
represents one of the latest innovations in minimally invasive surgery and has several potential
applications in gynecologic oncology surgery
[6, 7]. It is an evolving surgical approach aimed
at further minimizing the invasive nature of surgery. Rather than using multiple incisions, as in
traditional or robotic-assisted laparoscopy, procedures are performed through a single, small
incision positioned at the base of the umbilicus
(Fig. 15.11). Experience using LESS for both
benign and malignant gynecologic conditions is
rapidly expanding. Recently, the United States
Food and Drug Administration approved the
robotic single-site platform for cholecystectomy and benign hysterectomy. By operating
with pseudoarticulated instrumentation through
a single incision and a multiport device in the
umbilicus, the platform is compatible with the da
Vinci Si robotic system. We await further study
to determine the safety, feasibility, and indications for this surgical platform.

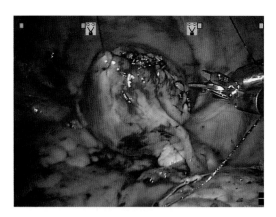

Fig. 15.10 Suturing a uterine defect during a robotic-
assisted myomectomy procedure

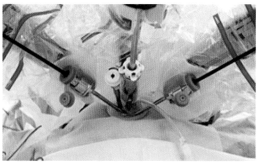

Fig. 15.11 Set up and docking of the robotic single-site
platform

References

1. Satava RM. Robotic surgery from past to future. Surg Clin North Am. 2003;83:1491–500.
2. Kho RM, Hilger RS, Hentz JG. Robotic hysterectomy: techniques and initial outcomes. Am J Obstet Gynecol. 1997;2007:113.e1–4.
3. Herron DM, Marohn M, SAGES-MIRA Robotic Surgery Consensus Group. A consensus document on robotic surgery. Surg Endosc. 2008; 22:313.
4. Advincula A, Falcone T. Laparoscopic gynecologic robotic surgery. Obstet Gynecol Clin North Am. 2004;31:599–601.
5. Gala RB, Margulies R, Steinberg A, Murphy M, Lukban J, Jeppson P, et al. Systematic review of robotic surgery in gynecology: robotic techniques compared with laparoscopy and laparotomy; Society of gynecologic surgeons systematic review group. J Minim Invasive Gynecol. 2013. pii: S1553–4650(13)01377–0.
6. Fader AN, Rojas-Espaillat L, Ibeanu O, Grumbine FC, Escobar PF. Laparoendoscopic single-site surgery in gynecology: a multi-institutional evaluation. Am J Obstet Gynecol. 2010;203:501.e1–6.
7. Escobar PF, Fader AN, Pariaso M, Kaouk JH, Falcone T. Robotic-assisted laparoendoscopic single-site surgery in gynecology: Initial report and technique. J Minim Invasive Gynecol. 2009;16:589–91.

Robotic-Assisted Laparoscopic Myomectomy

16

Michael C. Pitter

Approximately 600,000 hysterectomies are per-formed each year in the United States. Uterine fibroids are the leading indication for this proce-dure. Some patients choose a more conservative approach. Approximately 81 % of patients who undergo myomectomy have a resolution of their symptoms, but the risk of regrowth of myomas and possible reoperation must be discussed with the patient. Of the almost 40,000 myomectomies performed each year in the United States, only a small fraction are performed in a minimally inva-sive fashion. The new robotic platform, the da Vinci surgical system (Intuitive Surgical, Inc.; Sunnyvale, CA), was approved by the U.S. Food and Drug Administration in April 2005, allowing the surgeon the advantage of a three-dimensional view of the operative field and the ability to use wristed instruments with 7 degrees of motion, thereby providing a new viable option for patients. This chapter reviews the robotic-assisted laparoscopic myomectomy while providing the most current data.

16.1 Introduction

Uterine fibroids (Fig. 16.1) represent the leading indication for hysterectomy in the United States and are the most common benign tumors in women [1, 2]. This condition affects up to 30 % of women between the ages of 30 and 60 years, and 70 % of white women and 80 % of African American women have this diagnosis by age 50. The symptoms vary and are present in 20–50 % of cases [3]. These include menorrhagia (29–59 %) and pelvic pain and pressure (34 %), but most women are asymptomatic (50 %). The vast majority of women with uterine fibroids are treated by definitive surgical therapy such as hys-terectomy. In fact approximately 600,000 hyster-ectomy procedures are performed annually in the United States, making it the most common surgi-cal procedure second only to cesarean section.

A certain subset of patients, however, choose a more conservative approach to the treatment of uterine fibroids whether or not fertility-sparing concerns are an issue. Approximately 81 % of patients who undergo myomectomy have reso-lution of their symptoms [4], but they must be counseled on the risks of regrowth of myomas and the possibility of reoperation, whether it's another myomectomy or a hysterectomy. For a single myoma, 27 % of patients will experience regrowth, with 11 % requiring hysterectomy. For multiple myomas, the regrowth rate is 59 % or more, with 26 % needing repeat myomecto-mies [5–7]. Approximately 40,000 myomec-tomy procedures are performed each year in the

M.C. Pitter, MD, FACOG
Division of Minimally Invasive
and Gynecologic Robotic Surgery,
Department of Obstetrics and Gynecology,
Newark Beth Israel Medical Center,
201 Lyons Avenue, Suite L-2,
Newark, NJ 07112, USA
e-mail: mail@drpitter.net

P.F. Escobar, T. Falcone (eds.), *Atlas of Single-Port, Laparoscopic, and Robotic Surgery*,
DOI 10.1007/978-1-4614-6840-0_16, © Springer Science+Business Media New York 2014

197

United States, and of those only a small fraction are performed in a minimally invasive fashion. Laparoscopic myomectomy was first described at the end of the 1970s, exclusively for subserous myomas [8]. At that time it was thought that for intramural myomas, the technique of traditional laparoscopic myomectomy was challenging and technically difficult, resulting in longer operative times and increased blood loss and risk of conversion to laparotomy.

The da Vinci surgical system was approved by the U.S. Food and Drug Administration in April 2005 as a direct result of work done by Advincula and coworkers [9], who examined the performance of robotic-assisted laparoscopic myomectomy. This computer-enhanced system of telemanipulation provided some distinct advantages over traditional laparoscopic myomectomy in that the surgeon had a three-dimensional view of the operative field in addition to the ability to use wristed instruments with 7° of motion more than the capability of the human hand. Not only were the instruments wristed but their movements were intuitive, which was not typical of regular laparoscopic devices. In that pivotal study it was demonstrated that for a suture-intensive operation such as a laparoscopic myomectomy,

this new robotic platform might provide some advantages. Since the initial study in 2004, a number of articles have been published investigating various aspects of robotic myomectomy, including on pregnancy outcomes following robotic myomectomy [10]. This chapter contains a step-by-step tutorial on robotic-assisted laparoscopic myomectomy and presents the most current data on this topic.

16.2 Indication

The indication for robotic myomectomy is to transform abdominal myomectomy into a laparoscopic myomectomy. This may be accomplished by using wristed instruments and a three-dimensional view of the operative field to improve on the benefits afforded by the laparoscopic approach but applied to more complex pathologic conditions such as deeply infiltrating intramural myomas, type 1 and type 2 submucosal myomas larger than 5 cm in diameter, broad ligament myomas, and large parasitic myomas. In other words, the principal goal is to perform open surgery through laparoscopy [10]. If a patient is a candidate for laparoscopic surgery, then she is a candidate for robotic surgery.

16.3   Preoperative Evaluation

In addition to obtaining a thorough history of the patient's symptoms, a physical examination, and perhaps a pelvic ultrasound, and the use of magnetic resonance imaging (MRI) can be invaluable tools in determining who is an appropriate candidate for robotic myomectomy. Given the fact that one of the limitations of the robotic platform is the lack of haptics, it is imperative to use whatever tool is available to provide a road map of the locations of all myomas present in the uterus before the surgery. Not only will the study yield information about the number of myomas but it can also detect adenomyosis. Knowing that a patient has diffuse adenomyosis or a large adenomyoma may alter the decision to exercise a conservative surgical approach. The surgeon may even choose to defer surgery, especially if the desired outcome from a myomectomy is pregnancy, given the potential damage to the myometrium and endomyometrial junctional zone that can occur. The MRI images may even be projected into the surgeon's console during the operation using a feature known as TilePro (Intuitive Surgical Inc.; Sunnyvale, CA), making it easier for him or her to view the location of the myomas with selected T2-weighted images without leaving the robotic master controller environment (Fig. 16.1).

Some studies have also shown that preoperative MRIs as well as serum lactate dehydrogenase (LDH) determinations can be useful in helping to screen for rare variants such as leiomyosarcomas [11]. When central necrosis in a myoma is seen on MRI and total LDH is elevated along with an elevation in LDH isoenzyme 3, there is a high positive predictive value that the patient may have a leiomyosarcoma [11]. Clearly there is no test that will absolutely predict the presence or absence of uterine cancer. A tissue diagnosis in the end is the only definitive tool, but having some foresight about a possible problem will help the surgeon in the decision-making process regarding whether the specimen should be morcelated or removed whole. Preoperative use of gonadotropin-releasing hormone analogues should be discouraged because it may alter the cleavage plane between the myoma and the normal myometrium. It can also cause some degeneration of the myomas. This, in turn, may make it more challenging to enucleate the myomas without leaving several fragments behind. In addition, an endometrial biopsy should be performed when clinically indicated.

A risk of any surgical procedure, including myomectomy, is hemorrhage. An analysis of the hematocrit reading is essential in planning for the potential for improving the patient's status by preoperative iron infusion therapy or transfusions, whether with directed donor blood or from the hospital's supply. Although a review of the literature on robotic-assisted laparoscopic myomectomy shows that when compared to open myomectomy there is less intraoperative blood loss, the size and number of the myomas, the collateral blood supply as seen with parasitic myomas, and the operator's experience must be taken into consideration and are critical for success.

It is difficult to determine an appropriate limit in terms of the number of myomas, the size of the myomas, and the size of the uterus that can be safely treated with robotic myomectomy. Barakat and colleagues [12], in a study comparing robotic, laparoscopic, and open abdominal myomectomy, documented almost equivalent tumor burdens in their experience with robotic myomectomy as compared with the traditional abdominal procedures. What is important is determining by MRI that there is a clear cleavage plane between the myomas and that the patient does not have "miliary disease." Miliary disease refers to the condition in which there are several myomas per square centimeter and very little intervening cleavage plane. That means that a patient with a 20-weeks size uterus (Fig. 16.2) with one to five large myomas is a good candidate for robotic myomectomy, whereas a patient with a 12-weeks size uterus with 25 myomas would not be a good candidate.

Fig. 16.1 MRI images in TilePro (*bottom*) and operative field (*top*)

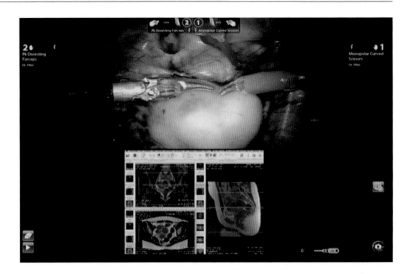

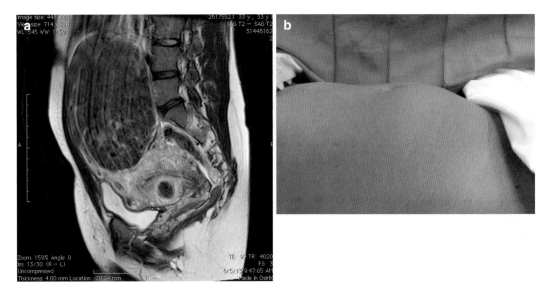

Fig. 16.2 (**a**) A 20–22-week size uterus with large fundal myoma on sagittal view MRI. (**b**) View of abdomen in same patient before surgery

16.4   Technique

16.4.1   Preparing the Operative Field

Robotic surgery starts like any other laparoscopic procedure, with the placement of a uterine manipulator and laparoscopic ports. The location of the trocar incisions depends on the size and number of the myomas and the number of robotic instruments used to carry out the procedure. The number of ports can vary. One can use five ports if all robotic instruments are used,

including the third instrument arm and an assist port; four if only two robotic instruments are used with one accessory port; and three (without an assist port) and even two ports if reduced port robotic myomectomy techniques are employed (Fig. 16.3a–d). Operator experience and the size of the pathologic tumor being addressed basically determine which modality is leveraged. In addition, the patient's concerns regarding cosmesis may influence the decision in terms of how many ports are placed and if the camera port or the largest port is placed in the umbilicus.

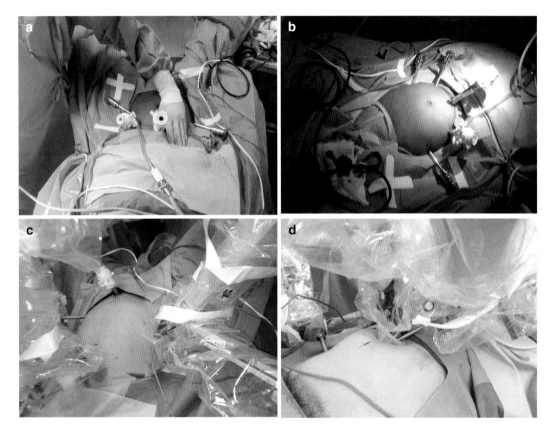

Fig. 16.3 (**a**) Multiport robotic surgery—instrument ports spaced one hands-breadth apart. (**b**) Multiport robotic surgery—two instruments on the right side. (**c**) Reduced port robotic surgery with supra pubic assistant trocar. (**d**) Single umbilical incision plus 5 mm robotic instrument right lower quadrant. (**e**) Supra pubic assistant trocar

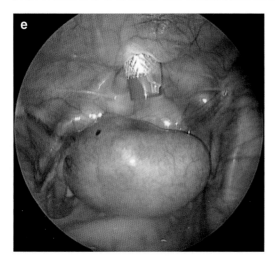

Fig. 16.3 (continued)

16.4.2 Step-by-Step

Prior to starting the procedure, attention must be paid to ensuring some modicum of hemostasis during the operation for a uterus that is still well vascularized. A number of techniques have been described that preemptively reduce pulse pressure to the area surrounding the myoma or myomas to be removed. These include (1) constricting the blood flow from the uterine arteries via a tourniquet by opening up the leaves of the broad ligament bilaterally and applying either sutures placed endoscopically or a Penrose drain. (2) Another technique involves the injection of a dilute solution of vasopressin into the area surrounding the intended hysterotomy incision, allowing the effects of the fluid to both create a plane for the enucleation of the fibroid and effecting vasoconstriction of the vessels supplying the myoma(s). In some countries (outside of the U.S.), however, the use of vasopressin is not allowed because of reports of serious and potentially fatal side effects of the drug. Therefore it is important to avoid direct intravascular injection of the mixture.

This can be accomplished by (1) introducing a catheter with a needle through one of the trocars and directing the medication to the intended area, or (2) a method preferred by the author that involves direct transcutaneous transabdominal instillation of the drug using a 22-gauge, 5-in (or 7-in) spinal needle and robotic instruments to guide the process (Fig. 16.4). The surgeon or assistant should first aspirate; then once it is evident that the intravascular space is not breached, the vasopressin may be injected in small aliquots. A typical mixture would be 20 U of vasopressin placed in 60 mL of normal saline. No more than 60 mL of the solution should be administered. If more is required, an interval exceeding the half-life of the drug should be used as a guide in terms of timing.

There are four basic steps to accomplishing a robotic myomectomy:
1. Hysterotomy incision(s)
2. Enucleation of the myoma(s)
3. Repair of the defect(s)
4. Extraction of the myoma(s).

After securing a method of prophylactic hemostasis, the hysterotomy incision may be created. The decision of creating a transverse versus a vertical versus an elliptical incision depends on the location and type of the fibroid. For broad-based exophytic myomas it may be preferable to perform an elliptical incision at a level from the base to allow for room for adequate myometrium for the repair of the defect. Transverse hysterotomy incisions (Fig. 16.5), especially on anterior myomas, may be preferable given the historical data on the strength of the closure from the experience from low transverse cesarean sections and the potential for uterine rupture rates versus vertical hysterotomy incisions during subsequent pregnancies. It must be noted, however, that there is an association between anterior hysterotomy incisions, large myomas, and the incidence of preterm labor for patients who become pregnant following robotic myomectomy [10].

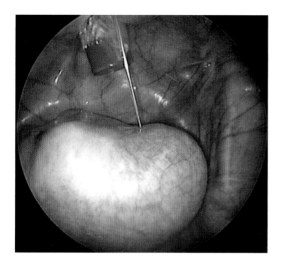

Fig. 16.4 Injecting vasopressin prior to hysterotomy incision

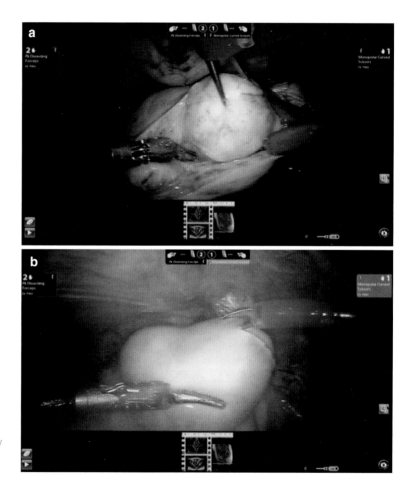

Fig. 16.5 (**a**) Enucleation using mechanical forces. (**b**) A transverse hysterotomy incision with "pure cut" energy setting

16.4.2.1 Hysterotomy Incision

The instrument of choice for the hysterotomy incision is usually monopolar curved shears. Other monopolar robotic instruments may be used, but whatever tool is chosen should be used efficiently, leveraging the principles of electrosurgery such as power density. This means that the energy delivered by the tip of the instrument is inversely proportional to its diameter, and a relatively low power setting in terms of wattage can be used to effectively cut through the serosa with the least amount of lateral thermal spread. Obviously the use of a CO_2 laser and/or a harmonic scalpel can result in less lateral thermal spread, but the difference may not be clinically significant. In addition the harmonic scalpel is not a wristed instrument and poses some challenges when used with other robotic instruments. The recommended energy settings are dependent on the generator's being used and the available data from the manufacturer.

Once the hysterotomy incision is created, it must be made at a uniform depth to the level of the pseudocapsule of the myoma and not protrude into the myoma itself. This may be accomplished by using a curved dissecting bipolar device such as the PK Dissector (Intuitive Surgical, Inc.; Sunnyvale, CA). The fenestrated bipolar device does not lend itself to fine dissection for robotic myomectomy. A list of recommended instruments is shown in Table 16.1.

Table 16.1 List of instruments used for robotic myomectomy

1. Uterine manipulator (e.g., HUMI Harris-Kronner Uterine Manipulator Injector; Cooper Surgical Inc., Trumbull, CT)

2. Bipolar device (e.g., PK Dissector [Intuitive Surgical, Inc., Sunnyvale, CA]; Gyrus ACMI (Olympus; Southborough, MA).

3. Hot shears (e.g., Monopolar Curved Shears (Intuitive Surgical; Sunnyvale, CA).

4. Robotic tenaculum (Intuitive Surgical; Sunnyvale, CA)

5. Needle drivers (e.g., Mega Suture Cut, Intuitive Surgical; Trumbull, CT)

6. ProGrasp forceps (Intuitive Surgical; Sunnyvale, CA)

7. Optional (Harmonic scalpel, Omni Guide CO2 laser [OmniGuide, Inc.; Cambridge, MA])

16.4.2.2 Enucleation

After making an adequate hysterotomy incision, the enucleation should be performed making use of mechanical forces in a push-spread fashion and minimizing the use of thermal energy. The analogy often used to describe this action is pushing the uterus away from the uterine fibroid rather than trying to extract the fibroid with the robotic tenaculum. Excessive thermal injury has been implicated in uterine rupture in pregnancy when either laparoscopic or robotic myomectomy procedures were performed [10]. Caution must be used to avoid entry into the endometrial cavity, and this can be achieved by relying on the information provided by the preoperative MRI.

16.4.2.3 Repair of the Hysterotomy Incision

Once the myoma is removed, it can be secured with the use of sutures to track the uterine fibroids and prevent loss of a myoma placed under the folds of the small and large intestines with the patient in the Trendelenburg position. This is known as the "string of pearls" technique (Fig. 16.6). The hysterotomy incisions may be closed in layers, depending on the depth, as soon as the enucleation process is complete. This minimizes intraoperative blood loss. If bleeding is fairly well controlled and the procedure is progressing very quickly, several myomas may be removed before the decision is made to close the incisions.

With the advent of barbed sutures, the closure of the hysterotomy incision may be accomplished much faster than with traditional sutures. Delayed absorbable polydioxanone type sutures are now available for that purpose. The layered closure is preferable because it more closely mimics the same closure that would be performed if the patient had an open abdominal myomectomy. After the hysterotomy closure is complete, the use of an adhesion barrier is recommended although no one method has been shown to be superior over another (Figs. 16.7 and 16.8).

Fig. 16.6 (**a**) String of fibroids (pearls) on a barbed suture. (**b**) Starting the string of pearls technique by placing a suture through the fibroids. (**c**) Securing the string pelvic wall, tethering the needle out of the way in the peritoneum

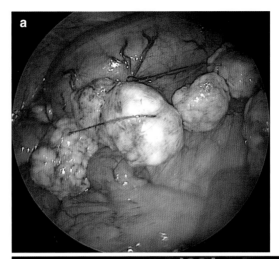

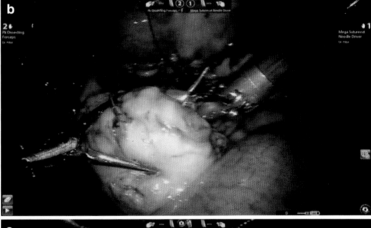

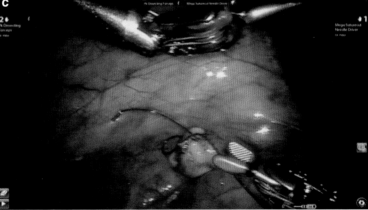

Fig. 16.7 Repair of
hysterotomy incision

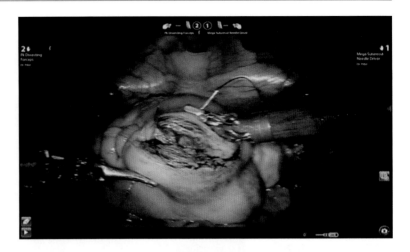

Fig. 16.8 Repair of
hysterotomy incision

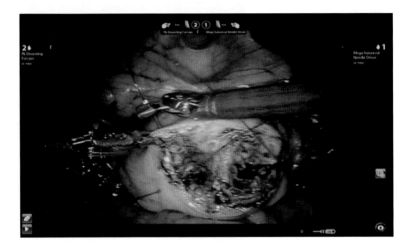

16.4.2.4 Extraction

The final phase of the myomectomy procedure is the extraction. This is typically accomplished via a mechanical morcellator. It is recommended that at least a 15-mm or, for better efficiency, a 20-mm diameter morcellating blade be used for efficient tissue extraction. A 5-mm endoscope placed more than 10 cm away should be used to visualize the entire process in order to minimize the potential for bowel and vascular injury. Each myoma that is removed at the time of the hysterotomy incision should be accounted for during the extraction process in a manner similar to the way instruments or needles are counted. The morcellation should also be done in the upper quadrants at the umbilical incision or close by because of the lower port placement of the morcellator, putting the patient at risk for bowel and vascular injury (Figs. 16.9 and 16.10).

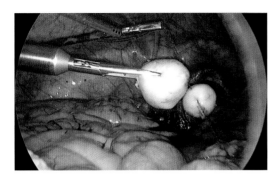

Fig. 16.9 Morcellating each fibroid one at a time from the string of pearls

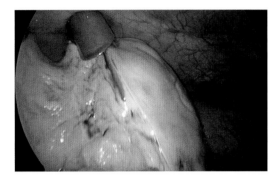

Fig. 16.10 Morcellation of large myomas under direct vision

16.5   Complex Robotic Myomectomy Techniques

Intraligamentary, cervical, and parasitic myomas present unique challenges for all approaches to myomectomy. Robotic myomectomy is no exception. Knowledge of pelvic anatomy, especially in the retroperitoneal spaces, is a prerequisite for safe removal of such tumors. The key to safe resection of intraligamentary or broad ligament myomas is identifying the course of the ureter and realizing that in the majority of cases the main blood supply to the fibroids arises from the uterine arteries or its branches, Therefore, whenever possible, the dissection should occur from lateral to medial, and caution should be used to properly outline the course of the ureter from the pelvic brim to the ureteric tunnel if necessary. Distending the bladder with water can also be helpful.

Parasitic myomas also present some unique challenges. In some cases recognition of the extra-uterine blood supply is relatively easy since it arises from the omentum. In other cases, these vessels arise from vessels in the retroperitoneal spaces. This requires more radical dissection and should only be undertaken by surgeons skilled in and knowledgeable about such techniques. Some hybrid techniques have been described in which the enucleation of the myomas is performed laparoscopically but the repair of the hysterotomy incision is done with computer-assisted laparoscopy. This technique bridges both modalities of traditional laparoscopic and robotic myomectomy, taking advantage of the haptic feedback obtained from one and the wristed suturing advantage from the other. When compared with standard laparoscopic myomectomy, the intraoperative blood loss only achieved marginal significance [13].

16.6 Summary

Robotic-assisted laparoscopic myomectomy appears to be a viable option for surgeons who are appropriately trained in such procedures. The technique has subtle differences from traditional laparoscopic myomectomy and many similarities to open surgery. Knowledge of pelvic anatomy is important for safe removal of intraligamentary myomas.

Finally, emerging technological advances such as single incision robotics may provide even more options in select uncomplicated cases in which patients may have their procedures performed with very few visible signs of surgical scars (Figs. 16.11, 16.12, 16.13, and 16.14). In this case a 2.5-cm umbilical incision and possibly a 5-mm right lower quadrant incision are all that is required. As technology improves, a single umbilical incision may become the norm. Additional data are forthcoming regarding pregnancy rates from much larger cohorts of patients than previously described.

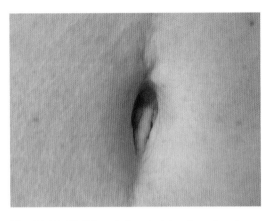

Fig. 16.11 Umbilicus before incision for reduced port robotics

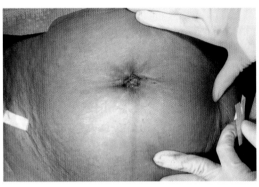

Fig. 16.13 Umbilicus after single umbilical port is removed, 5 mm right lower quadrant port added

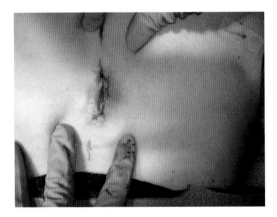

Fig. 16.12 Umbilicus after single umbilical port is removed

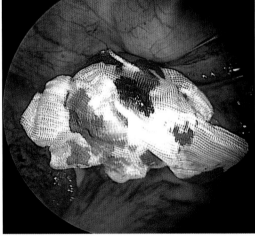

Fig. 16.14 Intercede after myomectomy, placing an adhesion barrier after myomectomy

References

1. Farquhar CM, Steiner CA. Hysterectomy rates in the United States 1990–1997. Obstet Gynecol. 2002; 99:229–34.
2. Merrill RM. Hysterectomy surveillance in the United States, 1997 through 2005. Med Sci Monit. 2008; 14:CR24–31.
3. Baird DD, Dunson DB, Hill MC, Cousins D, Schectman JM. High cumulative incidence of uterine leiomyoma in black and white women: ultrasound evidence. Am J Obstet Gynecol. 2003;188:100–7.
4. Buttram Jr VC, Reiter RC. Uterine leiomyomata: etiology, symptomatology, and management. Fertil Steril. 1981;36:433–45.
5. Wallach EE, Vlahos NF. Uterine myomas: an overview of development, clinical features, and management. Obstet Gynecol. 2004;104:393–406.
6. Candiani GB, Fedele L, Parazzini F, Villa L. Risk of recurrence after myomectomy. Br J Obstet Gynaecol. 1991;98:385–9.
7. The American Congress of Obstetricians and Gynecologists. ACOG practice bulletin. Alternatives to Hysterectomy in the Management of Leiomyomas. Obstet Gynecol. 2008;112:387–400.
8. Semm K, Mettler L. Technical progress in pelvic surgery via operative laparoscopy. Am J Obstet Gynecol. 1980;138:121–5.
9. Advincula AP, Song A, Burke W, Reynolds RK. Preliminary experience with robot-assisted laparoscopic myomectomy. J Am Assoc Gynecol Laparosc. 2004;11:511–8.
10. Pitter MC, Gargiulo AR, Bonaventura LM, Lehman JS, Srouji SS. Pregnancy outcomes following robot-assisted myomectomy. Hum Reprod. 2013;28:99–108.
11. Goto A, Takeuchi S, Sugimura K, Maruo T. Usefulness of Gd-DTPA contrast-enhanced dynamic MRI and serum determination of LDH and its isozymes in the differential diagnosis of leiomyosarcoma from degenerated leiomyoma of the uterus. Int J Gynecol Cancer. 2002;12:354–61.
12. Barakat EE, Bedaiwy MA, Zimberg S, Nutter B, Nosseir M, Falcone T. Robotic-assisted, laparoscopic, and abdominal myomectomy: a comparison of surgical outcomes. Obstet Gynecol. 2011;117(2 Pt 1):256–65.
13. Gargiulo AR, Srouji SS, Missmer SA, Correia EF, Velinga T, Einarsson JI. Robot assisted laparoscopic myomectomy compared with standard laparoscopic myomectomy. Obstet Gynecol. 2012;120(2 Pt 1):284–91.

Robotic-Assisted Total Laparoscopic Hysterectomy

17

Mona Orady

Robotic-assisted total laparoscopic hysterectomy has helped advance minimally invasive hysterectomy techniques by extending the candidacy of this procedure, offering patients with more complex pathology the option of having a minimally invasive procedure for their problem. Robotic surgery presents specific challenges and complexities that are unique to this type of surgical procedure. From patient selection to operating room setup and the approach to the procedure, subtle factors can contribute to the efficiency and success of the surgery. This chapter describes the technique of the robotic hysterectomy procedure and outlines details of patient selection criteria, operating room setup, optimization of the operative team, surgical tools, and port placement. The robotic hysterectomy procedure is broken down into segments and tips for approaching difficult hysterectomies, such as those in patients with an extremely enlarged uterus or severe adhesions. Postoperative care is also important in achieving fast recovery and a shorter hospital stay (the main advantage of minimally invasive procedures), so methods of optimizing postoperative care are also addressed.

17.1 Introduction

The da Vinci Surgical System (Intuitive Surgical, Inc.; Sunnyvale, CA) was first used in 1999 for urologic pelvic surgery. Its adoption curve was exponential, quickly reaching the point of majority in prostatectomy procedures. Soon after, in 2001, the first robotic-assisted laparoscopic hysterectomy was performed. After US Food and Drug Administration approval for use in gynecology in 2005, a similar adoption curve in hysterectomy was seen, as many gynecologic surgeons began training all over the United States. Even initial case series reported outcomes and benefits similar to those reported for laparoscopic hysterectomy [1–5]. The benefits of robotic-assisted laparoscopic surgery include three-dimensional magnification, high-definition vision, and wristed instrumentation that offers seven degrees of movement and intuitive direct mimicking of the surgeon's hand, affording the surgeon more control for easier and more precise dissection [6]. Clinical outcomes noted included the benefits of traditional laparoscopy, including minimal pain, small scars, fast recovery, a short hospital stay, and decreased blood loss, without increased complication rates. In fact, some comparative studies showed less pain, blood loss, and lower conversion rates than laparoscopy without robotic assistance [5, 7–9]. The thought of utilizing robotic assistance for more complex procedures led to several studies showing a benefit for use in more complex surgeries, such as in patients with a large uterus, a high body mass index (BMI),

M. Orady
Benign Gynecology Section,
Women's Health Institute, Cleveland Clinic,
9500 Euclid Avenue, A-81, Cleveland,
OH 44195, USA
e-mail: oradym@ccf.org

P.F. Escobar, T. Falcone (eds.), *Atlas of Single-Port, Laparoscopic, and Robotic Surgery,*
DOI 10.1007/978-1-4614-6840-0_17, © Springer Science+Business Media New York 2014

severe endometriosis, or extensive adhesions [10–13]. The recent decline in laparotomy rates for hysterectomy is thought to be due to the ease of use of the robotic instrument for dissection, as well as a faster learning curve than that for total laparoscopic hysterectomy, leading to increased utilization of the robotic-assisted approach rather than laparotomy [14].

This technology does present several disadvantages, however. First, in order to maintain shorter operating room times, efficient turnover, and cost-effectiveness, there is a need for a well-trained team and bedside assistant to assist with troubleshooting and to keep surgery moving efficiently. Cost also must be considered. In addition to the capital cost of the robotic surgical system, there is a maintenance cost as well as the cost of robotic instruments (each of which expires after 10 uses) and special drapes for the robotic arms and camera. Thus, the potential cost must be balanced with the benefits of offering the patient a minimally invasive procedure that results in a much faster recovery and return to work as compared to laparotomy.

17.2 Candidates for Robotic Surgery

Any patient who is a candidate for laparoscopic surgery may be a candidate for surgery performed with robotic assistance, but given the cost and resource considerations for robotic-assisted surgery, traditional laparoscopy may be the preferred approach for patients without high risk of conversion or complications. The greatest utility for the device arises in more complex hysterectomy procedures, with the intention of avoiding laparotomy. Therefore, a patient who would be considered a candidate for hysterectomy via laparotomy or who has a higher risk of conversion to laparotomy secondary to the complexity of the procedure is a potential candidate for robotic hysterectomy because the instrumentation allows for greater control and stability of instruments, improved visualization, and more precise dissection (Fig. 17.1). Surgeons should choose candidates carefully and gradually increase the level of difficulty of the procedures performed as they gain experience with robotic assistance.

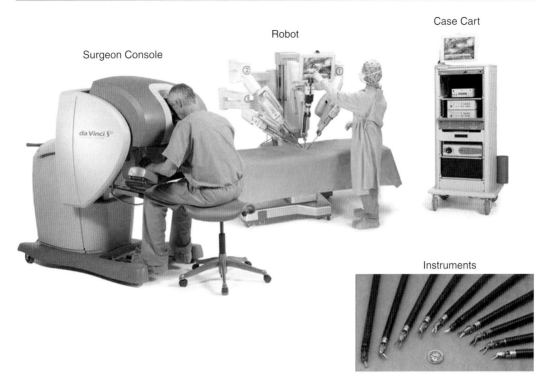

Fig. 17.1 Da Vinci Surgical System (Intuitive Surgical Inc., Sunnyvale, CA). The system consists of the tower, surgeon console, and robotic instrument. The camera arm cradles a 12- or 8-mm three-dimensional 10× high-definition camera with two to three additional robotic arms, which cradle interchangeable, wristed robotic surgical instruments

17.2.1 Large Fibroid Uterus

Large fibroid uteri often pose a laparoscopic challenge, primarily because difficulty navigating around large fibroids limits the surgeon's ability to dissect and access uterine vasculature and the colpotomy sites with straight instruments. A large uterus also requires more aggressive manipulation and more extensive retroperitoneal dissection because the anatomy is often extremely distorted and accessory vasculature may be present. Robotic assistance adds enhanced vision, which helps with dissection in deep spaces and easier control of bleeding, and the control of the camera, instruments, and uterus with the fourth arm allows for stability and precision in the dissection. In addition, the wristed instruments allow for navigation around bulky fibroids and the uterus, reaching for structures not in the direct line of the port, so that even cases such as that shown in Fig. 17.2 can be successfully accomplished with this approach.

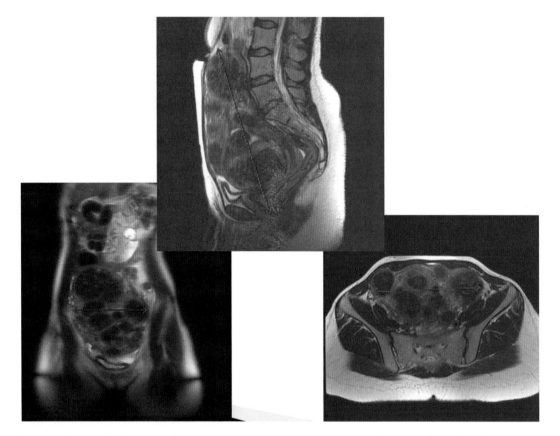

Fig. 17.2 Large fibroid uterus. The enhanced vision and instrument control in robotic-assisted laparoscopic hysterectomy increase the likelihood of a successful procedure

17.2.2 Endometriosis

Endometriosis (Fig. 17.3) often causes severe fibrosis and scarring, greatly distorting anatomic landmarks and tissue planes. The enhanced vision and ease of dissection while using robotic instruments can assist in navigating the pelvis, allowing more precise excision of the endometriotic lesions.

17.2.3 Obesity

With the increasing epidemic of obesity, Docked robotic instrumentation allows for better control and easier use of instruments despite the thickness of the abdominal wall, which often restricts movement of traditional laparoscopic instruments (Fig. 17.4). In addition, the benefits of laparoscopic surgery greatly decrease laparotomy complications, which are more prevalent in obese patients.

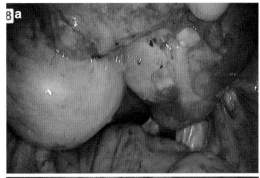
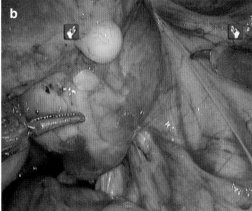

Fig. 17.3 Endometriosis. (**a**, **b**) Robotic instruments can more precisely excise these lesions

X

Clearing.

Fig. 17.4 Obesity. Laparoscopic procedures with robotic assistance are more likely to be successful in obese patients, thereby avoiding the need for laparotomy and its complications

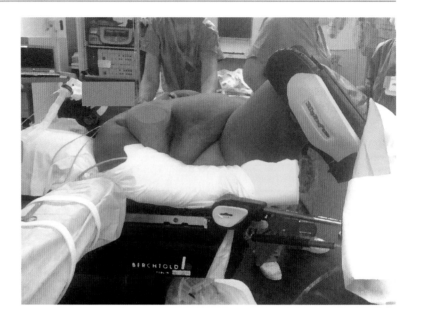

17.2.4 Pelvic Adhesive Disease

Extensive adhesions are most commonly associated with previous surgery, especially laparotomy. With cesarean section, as one of the most common surgical procedures performed in women and often performed more than once during the woman's lifetime, adhesions encountered at time of laparoscopic hysterectomy are a frequent cause for conversion. Similar to its utility for adhesions associated with endometriosis, robotic instrumentation can assist in adhesiolysis for adhesions near the abdominal wall (Fig. 17.5) or more extensive adhesions surrounding the uterus, such as those encountered after previous myomectomy, prior severe pelvic inflammatory disease, or other previous surgeries.

17.3 Preoperative Assessment

Appropriate and thorough preoperative assessment is essential for adequate decision-making and surgical planning. A thorough history and physical examination should be performed. Appropriate imaging modalities should be used to confirm the extent of pathology and assess anatomy for surgical planning. The possibility of malignancy needs to be ruled out, so assessment of cervical pathology and endometrial biopsy should be considered. Endometrial sampling is especially recommended if morcellation is likely in patients over age 35, or in those with risk factors such as those listed in Table 17.1, in order to rule out underlying hyperplasia or cancer.

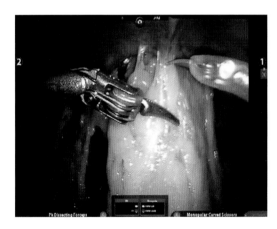

Fig. 17.5 Pelvic adhesive disease. Robotic instrumentation can assist in adhesiolysis for adhesions near the abdominal wall, as shown, or more extensive adhesions surrounding the uterus

Table 17.1 Risk factors for endometrial hyperplasia, endometrial cancer, or carcoma

Endometrial hyperplasia/endometrial cancer
Age older than 35 years
White race
Nulliparity
Older age at menopause
Early menarche
Obesity
Family history of ovarian, colon, or uterine cancer
Use of tamoxifen or unopposed estrogen
History
Diabetes mellitus
Polycystic ovary syndrome
Gallbladder disease
Thyroid disease
Cigarette smoking
Sarcoma
Prior pelvic radiation
Treatment with tamoxifen for breast cancer
African-American race
Retinoblastoma (*RB1*) gene

If concern about the size or location of fibroids or other pathology remains after a thorough evaluation and imaging, causing doubt about the ability to approach the patient with a robotic approach, an examination under anesthesia or diagnostic laparoscopy at the beginning of the case will help in the decision to proceed with the surgery as planned, versus converting to laparotomy. Table 17.2 illustrates assessment methods used in the preoperative evaluation.

Table 17.2 Preoperative evaluation for candidacy for robotic hysterectomy

Assessment method	Improves candidacy	Decreases candidacy
History	Bulk symptoms, intractable bleeding and pain not responding to medical therapy	Unevaluated postmenopausal bleeding
	For menorrhagia or mild bulk symptoms, alternative management options should be discussed (levonorgestrel-releasing intrauterine system and uterine fibroid embolization)	Rapid enlargement of abdominal mass
	Prior surgical history indicating likelihood of adhesions and need for dissection, or history of endometriosis	Adnexal pathology suspicious for malignancy
Physical examination	Assessment of abdominal scars	Multiple abdominal scars (must be assessed to plan access method)
	Access to and mobility of the cervix (at least 1 cm length)	Immobile, fixed uterus
	Lateral mobility of the uterus	Fibroids filling abdomen, leaving no room for ports
	Patent vagina with room for manipulator and extraction of uterus	Severe cervix deviation, prolapsing fibroids, cervical mass or fibroid
Pathology and laboratory evaluation	Assessment of anemia	Risk factors for sarcoma or suspicious for sarcoma
	Assessment of cervical pathology	Endometrial hyperplasia with large uterus
	Assessment of endometrial pathology	
Imaging (triaxial CT or MRI)	Narrower lower uterine segment	Fibroids filling pelvic cavity
	Well-delineated cervix	Severely deviated or obliterated cervix
	Lateral side walls and posterior cul-de-sac free of fibroids	Extensive lateral fibroids
Examination under anesthesia or diagnostic laparoscopy	Mobility of the uterus from below with the uterine manipulator	Prolapsed fibroids
	Mobility from above with instruments	Cervical fibroids
	Access to the retroperitoneal space	Lack of mobility of uterus
	Delineation of the colpotomy site or cervix	Lack of lateral access for retroperitoneal dissection
		Lack of space for port placement
		Suspected malignancy

Extensive discussion with the patient regarding treatment options and the risks and benefits of each treatment or surgical approach should be undertaken preoperatively, with a thorough explanation of the minimally invasive approach and factors that would cause conversion. Patients with complex pathology are usually willing to undergo an attempt at a minimally invasive procedure, even with a higher risk of conversion, rather than proceeding directly to laparotomy. Adequate preoperative counseling should include a discussion regarding general surgical risks and the risks and benefits specific to laparoscopic or robotic surgery. Risks of visceral injury, including unrecognized injury to bowel or the urinary tract, should also be discussed, and every patient must be counseled in regards to the risk of conversion to laparotomy. Preoperative preparation and the plan for postoperative care should be reviewed. It is important to set expectations for postoperative care and recovery. Many patients have experience with friends or family members who have undergone abdominal hysterectomy with less expedient recovery, so the early ambulation and discharge common after robotic-assisted hysterectomy may be unexpected.

Imaging can assist with assessment and surgical planning. In general, pelvic ultrasound can provide adequate assessment for uteri less than 16 weeks size. However, if fibroids are large or if the uterus is very bulky, the addition of either a triaxial CT scan or pelvic MRI is helpful for surgical planning. These images are especially important for uteri with decreased mobility or lateral fibroids on examination, because the shape of the uterus, the presence or absence of hydronephrosis, and the location of the bladder relative to the uterus are necessary additional information. For example, in the presence of very large fibroids or a low cervical fibroid, a myomectomy may be needed to debulk the uterus first at the time of hysterectomy. The general shape of the uterus, which can be assessed on triaxial CT scans or MRI, indicates the possibility of elevating the uterus out of the pelvis, the location of fibroids relative to the bladder, and the ease of access to uterine vasculature. Thinner lower uterine segments and a longer cervix indicate more accessible uterine vessels, which come in at the junction between the cervix and the uterus. Figure 17.6 illustrates a case amenable to the robotic approach despite a large, bulky, fibroid uterus.

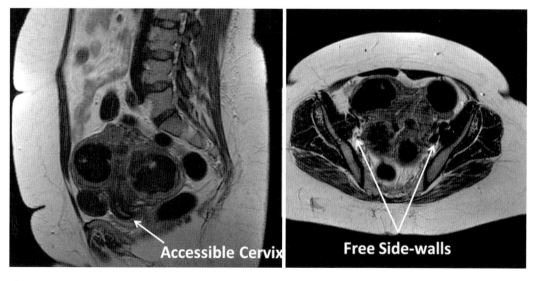

Fig. 17.6 Favorable features for robotic hysterectomy on imaging. In this MRI, the accessibility of the cervix and free pelvic side walls indicate that this case is amenable to the robotic approach despite the large, bulky, fibroid uterus

17.4 Preparation for the Procedure: Setup and Equipment

17.4.1 Operating Room Setup and the Operative Team

In the operative suite, a team effort is essential in all surgical procedures, but it is especially critical in robotic-assisted procedures. Involvement of the anesthesia staff, assistants, nurses, and scrub technicians is required in order to provide expedient and efficient care. Protocols that include multitasking and parallel-tasking of all team members allow for increased efficiency and accuracy. As depicted in Fig. 17.7, parallel rather than sequential tasks are assigned to all members of the operating room team, including anesthesia and the surgeon. If possible, a stable and consistent team implementing such a repetitive protocol maximizes efficiency

of the surgery and turnover, thus reducing the cost of the procedure. It is also important for all team members and the assistant to have detailed knowledge and practice of quick troubleshooting of the robotic system. They should be trained in the skills laboratory and mock drills and should have checklists that help keep the system working properly and ensure expedient resolution of any problems. The camera and instruments should be checked prior to the start of the procedure so that any problems can be resolved before the patient undergoes anesthesia. While the scrub technician and nursing staff are ensuring the availability and readiness of the equipment, the surgeon and assistant can take care of positioning the patient, while the anesthesia team, often needing two intravenous access sites, places the additional lines. All team members should also pay careful attention to the proper positioning and padding of the patient to prevent injury.

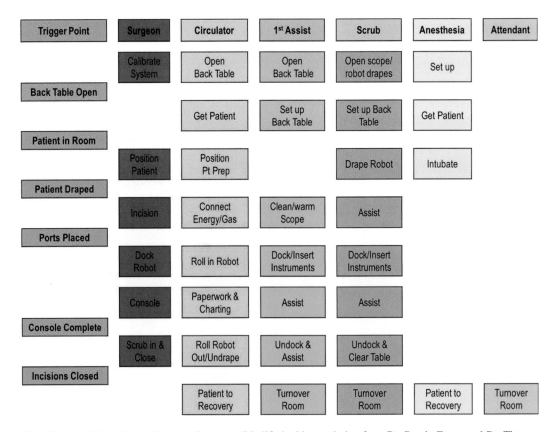

Fig. 17.7 Parallel tasking in the operating room (Modified with permission from Dr. Randy Fagen and Dr. Thomas Payne, Texas Institute for Robotic Surgery, Austin, TX.)

Operating room setup helps to ensure clear communication and the swift execution of needed tasks. By placing the surgeon console near the anesthesia team and scrub technician or assistant, as shown in Fig. 17.8, communication can be improved, as the microphone at the console amplifies the surgeon's voice. The plan, approach, and necessary instruments should be communicated clearly by the surgeon. Communication with the anesthesia staff regarding expected blood loss, length of surgery, and restriction of fluids should be ongoing. The robot can be docked on either side of the patient, and the assistant should be placed opposite the robot column, in order to give more room to operate. The vision cart and monitors should allow both the assistant and scrub technician to view the screen. The scrub technician should be placed either at the feet of the patient or on the opposite side in order to easily pass instruments or help with instrument exchanges from side to side. Selection of an appropriate bedside assistant and proper placement allowing access to both the uterine manipulator and assistant port is extremely important for an efficient and safe surgical procedure. For difficult cases, the bedside assistant may be one of most important factors determining success, because the surgeon is not scrubbed and is thus not directly available at the patient side, making the surgeon dependent on the skill of the assistant.

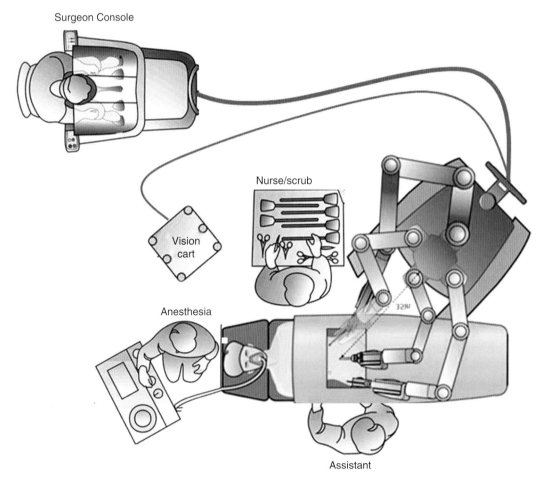

Fig. 17.8 Operating room setup. The surgeon console is placed near the anesthesia team and scrub technician or assistant. The robot can be docked on the patient's left side (**a**) or the right side (**b**) (Modified with permission from Dr. Arnold Advincula, Global Robotic Institute, Florida Hospital, Celebration, FL.)

Surgeon Console

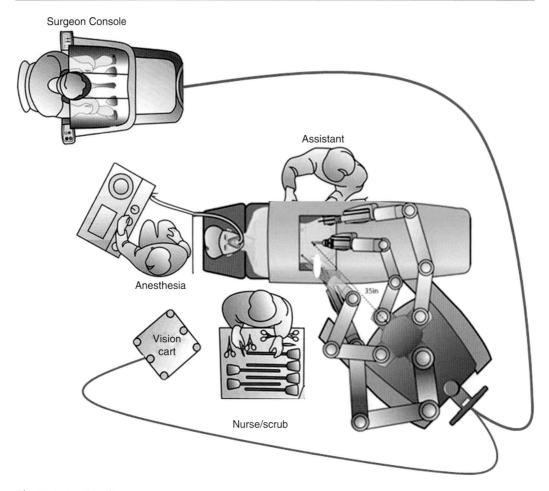

Assistant

Anesthesia

Vision
cart

Nurse/scrub

35in

Fig. 17.8 (continued)

17.4.2 Patient Positioning

As with laparoscopic procedures, patients are positioned in the dorsal lithotomy position, in Trendelenburg with both arms tucked at the sides in anatomic positioning. Padding and proper positioning avoid risk of nerve injuries. As patients are often in a Trendelenburg position (20–30°) for a prolonged period during surgery while the robot is docked, vaginal access must be maintained and it is extremely important to take measures to prevent the patient from slipping in the caudad direction on the operating room bed. There are a few mechanisms that have been described to prevent sliding in Trendelenburg, including shoulder braces, strapping, egg-crate foam (Fig. 17.9), and bean bag. Each approach has advantages and disadvantages. With shoulder braces, there is concern for brachial plexus injury; straps across the chest can restrict ventilation; the bean bag is quite firm and can cause bruising or neuropathy if not properly placed; gel pads can cause friction burns on heavy patients; while foam must be replaced with each patient and makes moving the patient into position after intubation difficult because of the lack of a draw sheet. Each surgeon must find his or her own comfort level with these measures. Egg crate foam and is the preference of some surgeons, as one study has linked its use to persistent success, with less than 2 in. of slide [15].

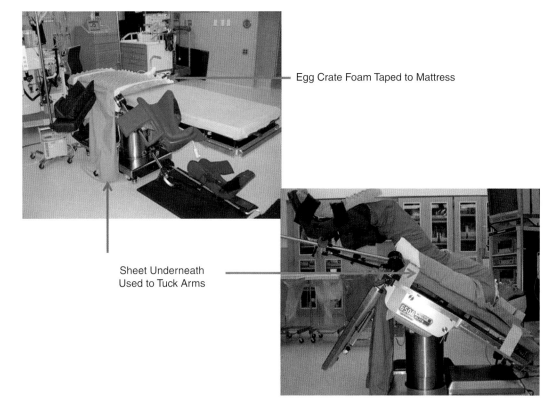

Egg Crate Foam Taped to Mattress

Sheet Underneath
Used to Tuck Arms

Fig. 17.9 Methods of preventing sliding in Trendelenburg include the use of egg crate foam (Modified with permission from Dr. Arnold Advincula, Global Robotic Institute, Florida Hospital, Celebration, FL.)

While positioning a patient's legs in the stirrups, meticulous attention should be given to correct placement and padding and to the angles of the hip, knee, and ankle joints in the stirrups in order to prevent nerve injury (Fig. 17.10). As the stirrups will be dropped for docking, the legs should be positioned with the stirrups already dropped maximally; after positioning, they may be elevated slightly in order to prevent femoral nerve stretch injuries when the legs are moved under the drape.

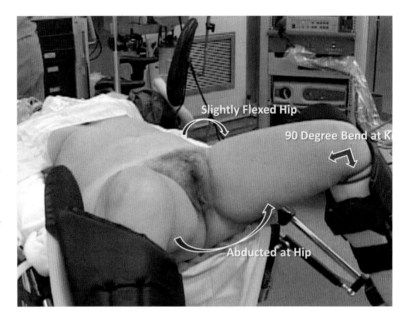

Fig. 17.10 Leg positioning requires meticulous attention to correct placement and padding and to the angles of the hip, knee, and ankle joints in the stirrups, in order to prevent nerve injury (Modified with permission from Dr. Arnold Advincula, Global Robotic Institute, Florida Hospital, Celebration, FL.)

Similarly, while tucking the arms, attention should be paid to proper padding at the elbows and wrists while watching the position of the thumbs and hands; padding around the hands and wrists will prevent catching them in the stirrups (Fig. 17.11). The team should ensure adequate preparation of surgical sites, including a wide prep on legs, buttocks, and inner thighs, as vaginal access for vaginal morcellation may be needed.

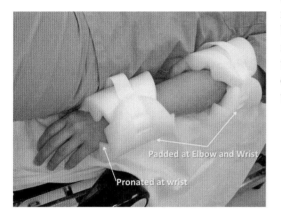

Fig. 17.11 Arm positioning requires attention to proper padding at the elbows and wrists, care with the position of the thumbs and hands, and padding around the hands and wrists to prevent them from catching in the stirrups (Modified with permission from Dr. Arnold Advincula, Global Robotic Institute, Florida Hospital, Celebration, FL.)

17.4.3 Specialized Equipment

The uterine manipulator has two purposes: (1) to elevate the uterus up and out of the pelvis and thus elevate the uterine vasculature away from the ureters, presenting tissue for dissection, sealing, and cutting; and (2) to delineate the vaginal fornices for colpotomy, or to help identify an appropriate location for supracervical hysterectomy. The colpotomy ring acts additionally as a homing device, allowing delineation of anatomy relative to it in the face of distorted anatomy, bulky fibroids, or extensive adhesions. All uterine manipulators share the ring concept, something to push the uterus upwards, and some manner of colpotomy delineation. Figure 17.12 shows the two most commonly used manipulators.

a   v-Care ® Uterine Manipulator

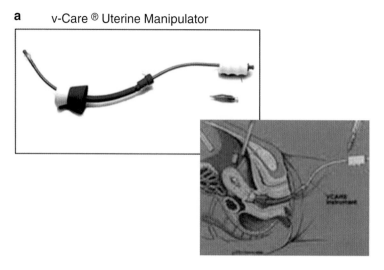

b   Rumi and Arch Uterine Manipulator

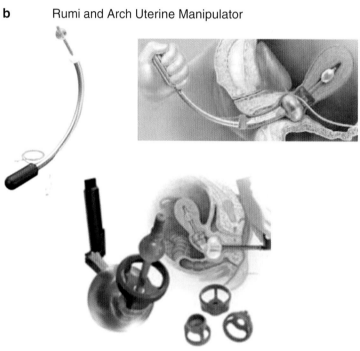

Fig. 17.12 The two most commonly used uterine manipulators are the (**a**) VCare (ConMed; Utica, NY) and the (**b**) KOH Colptomizer System (Cooper Surgical; Trumbull, CT), attached to either the RUMI Advanced Uterine Manipulation System (Cooper Surgical; Trumbull, CT) or the Advincula Arch (Cooper Surgical; Trumbull, CT). (**a**) The plastic VCare device has an S-shaped curve. The colpotomy ring has the advantage of having a groove for colpotomy, but it is somewhat soft and the ring is not fenestrated, making it a little more difficult to identify the fornix. In addition, as the device is plastic, it can easily bend, making it difficult to push up and manipulate a larger uterus. As it is one piece, it cannot be left in vaginally and may be a bit easier to place. (**b**) The older RUMI Avanced Uterine Manipulation System (Cooper Surgical; Trumbull, CT) and newer Advincula Arch are made of Metal. The Arch is the same shape as the Aumi or Humi manipulators (both by Cooper Surgical; Trumbull, CT) and have the advantage of not bending or breaking with a large uterus. In addition, its arched configuration helps to push the uterus up and out of the pelvis, providing access to uterine vasculature and colpotomy around large fibroids and making it possible to identify the colpotomy site in a setting of dense endometriosis or adhesions. The firm KOH Colpotomizer™ (Cooper Surgical; Trumbull, CT) attached to the Rumi or Arch has fenestrations and a uniform shape that allows easy identification and palpation of the ring and acts to push ureters more laterally, away from uterine vessels (Images from Cooper Surgical, Trumbull, CT, and ConMed, Utica, NY)

Two uterine manipulators, the RUMI Advanced Uterine Manipulation System and the Advincula Arch (both by Cooper Surgical; Trumbull, CT), have the advantage of being able to be mounted on the Uterine Positioning System (UPS; Cooper Surgical; Trumbull, CT). This device attaches to the OR bed and uses a hydraulic system to hold the uterine manipulator in place. The surgeon can position the uterus as desired and the device holds the position steady during the operation. For more complex surgeries, the surgeon should strongly consider using the UPS. With more prolonged dissection, especially for a large uterus or dense adhesions, assistants often fatigue, causing the uterus to drift. By holding the uterus in place, the UPS helps to hold things stable, keeping the target in view. The surgeon can adjust the position for optimal surgery, thus reducing the load on the assistant, who can then focus on bedside assistance.

Uterine Positioning System™

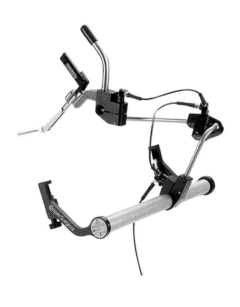
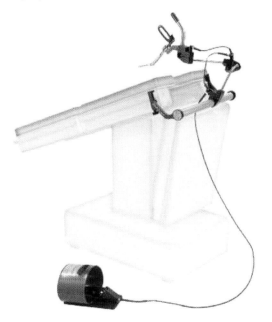

Fig. 17.13 The Uterine Positioning System™ (UPS; Cooper Surgical; Trumbull, CT) attaches to the bed and uses a hydraulic system to hold the uterine manipulator in place. Its use is especially helpful for complex surgeries (Images from Cooper Surgical, Trumbull, CT, and ConMed, Utica, NY)

17.5   The Surgical Procedure

17.5.1 Peritoneal Access and Port Placement

Careful planning for port placement location is indispensable for surgery on a patient with a large uterus of variable size and shape. After initial entry into the peritoneal cavity, whether by direct entry, Hassan, or Veress insufflation techniques, the location of the camera trocar should be determined, followed by placement of the accessory trocars, dependent on where the two working arms will be placed. Both the size and shape of the uterus must be considered for port placement planning. If most of the bulk of the uterus is above the ovaries and there are no adhesions or minimal need for access posteriorly, the camera may be placed lower down, close to or at the umbilicus, as most of the work of the procedure will be performed in the lower segment of the uterus. Otherwise, it is more prudent to place the camera higher up in the supraumbilical region, to one side of the falciform ligament. Initial entry into the peritoneal cavity may be performed with a camera port or a lateral port. Some advocate a left upper quadrant entry with 5-mm visual entry trocar, with or without insufflation with a Veress needle, for initial assessment. This may then be replaced by a working robotic trocar or maintained as the accessory port. Working arms then can be introduced. If the uterus is broad, they should be placed ultralaterally and low, so one arm can just reach over the lower uterine segment to the opposite side and a more medial fourth arm for manipulation of the uterus may be utilized as needed. For a uterus that is large but narrow, a more medial working arm allows reach over the bulk of the uterus and access to both sides with a lateral manipulating fourth arm added as needed.

For a larger uterus or complex pathology, the typical 25-10 rule for port placement may not apply (Fig. 17.14). The key to adjusting port sites is remembering that the uppermost "target organ" is not really the fundus, but rather the utero-ovarian ligaments or ovaries. This "target organ" is the highest structure that must be accessible for sealing and cutting with the robotic instruments, and this incision will be the highest incision made for the hysterectomy by sealing and cutting either the infundibulopelvic (IP) ligament or the utero-ovarian ligament, if ovaries are removed or preserved. These initial incisions will then be extended into the broad ligaments and carried inferiorly toward the uterine arteries, which are the other vascular bundles that must be accessed in order to accomplish the hysterectomy. Port placement must allow robotic instruments to access both the utero-ovarian ligaments and the uterine arteries. Access to the colpotomy ring is less critical, as performing the supracervical hysterectomy first can always allow access for the colpotomy ring.

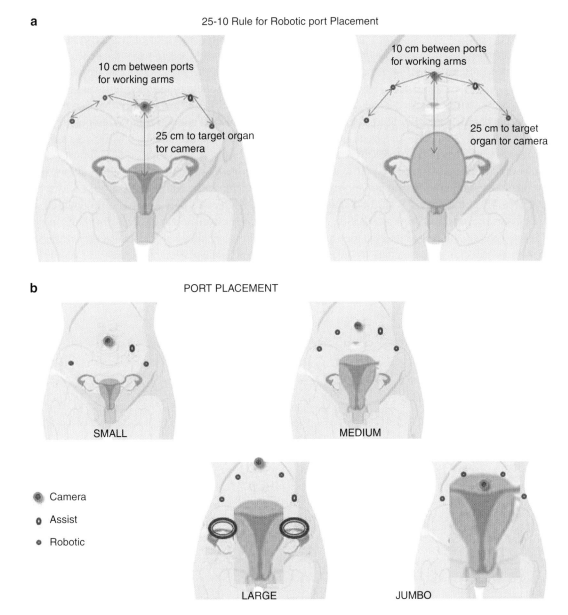

Fig. 17.14 The typical 25-10 rule for port placement (25 cm above the target organ for the camera and 10 cm between ports and above the target) may not apply if the patient has a large uterus or complex pathology, as there may not be enough room (**a**). Port placement should thus be adjusted for each individual case, depending on patient characteristics and pathology (**b**)

17.5.2 Docking and Instruments

Once ports are placed, docking should be undertaken. An experienced team can generally accomplish docking in less than 5 min. The robot may be either center docked or side docked (Fig. 17.15). Center docking was initially utilized extensively and is helpful if ports are very high, or in very narrow patients, where ports are closer together. However, it severely limits vaginal access for uterine manipulation or for vaginal morcellation and removal of the uterus. With the S and Si da Vinci systems (Intuitive Surgical, Inc; Sunnyvale, CA), which have longer arms than the standard system, side docking is easier and is now utilized routinely by most gynecologic robotic surgeons because it allows for better vaginal access for uterine manipulation, vaginal morcellation, or cystoscopy while the robot is docked. Left-side docking puts the assistant on the patient's right side, forcing them to use their left hand for laparoscopic assistance and the right hand for uterine manipulation. Patient's right side-docking puts the assistant on the patient's left allowing a right-handed assistant to use his or her dominant hand for uterine manipulation. This also allows two instruments to be under the control of a right-handed surgeon's dominant hand. In addition, if left upper quadrant entry is performed, the initial port used for entry may remain in the left upper quadrant as the assistant port.

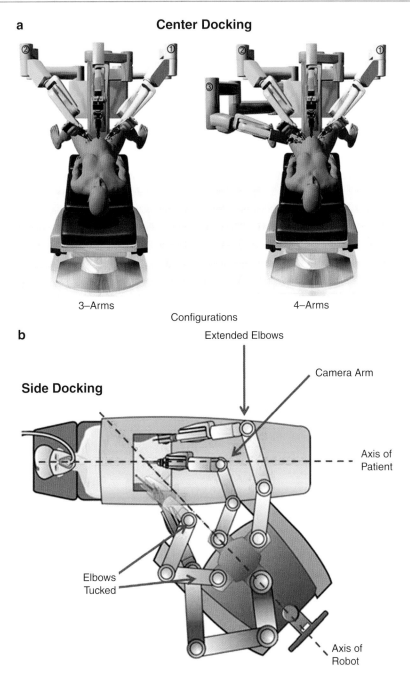

Fig. 17.15 Docking options. (**a**) Center docking can be helpful in some situations, but it severely limits vaginal access. With the S and Si da Vinci systems (Intuitive Surgical, Sunnyvale, CA), which have longer arms than the standard system, side docking is easier and is now routinely used by most gynecologic robotic surgeons because it allows better vaginal access. (**b**) Left-side docking puts the assistant on the patient's left, so a right-handed assistant can use his or her dominant hand for uterine manipulation. This also puts tow instruments under the control of a right-handed surgeon's dominant hand. Docking on the left side places the assistant on the patient's right side forcing him to use his left hand to assist with. (Modified with permission from Dr. Arnold Advincula, Global Robotic Institute, Florida Hospital, Celebration, FL.)

A selection of different instruments can be considered for performance of hysterectomy. Instruments such as monopolar scissors or monopolar hook are generally placed in the dominant hand and utilize monopolar energy for cutting or coagulation. The scissors have the advantage over the hook in that they can be used for spreading in fine dissection. Instruments such as a plasmakinetic (PK) dissector, bipolar fenestrated grasper, or Maryland bipolar forceps are generally placed in the opposite or left hand. These are used for both coagulation and vessel sealing, as well as for spreading and dissection. The PK dissector has a finer tip and thus can be used for finer dissection, but because it is thinner, it may not grasp as well as the fenestrated instruments. Gyrus plasmakinetic energy (Southborough, MA) used for the PK dissector creates less charring and is a better vessel sealer with less thermal spread than bipolar energy. The third, or accessory, arm generally has a grasping or manipulation instrument such as fenestrated ProGrasp forceps (Intuitive Surgical,

Sunnyvale, CA); longer, thinner "long-tip" forceps; or a single-toothed tenaculum that does not have energy associated with it. Different grasping instruments may be chosen depending on the type of tissue that needs to be manipulated. The tenaculum is more useful for myomectomy procedures or larger hysterectomies, whereas the ProGrasp forceps (Intuitive Surgical, Sunnyvale, CA) are great for retraction and can be used gently on bowel or adnexal tissue. Newer instruments include the robotic suction-irrigation device or the ligature seal-and-cut device, which may be useful in certain situations. The usefulness of each instrument must be balanced with the extra expense. Four types of needle drivers may be used in hysterectomy: a smaller "large needle driver," a heavier "mega needle driver," and two similar-sized instruments with a suture scissor at the base, called a suture-cut needle driver. For vaginal cuff closure in hysterectomies, most surgeons use the mega needle drivers because they are wider and thus can more easily handle thicker tissues.

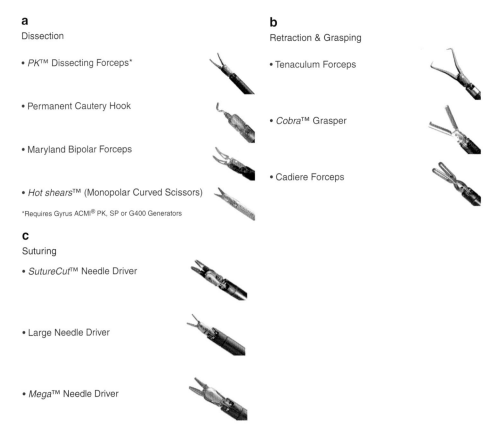

a
Dissection

• *PK*™ Dissecting Forceps*

• Permanent Cautery Hook

• Maryland Bipolar Forceps

• *Hot shears*™ (Monopolar Curved Scissors)

*Requires Gyrus ACMI® PK, SP or G400 Generators

b
Retraction & Grasping

• Tenaculum Forceps

• *Cobra*™ Grasper

• Cadiere Forceps

c
Suturing

• *SutureCut*™ Needle Driver

• Large Needle Driver

• *Mega*™ Needle Driver

Fig. 17.16 (**a–c**) EndoWrist instruments (Intuitive Surgical, Sunnyvale, CA) typically utilized in robotic hysterectomy (Modified with permission from Dr. Arnold Advincula, Global Robotic Institute, Florida Hospital, Celebration, FL.)

17.5.3 Hysterectomy Procedure

The key to the approach to the large uterus or complex hysterectomy procedure is finding the anatomy in the face of extreme distortion and displacement of important structures. After docking, an initial survey should be performed, any adhesions lysed, and the bowel swept upwards. A survey of the general shape and configuration of the uterus and the presence of fibroids should be performed, noting the size and location of fibroids and assessing the mobility of the uterus in both the caudal direction and laterally. Initial upwards mobility is most important, as even a very broad uterus will gain lateral mobility once the round ligaments are transected and the retroperitoneal space is entered.

To then plan the approach, one must understand the anatomy of a hysterectomy, which can be simplified into three phases, as described in Fig. 17.17. The process of hysterectomy includes securing the necessary vessels and detaching the uterus from its attachments. Vessels and attachments occur at two locations each. Vascular entry points occur on each side at the utero-ovarian ligaments and at the uterine vessels. Ascending vessels ascend laterally along the uterine wall between these two entry points. After uterine fibroid embolization, lateral accessory vessels tend to form in this intermediate location. Similarly, ligamentous attachment points occur at the same locations: at the round ligaments, with broad ligaments extending from that point downward, and at the fornices at the top of the vagina, with lateral cardinal and uterosacral attaching at the angles.

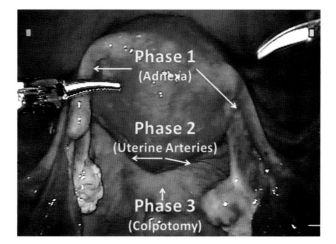

Fig. 17.17 A simplified approach to a robotic hysterectomy can be divided into three phases: (1) securing and transecting ovarian vasculature and the round ligaments, and performing lateral dissection; (2) securing the uterine vasculature; and (3) performing colpotomy. Once landmarks for each phase are identified, the hysterectomy procedure can be broken down into smaller parts, thus making a difficult hysterectomy less daunting. The initial approach therefore, should consist of identification of phase 1 landmarks (*ie*, round ligament, utero-ovarian ligaments, and ureters), then moving downwards towards phase 2 landmarks, skeletonizing uterine vasculature and dissecting down to the vaginal fascia along the colpotomizer ring and identifying the uterosacral ligaments. Phase 3 involves detaching the uterus, either by amputation at the level of the cervix for a supracervical hysterectomy, or at the level of the vaginal fornices for a total laparoscopic hysterectomy

17.5.3.1 Adnexa

With a large uterus, dissection of the adnexa may be difficult, as the ovaries may be pushed upwards above the pelvic brim by large fibroids, and cornual fibroids may obliterate the utero-ovarian ligaments completely. If displaced away from the ovary, salpingectomy may help to clear and isolate ovarian blood supply. If the plan is to preserve the ovaries, care must be taken to start at the infundibulopelvic ligament and identify ovarian vasculature as it ascends upwards from the region of the round ligament attachment towards an ovary that may be pushed superiorly by the underlying fibroids (Fig. 17.18). Otherwise, ovarian vasculature may be inadvertently transected or compromised, resulting in an undesired oophorectomy.

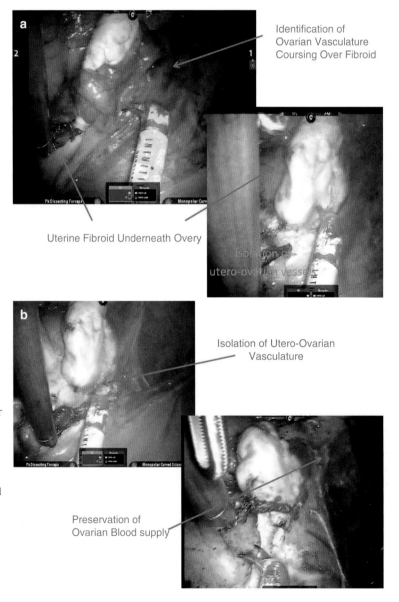

Fig. 17.18 Ovarian isolation in case of distorting fibroids. (**a**) Identification of the course of the ovarian artery must be performed prior to isolation of the ovary. The retroperitoneal space may be entered between the round ligament and infundibulopelvic (*IP*) ligament; then it can be followed upwards, separating it from the uterus and finally isolating the ovary in a retrograde fashion in order to separate it from the uterus (**b**). An underlying fibroid may also be dissected to help lift the ovary up and away from it. Sometimes after separation, the ovary may be left on a long, stretched-out IP ligament and should be secured to the round ligament after the hysterectomy is performed in order to suspend it away from the vaginal cuff and prevent torsion, while also ensuring that there is no peritoneal window large enough to admit a loop of bowel that may cause obstruction

17.5.3.2 Ureter

The importance of identification of the ureter (Fig. 17.19) cannot be overemphasized, especially when dealing with a very large uterus, broad ligament fibroids, or endometriosis. The location of the ureter can be quite distorted by fibrosis in surrounding tissue, or adherence to fibroids can draw the ureter more superior and medial to its usual location, thus making it more prone to injury. As it also takes more energy to seal the much larger uterine vessels feeding a large fibroid uterus, there is greater thermal spread, making it even more important to ensure that the ureter is far away from the area of energy application.

When trying to identify the ureter and uterine vasculature (Fig. 17.20), it is most important to maintain the areolar nature of the tissue in order to identify correct tissue planes. Enter the retroperitoneal space (either superior to or inferior to the IP ligament) hemostatically, and avoid bleeding before it starts with prudent control of small vessels, refraining from irrigation, and suctioning any fluid that may be in the pelvis before it enters the retroperitoneal space. Peritoneal leafs are initially spread apart to open the space and then dissection should be carried out parallel to the ureter until it is identified.

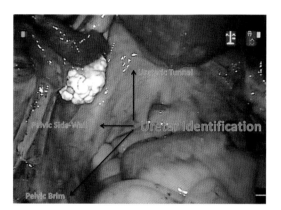

Fig. 17.19 Locations for ureter identification. There are generally three locations where the ureter may be identified: distally, as it dives beneath the uterine artery; centrally, just below the pelvic brim; or more proximally, above the pelvic brim in retroperitoneal space above the iliac vessels. The ureter is most easily seen at the pelvic brim, on the medial leaf of the peritoneal reflection beneath the IP ligament. It may then be followed inferiorly down to where it crosses under uterine vasculature to enter the bladder. Always dissect parallel, not perpendicular, to its course, starting at the peritoneum just beneath the IP ligament and working medially in order to locate it. With large fibroids, it is often dilated and easier to locate, but it is often difficult to locate in patients with high body mass index or severe endometriosis

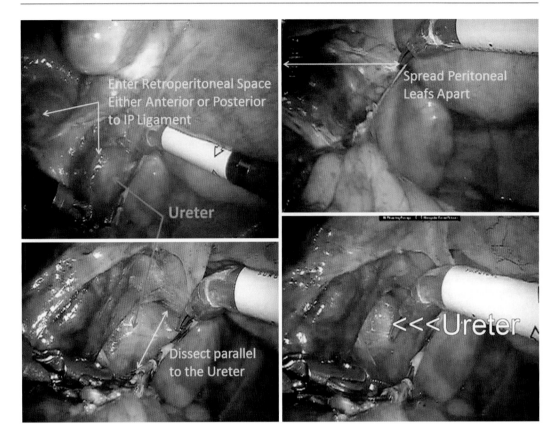

Fig. 17.20 Ureter dissection. Use the pneumoperito- raytec sponge into the peritoneal cavity and dissect with neum and gentle dissection to enter retroperitoneal space gentle blotting motions in order to find the appropriate hemostatically; avoid bleeding before it starts with pru- planes, making it easier to see the ureter. Retroperitoneal dent control of small vessels, refraining from irrigation, space may be entered either superior to or inferior to the and suctioning any fluid that may be in the pelvis before IP ligament. Peritoneal leafs are initially spread apart to it enters the retroperitoneal space. If bleeding or fluid open the space, and then dissection should be carried out obscures the planes prematurely, introduce a cottonoid or parallel to the ureter until it is identified

17.5.3.3 Broad Ligaments and Uterine Vasculature

After the ovarian vasculature is controlled, the round ligaments are transected, and retroperitoneal space has been entered to identify the ureter, phase 1 of the hysterectomy is essentially completed. For phase 2, the major tasks are the identification of the colpotomy ring, and securing of the uterine blood supply. Three approaches to the uterine arteries may be used: anterior, posterior, or lateral. The approach taken depends on what the surgeon can see and what is accessible; different cases require different approaches. By knowing the goals for phase 1 and phase 2 of the hysterectomy, multiple approaches may be taken to achieve the same result, using the landmarks as the guide. The ultimate destination is the colpotomy ring, and the two forks in the road are the ovarian and uterine vasculature. If those can be isolated and controlled, the remainder of the hysterectomy is simple.

Once the uterine artery is identified, it can be isolated and ligated at three points, as shown in Fig. 17.21:

- at the level of the internal cervical os, for supracervical hysterectomy
- at the level of the colpotomy ring, for total laparoscopic hysterectomy
- laterally at its origin, if large fibroids or endometriosis make isolation difficult

The anterior approach (Fig. 17.22) is most useful for the obliterated cul-de-sac, large posterior fibroids, or an extremely wide uterus.

The lateral approach to the uterine artery (Fig. 17.23) is most useful for lateral broad ligament fibroids or extensive endometriosis with an obliterated cul-de-sac.

The posterior approach to the uterine artery (Fig. 17.24) is best used for bulky fibroid uteri with large anterior or lower uterine-segment fibroids, or in uteri with extensive anterior adhesions from prior cesarean section or myomectomy.

Fig. 17.21 Locations for isolation of uterine vasculature. Once the uterine artery is identified, there are three points at which it can then be isolated and ligated: at the level of the internal cervical os, for supracervical hysterectomy; at the level of the colpotomy ring, for total laparoscopic hysterectomy; or laterally at its origin in cases of large broad ligament or cervical fibroids or difficult isolation secondary to endometriosis

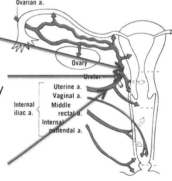

Skeletonization and Control of Uterine Vasculature

▹ **Control at level of internal cervical os for supracervical hysterectomy**

▹ **Control just above vaginal fornix (outlined by colpotomy ring) for total laparoscopic hysterectomy.**

▹ **Control laterally at it's origin for large broad ligament fibroids.**

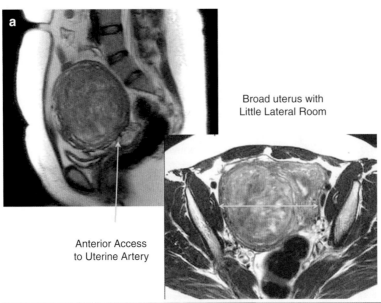

Broad uterus with
Little Lateral Room

Anterior Access
to Uterine Artery

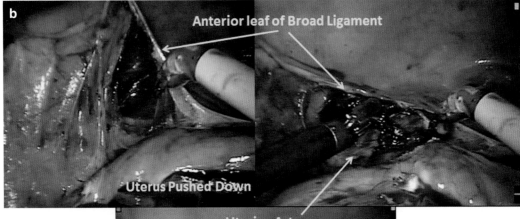

Anterior leaf of Broad Ligament

Uterus Pushed Down

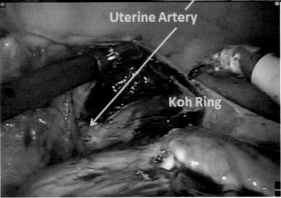

Uterine Artery

Koh Ring

Fig. 17.22 Anterior approach to uterine vessels. (**a**) In this approach, after transection of the round ligaments, the anterior broad ligament is opened, creating the bladder flap utilizing principles of careful hemostatic dissection. The bladder is then dissected down below the colpotomy ring (**b**), which in turn is pushed in maximally, elevating the uterine arteries. Starting in the midline, the tissue is gradually dissected in layers, working medially to laterally until the uterine arteries are exposed. They may be partially sealed above the uterocervical junction to reduce blood supply to the uterus until posterior fibroids can be removed, or further dissection can be performed. By then opening up the posterior leaf, the ureters can be pushed more laterally and inferiorly away from the uterine artery. Opening the posterior leaf of the broad ligament releases the ureters further, allowing the uterine arteries to be further skeletonized, sealed, and cut

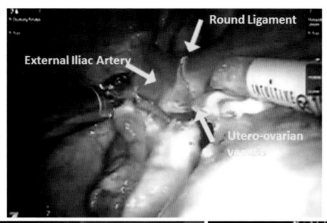

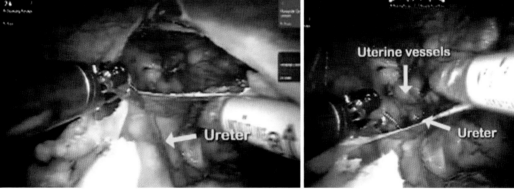

Fig. 17.23 Lateral approach to uterine vessels. In this approach, the critical triangle between the round ligament, the utero-ovarian ligament, and the external iliac artery is entered and dissection is begun more laterally and inferiorly along the path of the ureter. The obliterated umbilical ligament can also be followed down to the hypogastric artery bifurcation, where the uterine artery can be isolated and clipped, tied, or cautery sealed. The uterine artery can then be followed medially, dissecting out the ureter and separating it from any broad ligament fibroids, which can then be carefully separated from the retroperitoneal space, elevating them and pushing them medially away from the lateral side wall. Again, if accessible, the uterine vasculature can be resealed at the angles before colpotomy is made, and then the uterus can be transected or the fibroid removed by myomectomy in order to access the colpotomy ring for colpotomy

Fig. 17.24 (**a**, **b**) Posterior approach to uterine vessels. After the uterus is pushed up and anteverted maximally and the location of the ureter is noted, the posterior peritoneum is entered above the ureters, with the peritoneal incision carried down, outlining the uterus from beneath the utero-ovarian ligament down to just above the insertion of the uterosacral ligaments. The retroperitoneal space is then entered and the ureters are dissected inferiorly. Then the uterine arteries can be isolated at the colpotomy ring just lateral and superior to the uterosacral ligaments. Once the uterine vasculature is controlled, myomectomy may be performed and dissection can be carried laterally and then anteriorly to lyse any adhesions or dissect the adherent bladder

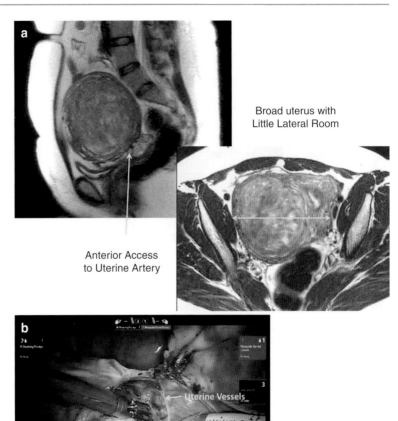

17.5.3.4 Bladder Flap

The bladder flap can be approached either before or after the uterine vasculature is isolated, depending on the approach used. Proper identification of planes and careful dissection will avoid injury, even in the case of a tethered uterus or extensive anterior bladder adhesions (Fig. 17.25). As layers are dissected, the uterine arteries are exposed and skeletonized so that they can be sealed, staying above the colpotomy ring towards the cervicovaginal junction. Large vasculature should be well skeletonized down to the vessel wall in order to allow adequate sealing with application of bipolar or PK cautery. The vessels should then be cut sharply to avoid disruption of the seal, which can occur with application of monopolar energy to a sealed vessel. The vessels then can fall laterally away from the site of a future angle incision, clearing the colpotomy ring.

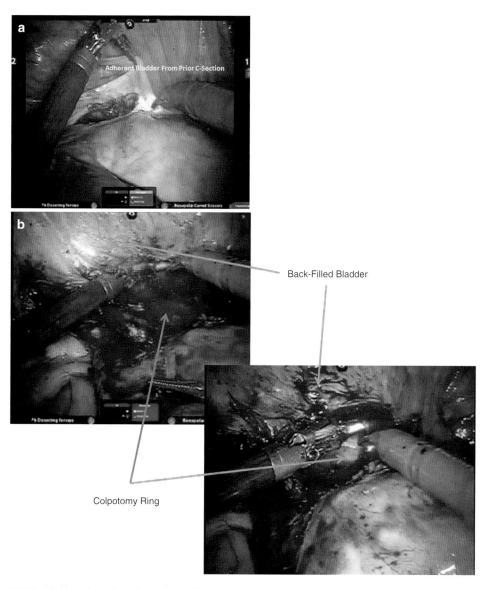

Fig. 17.25 Bladder flap dissection. Back-filling the bladder with approximately 150–200 mL of blue stained saline often assists with this dissection. The colpotomy ring acts as the landmark that delineates the vaginal margin. Starting more laterally, the correct tissue plane can be identified and taken down with fine dissection in layers, utilizing the PK dissector to elevate the layers and incising them with the monopolar scissors. Once the correct tissue plane is identified, gradual medial dissection can be performed as adhesions are identified and cut, in order to release the bladder and dissect it down to 1–2 cm below the colpotomy ring

17.5.3.5 Colpotomy

Different approaches to colpotomy can be undertaken (Fig. 17.26). Anterior and posterior colpotomy may be started first, sparing the angles for last. Alternatively, one may start at the angles and then perform posterior and anterior colpotomy once hemostasis at the angles is assured. This is the best approach for a large uterus in particular, because if colpotomy is started anteriorly, the weight of the uterus will often pull the uterus away and possibly off the uterine manipulator, making it difficult to extend the incision posteriorly. By severely anteverting and elevating the uterus out of the pelvis, however, colpotomy incisions started at the angles can easily be extended posteriorly, first on one side and then the other, back and forth until posterior incision is complete. The weight of the uterus then works in favor of the surgeon, as the uterus is pushed up further and angled towards the sacrum and the anterior colpotomy site is stretched, making for a more efficient and easy anterior colpotomy. A 30° angled camera turned 90° can visualize the angles directly and will help to visualize the posterior colpotomy site in the face of a large uterus. This angled lens also helps to look over the uterus to access the anterior colpotomy site after posterior colpotomy is made. If the uterus is so bulky that the posterior colpotomy site is not visible even with one arm elevating the uterus and a 30° upward lens placed, an alternative approach would be to perform a supracervical hysterectomy, amputating the bulk of the uterus first by pulling the manipulator slightly out of the uterus until the cervical os is reached and then reinserting it and completing the amputation. Once the amputation is performed, the colpotomy is then much simplified and can be performed with maximal upward traction allowing a swift cut around the cervix.

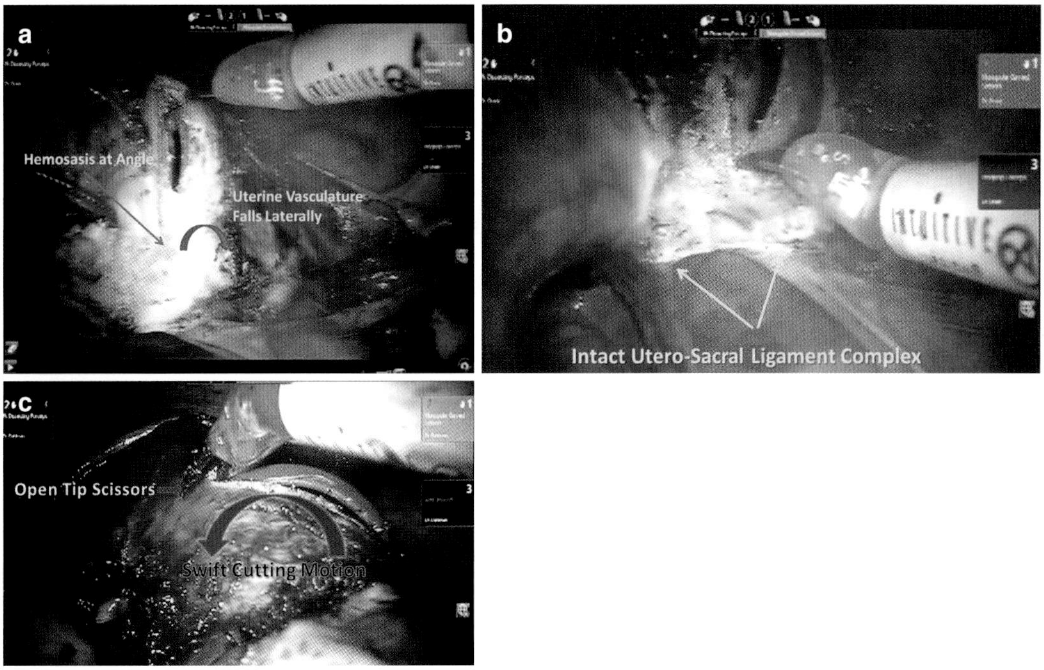

Fig. 17.26 Principles of colpotomy. (**a**) Incision towards the internal cervical os and then inferiorly towards the angle ensures that uterine pedicles fall laterally and are released away from the uterus and colpotomy edge. The incision can then be carried through the full thickness of the vagina to the colpotomizer edge. (**b**) If accessible, it is preferable to first extend angle incisions posteriorly to the beginning of the uterosacral ligaments before turning attention anteriorly. The peritoneum is then scored above the uterosacral ligaments, and this incision is carried down towards the colpotomizer, allowing the uterosacral ligaments to remain intact and attached to the posterior vaginal cuff for support. By using full force with the uterine manipulator to tent the uterus upwards and severely anteverted, this region is exposed and the vaginal fornix is tented up, allowing for efficient, swift extension of the colpotomy posteriorly. (**c**) When performing the colpotomy, it is important to minimize the energy applied to the vaginal cuff in order to maximize healing and thus minimize necrosis and the risk of cuff dehiscence. By opening monopolar scissor tips and moving swiftly across the tissue, the energy application is reduced. On Si da Vinci systems (Intuitive Surgical, Sunnyvale, CA) the monopolar cut mode of cautery also may be used to decrease the energy effect on vaginal cuff tissue

17.5.3.6 Colpotomy Repair

The goals of appropriate colpotomy repair (Fig. 17.27) include adequate closure, reapproximation of vaginal mucosal edges to prevent granulation and dehiscence, hemostasis at the angles and the cuff, closure of vaginal fascia to prevent dehiscence and enterocele, and suspension of the vagina to prevent future prolapse. With the introduction of robotic hysterectomy, there was initial concern about a possible high rate of vaginal cuff dehiscence, which was theorized to be caused by prolonged application of monopolar energy to the cuff, devitalizing the tissue, as well as by inadequate tissue bites during cuff closure secondary to the extremely magnified view provided by the robotic camera. As experience with this technique increased, further reports of complications from case series showed no increased risk of vaginal cuff dehiscence as compared with total laparoscopic hysterectomy; rates were under 1 %. The method of cuff closure was never implicated in increased dehiscence rates, and no technique or suture choice has been shown to be superior in this regard. Thus, it is more important to maintain healthy vaginal cuff tissue by minimizing energy application during colpotomy, allowing the maintenance of the vascular blood supply to the tissue and promoting good tissue healing. During cuff closure, it is more important to incorporate adequate margins of both mucosa and fascia into the closure suture, rather than relying on a particular type of suture to secure the closure (Fig. 17.28). After the vaginal cuff is closed, a vaginal exam should be done to assess for bleeding and adequate closure of the cuff, and cystoscopy should be performed to assess for kinking of a ureter or passage of sutures through the bladder, especially on wider, larger vaginal cuffs.

Fig. 17.27 Principles of colpotomy repair. (**a**) Attention to the colpotomy repair actually begins with the creation of the bladder flap. Care must be taken to take the bladder to at least 1–2 cm below the colpotomizer edge all the way out to the angles, in order to avoid incorporating bladder into the stitches and making room for adequate bites of the vaginal fascia and mucosa. (**b**) When performing the colpotomy repair, each suture should take adequate bites at least 1 cm in depth, incorporating the vaginal fascia into the bite (not just mucosa), allowing mucosal edges to be everted and approximating mucosal edges together. Posteriorly while performing the colpotomy, the colpotomizer cup should be tented upwards and the incision begun above the uterosacral ligaments, carrying the incision downwards toward the colpotomy cup, thereby maintaining attachment of the uterosacral complex to the posterior vaginal cuff. Cuff closure sutures will then secure them further to the top of the cuff. (**c**) In addition, the angle sutures can tighten and slightly shorten the uterosacral ligaments, bringing them closer to the midline and securing them to the vagina. These sutures will thus suspend the vaginal cuff at all levels, helping to prevent future prolapse. Thus the main principles of cuff closure are careful colpotomy, reapproximation of mucosal edges, and incorporation of vaginal fascia and uterosacral attachments into the stitches

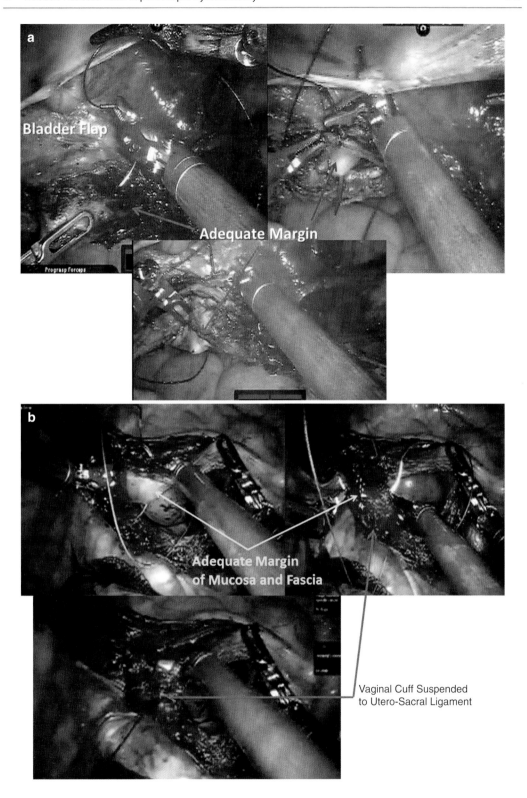

Fig. 17.27 (continued)

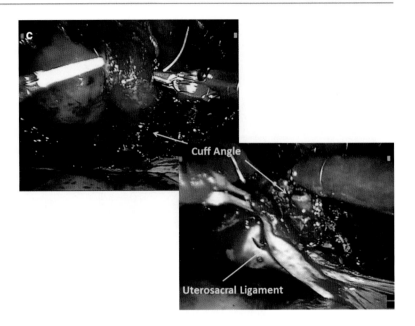

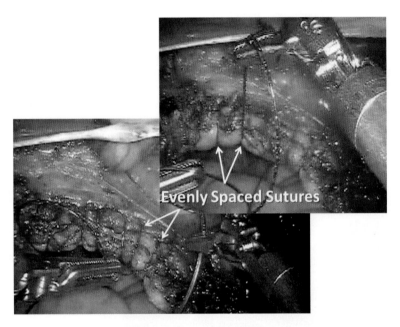

Fig. 17.28 Vaginal cuff closure methods. The cuff may be closed with a single running layer, double layer, or interrupted figure-of-eight sutures. For running closures, longer-lasting 0-PDS (especially in running double-layer closures) or barbed 2-0 or 0-V-Loc™ suture (Covidien, Mansfield, MA) may be used. These sutures do tend to last much longer than more quickly absorbed 0-Vicryl suture, which is often used for figure-of-eight sutures. No matter the technique, special attention should be paid to the angles (achieving both hemostasis and suspension of the vaginal cuff to the uterosacral ligaments) and to even spacing of the sutures reapproximating mucosal and fascial edges

17.5.3.7 Extraction of the Uterus

If the uterus is large, a significant portion of the procedure can involve its extraction. The size, shape, and configuration of the uterus determine which options are available as methods of extraction. Possibilities include myomectomy during the hysterectomy to debulk the uterus; bivalving the uterus and cutting it into segments with the monopolar cut mode of energy, with the uterus in situ after the uterine vasculature is ligated; vaginal morcellation (Fig. 17.29a), mechanical morcellation (Fig. 17.29b), or morcellation through a minilaparotomy incision 3–4 cm in length (Fig. 17.29c). The most important determining factor is the surgeon's comfort with the technique, but the more options a surgeon has, the more easily the task can be completed, as multiple approaches can be taken in one case. It is easiest to morcellate a small uterus vaginally and a medium-sized uterus either vaginally (if a portion will pull into the vagina) or mechanically if it is more bulky or broad and an efficient mechanical morcellator is available. An extremely large uterus can be myomectomized, especially if only one to three large myomas are making the uterus bulky. Once the uterine vasculature and angles are cut, myomectomy may be performed, keeping track of the numbers of fibroids excised to ensure complete removal. These fibroids may then be individually extracted vaginally. Note that it is important to keep the uterus attached to the cuff when applying energy; providing surface area for grounding the monopolar current in order to prevent burns to the bowel or other nearby structures. Similarly, a very bulky uterus can be bivalved or sectioned into fragments. Fragments may then either be stringed for easier removal in a series vaginally, or may be removed individually by placing ring forceps through the vaginal occluder and colpotomy to grasp each fragment and remove it separately.

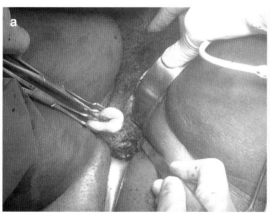 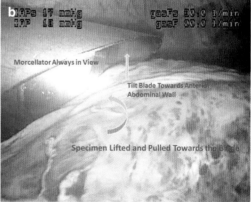

Fig. 17.29 Methods of extraction of a large uterus. (**a**) If the cervix and a part of the uterus can be pulled into the vagina, a long, weighted speculum may be placed to protect the rectum, with one or two vaginal retractors placed anteriorly or laterally to protect the bladder and lateral vaginal side walls. Two double-toothed or triple-toothed tenacula can then be used to place traction on the uterus, and a "paper roll" or "runway" technique can be used to morcellate the uterus with a scalpel, with myomectomies performed as well on the way, until the entire uterus is extracted. (**b**) Alternatively, a mechanical morcellator can be utilized through the camera port or a lateral port to extract the uterus after the vaginal cuff is closed. (**c**) If the uterus is extremely large (>1,000 g) or has severely calcified fibroids, a small (3–4 cm) minilaparotomy incision can be made in the suprapubic area, with the placement of an Alexis wound retractor (Applied Medical; Rancho Santa Margarita, CA). The uterus may then be removed through this small incision via a technique similar to vaginal morcellation

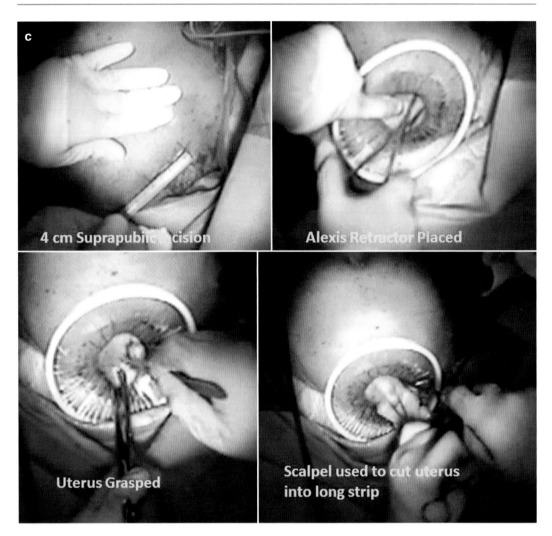

Fig. 17.29 (continued)

17.6   Postoperative Care

One of the main advantages of approaching a complex hysterectomy in a minimally invasive fashion is the remarkably fast postoperative recovery time. The average hospital stay after robotic hysterectomy less than 23 h, with some institutions even advocating same-day discharge as an outpatient procedure. Postoperative care should be the same as it would be for any other laparoscopic hysterectomy, with routine early ambulation, discontinuation of the Foley catheter, and early feeding, all of which encourage expedient recovery. Ambulation should be encouraged as soon after surgery as possible, and the Foley catheter may be discontinued within 6 h after the procedure. A prophylactic gastrointestinal regimen with scheduled intravenous famotidine, with or without the addition of scheduled Reglan (metoclopramide), in addition to early feeding, helps expedite the return of gastrointestinal function and discharge. Scheduled intravenous NSAIDs can greatly reduce the use of narcotic drugs, and patients should be switched to oral narcotics as soon as possible. Thus, the use of patient-controlled analgesia is not necessary; intravenous narcotics should be used only as needed during the initial postoperative period and for breakthrough pain. Table 17.3 summarizes methods of expediting discharge.

Table 17.3 Maximizing utility of a short hospital stay

Component	Expediting features	Modality
Patient expectation	Preoperative education	Preoperative nurse education
		Educational videos
		Written information on what to expect
Nursing	Facilitate early discharge	Nursing education as to postoperative care
		Nurse will reassure patient as to ability to function and encourage patient towards early feeding, ambulation, and voiding trials
Pain	Minimize pain	Schedule IV NSAIDs for baseline pain
		PRN IV narcotics for breakthrough pain
		Start PO narcotics as soon as possible
GI function	Early feeding	Prophylactic GI regimen
		Advance diet as tolerated
		Avoid IV narcotics
GU function	Voiding initiation	Reduce trauma to bladder during surgery
		Discontinue Foley 4–6 h postoperatively
Ambulation	Early ambulation	Encouragement from nurses
		Good pain control
		Early Foley removal
		Early discontinuation of IV fluid

GI gastrointestinal, *GU* genitourinary, *IV* intravenous, *NSAIDs* nonsteroidal anti-inflammatory drugs, *PO* by mouth, *PRN* as needed

References

1. Beste TM, Nelson KH, Daucher JA. Total laparoscopic hysterectomy utilizing a robotic surgical system. JSLS. 2005;9:13–5.
2. Reynolds RK, Advincula AP. Robot-assisted laparoscopic hysterectomy: technique and initial experience. Am J Surg. 2006;191:55–60.
3. Fiorentino RP, Zepeda MA, Goldstein BH, et al. Pilot study assessing robotic laparoscopic hysterectomy and patient outcomes. J Minim Invasive Gynecol. 2006; 13:60–3.
4. Kho RM, Hilger WS, Hentz JG, et al. Robotic hysterectomy: technique and initial outcomes. Am J Obstet Gynecol. 2007;197:113.e1–4.
5. Payne TN, Dauterive FR. A comparison of total laparoscopic hysterectomy to robotically assisted hysterectomy: surgical outcomes in a community practice. J Minim Invasive Gynecol. 2008;15:589–94.
6. Chen CC, Falcone T. Robotic gynecologic surgery: past, present, future. Clin Obstet Gynecol. 2009;52: 335–43.
7. Orady M, Hrynewych A, Nawfal AK, Wegienka G. Comparison of robotic-assisted laparoscopic hysterectomy to other minimally invasive approaches. JSLS. 2012;16:542–8.
8. Payne TN, Dauterinve FR. Robotically assisted hysterectomy: 100 cases after the learning curve. J Robot Surg. 2010;4:11–8.
9. Sarlos D, Kots L, Stevanovic N, Schaer G. Robotic hysterectomy versus conventional laparoscopic hysterectomy: outcome and cost analyses of a matched case-control study. Eur J Obstet Gynecol Reprod Biol. 2010;150:92–6.
10. Orady M, Nawfal AK, Wegienka G. Does size matter? The effect of uterine weight on robot-assisted total laparoscopic hysterectomy outcomes. J Robot Surg. 2011;5:267–72.
11. Payne TN, Dauterive FR, Pitter MC, et al. Robotically assisted hysterectomy in patients with large uteri: outcomes in five community practices. Obstet Gynecol. 2010;115:535–42.
12. Nawfal AK, Orady M, Eisenstein D, Wegienka G. Effect of body mass index on robotic-assisted total laparoscopic hysterectomy. J Minim Invasive Gynecol. 2011;18:328–32.
13. Boggess JF, Gehrig PA, Cantrell L, et al. Perioperative outcomes of robotically assisted hysterectomy for benign cases with complex pathology. Obstet Gynecol. 2009;114:585–93.
14. Lenihan Jr JP, Kovanda C, Seshadri-Kreaden U. What is the learning curve for robotic assisted gynecologic surgery? J Minim Invasive Gynecol. 2008;15:589–94.
15. Klauschie J, Wechter ME, Jacob K, Zanagnolo V, Montero R, Magrina J, Kho R. Use of anti-skid material and patient-positioning to prevent patient shifting during robotic-assisted gynecologic procedures. J Minim Invasive Gynecol. 2010;17:504–7.

Robotic-Assisted Management of Endometriosis

18

Camran Nezhat, Jillian Main, Elizabeth Buescher, Amanda Stevens, and Rose Soliemannjad

Endometriosis is a complex disease in which endometrial glands and stroma grow outside of the endometrial cavity. The classic symptoms of endometriosis consist of dysmenorrhea, dyspareunia, pelvic pain and infertility [1]. In the general reproductive-age population, the prevalence of endometriosis approaches 10 %, but in patients with infertility it can be as high as 50 % [2]. These numbers likely underestimate the true incidence of endometriosis since endometriosis is often undiagnosed or misdiagnosed.

Endometriosis is most commonly found on the pelvic organs or the peritoneal surface of the abdominopelvic cavity, but there are reports of endometriosis affecting many other organ systems. The only place where endometriosis has not been reported is in the spleen [1, 3]. It can involve the urinary tract, gastrointestinal tract, thoracic cavity, and even the heart. Extragenital endometriosis requires a high index of suspicion for diagnosis and a multidisciplinary approach to treatment.

Endometriosis can be treated medically or surgically. Minimally invasive techniques are now the gold standard for the diagnosis and treatment of endometriosis [4]. Because advanced laparoscopy requires a sophisticated skill set, enabling devices have been created to allow more surgeons to perform minimally invasive surgery. The da Vinci Surgical System ("robot," Intuitive Surgical; Sunnydale, CA) is one of these devices and it is an acceptable method for the treatment of endometriosis. For patients who wish to preserve their fertility, treatment is focused on removing endometriotic lesions, restoring normal anatomy, and optimizing fertility. For patients who no longer desire fertility, hysterectomy and bilateral salpingectomy with or without oophorectomy are recommended. Since Endometriosis is a complex disease, the treatment is an evolving process.

18.1 Pathogenesis of Endometriosis

The pathogenesis of endometriosis remains unclear, but there are three leading theories on the etiology: retrograde menstruation, metaplasia of coelomic stem cells, or hematologic and lymphatic spread of endometrial cells. The most popular theory, retrograde menstruation, is generally attributed to Sampson's work in 1927 [5]. Retrograde menstruation is the process by which a small amount of menstrual blood flows through

C. Nezhat, MD (✉) • J. Main, MD
R. Soliemannjad • E. Buescher, MD, MEd
A. Stevens, MD
Department of OBGYN, Center for Special Minimally Invasive and Robotic Surgery, Stanford University Medical Center, 900 Welch Road, Suite 403, Palo Alto, CA 94304, USA
e-mail: cnezhat@stanford.edu;
jillianmain@gmail.com; lizziebuescher@gmail.com;
mandistevensmd@gmail.com;
rsoleimannjad@gmail.com

P.F. Escobar, T. Falcone (eds.), *Atlas of Single-Port, Laparoscopic, and Robotic Surgery*,
DOI 10.1007/978-1-4614-6840-0_18, © Springer Science+Business Media New York 2014

the fallopian tubes and into the peritoneal cavity with each cycle. The theory suggests that the endometrial cells in the menstrual blood can implant on the peritoneum and form endometriosis. Pelvic surgery performed at the time of menses confirms that retrograde menstruation occurs [6]. The anatomic distribution of endometriotic lesions supports this theory as most lesions are in the dependent portion of the abdomino-pelvic cavity and favor the left hemi-pelvis. While this theory explains how endometrial cells are present outside the uterus, it does not explain why these cells escape immune system clearance, implant, proliferate and cause symptoms.

The second theory, coelomic metaplasia, arises because both endometrial and peritoneal cells are derived from coelomic cells. It is theorized that undifferentiated coelomic cells in the peritoneum undergo metaplastic change into endometrial cells. This theory is supported by reports of endometriosis in women with congenital absence of a uterus and in men undergoing high-dose estrogen treatment for prostate cancer [7, 8]. The trigger that causes this transformation is uncertain, but it is generally thought to be inflammation or hormonal stimulation [4].

The theory of lymphatic and hematologic spread helps explain the presence of endometriosis in areas remote from the abdominopelvic cavity, such as the eye or the brain. This theory postulates that endometrial cells are spread through the lymphatic or hematologic systems, much like the metastatic spread of cancer. There is known lymph spread from the endometrium to lymph nodes and endometrial cells have been found in the lymph nodes of 6.7 % of women at autopsy [9].

Although these present as three distinct theories, it is likely that all contribute to the pathogenesis of this enigmatic disease. However, the inciting event and process by which endometriosis is permitted to persist and proliferate is still elusive.

18.2 Prevalence of Endometriosis

The diagnosis of endometriosis requires a high index of suspicion and access to health care practitioners who are familiar with the disorder. The prevalence of endometriosis is likely underestimated because patients are often misdiagnosed as having "normal" menstrual pain, irritable bowel syndrome, recurrent infections, ovarian cysts or psychological disorders. Most clinicians consider endometriosis to have a prevalence of 6–10 % in the general reproductive aged population and 35–50 % in women with pain and/or infertility [2]. A diagnosis of endometriosis should be considered in patients with unexplained infertility and pelvic pain, as some practices report up to 90 % of these women have had pathology-proven endometriosis [4]. One of the difficulties in the understanding endometriosis is that the severity of symptoms does not always correlate with the stage of disease. Some women with advanced disease have only minimal symptoms while other women with early stage disease have significant pain and infertility issues. Additionally, there is evolving information about the correlation of endometriosis in women with fibroids, one of the most common gynecologic diagnoses. There is a recent study showing that 86 % of patients with uterine myomas also have endometriosis [10]. If the prevalence of fibroids reaches over 50 % by the age of 45, and a significant portion of these patients have concomitant endometriosis, the prevalence of endometriosis is likely much higher than the quoted values.

18.3 Treatment of Endometriosis: General Concepts

Endometriosis can be treated either medically or surgically, depending on the severity of symptoms and the patient's goals of fertility. The primary goal of medical treatment is to decrease the amount of systemic estrogen since endometriosis proliferates in the presence of estrogen. Combined estrogen-progesterone pills or progesterone pills are primarily used to suppress the estrogen surge that occurs in ovulation and promote decidualization of endometriotic lesions. Gonadotropin-releasing hormone (GnRH) agonists, which significantly decrease circulating estrogen, should only be used for short-term therapy due to the adverse side effects on bone and cardiovascular health seen with long-term use.

When patients present with pain that is refractory to medical management, infertility that is refractory to assisted reproduction techniques, or endometriotic ovarian cysts, surgical treatment is indicated. Medical therapy can then be used to keep the endometriosis in remission after surgery, provided that the patient does not desire immediate fertility. For young patients with infertility and endometriosis, natural conception after surgery has yielded promising results [11]. For older patients, in vitro fertilization may be necessary for fertility [12].

18.4 Treatment of Endometriosis: Computer-Enhanced Technology

Minimally invasive surgery is the gold standard for the diagnosis and treatment of endometriosis. Technological advances such as video-assisted laparoscopy and the robot help surgeons increase the proportion of minimally invasive surgical procedures they perform. Dr Camran Nezhat first reported video-assisted laparoscopic surgery for the treatment of extensive endometriosis in 1986 [13]. He reported that the limiting factor in laparoscopy is the skill and experience of the surgeon, and the availability of proper instrumentation [14]. Modern surgical tools have expanded the gynecologic surgeon's ability to treat endometriosis. These include the CO_2 laser, monopolar and bipolar electrocautery, the PlasmaJet (Plasma Surgical, Inc.; Roswell, GA), and the da Vinci Surgical System "robot" (Intuitive Surgical Inc., Sunnyvale, CA). These instruments allow for the resection or vaporization of endometriosis. Although this chapter focuses on the robot technology, the gynecologic surgeon should be adept at different modalities to treat endometriosis and the general principles of treatment remain the same. Conservative surgery should often be considered first, with the goal to remove all visible endometriotic lesions and restore normal anatomy. For women who have no desire for future fertility, there is a continued role for more radical surgery such as a hysterectomy.

In general, there is a need for enabling devices that allow surgeons to convert more open procedures to endoscopic procedures. There is also a need for instruments that allow surgeons to practice in a virtual setting, instead of learning on patients. Incorporation of computer-enhanced technology in surgery, such as the da Vinci robot, is one development that contributes to achieving these goals [15].

18.5 Computer-Enhanced Technology: The Robot

The introduction of the da Vinci robot in 1999 has enabled more surgeons to treat advanced endometriosis in a minimally invasive manner. Robotic-assisted surgery provides three-dimensional views and has articulating instruments that more closely resemble the movements of the human wrist. This articulation makes surgical techniques, such as suturing, running the bowel, and manipulation of delicate tissues, easier to master with the robot than with traditional laparoscopy. The robot also provides tremor filtration, allowing more precise movements, and a seated console, decreasing physician fatigue. This may have the potential benefit of allowing highly experienced physicians to continue operating later into their careers. As physicians and hospitals integrate the robot into patient care, it is important to dedicate a specific surgical team to help reduce operating times. Studies have shown that robotic surgeries take longer to complete than their laparoscopic counterparts, but the operating time decreases as more procedures are performed [16]. The primary advantage of the robot over laparoscopy is that the robot has a shorter learning curve, thereby enabling more physicians to provide their patients with minimally invasive surgical treatment [17]. Despite the numerous advantages of laparoscopy over laparotomy, the majority of major gynecologic procedures are still performed via laparotomy. Because robotic-assisted laparoscopic surgery has the potential to lower the incidence of laparotomy, it must be considered a major medical advance.

However, as with all surgical tools, the robot presents its own set of challenges and potential complications. The da Vinci robot does not have haptic perception, so the surgeon cannot feel the tension being placed on the tissues. In addition, there are limitations in the instrumentation offered by da Vinci at this time. This limitation will likely resolve as more innovations and instrumentation become available. Finally, one of the most cited drawbacks is that the cost of purchasing and maintaining the da Vinci robot is often prohibitively high [18]. This is an important consideration in the current state of the healthcare economy.

18.6   Surgical Technique: Robotic Set-up

Appropriate positioning to maximize exposure and minimize the risk of neuromuscular injury are even more important with the robot due to the size of the device and the remote console. The patient should be placed in the dorsal lithotomy position using Allen stirrups, which is the standard position for all gynecologic laparoscopic surgery. Care must be taken to avoid pressure points in positioning the arms and legs. A de-flatable beanbag can be helpful to maintain a gentle but secure position. Both arms are wrapped in protective padding and tucked at the patient's side. Tucking the arms is crucial for several reasons. First, during the laparoscopic portions of the procedure, the surgeon's movements will be limited if the arms are not tucked in. Second, because the surgeon is stationed at the console, he or she may inadvertently put pressure on an arm if it is not tucked. Additionally, care must be taken to assure proper protection for the patient's face and eyes because there is increased risk of corneal abrasion with robotic surgery [19].

The abdomen should be entered through the umbilicus, unless the patient has a mass such as a fibroid or ovarian cyst that extends superior to the umbilicus, or a prior midline vertical incision extending to above the umbilicus. In patients such as these, peritoneal access can be obtained through a left upper quadrant port or a port between the umbilicus and the xyphoid process. Lateral ports are placed two centimeters medial to the anterior superior iliac spine and several fingerbreadths above the iliac spine at approximately the same level. Trocar placement should depend on the specific pathology and body habitus of each patient. In general, the trocars are placed a few centimeters superior to the placement for laparoscopy. Each robotic trocar should be at least 8–10 cm from adjacent trocars, so that the robotic arms do not collide and limit movement. Because the robot does not have haptic perception, the surgeon cannot feel if the instruments are colliding from the console. This makes proper set-up even more important. An assistant port can be placed in the upper quadrant or suprapubically, depending on assistant comfort. The accessory ports should be placed under direct visualization to avoid injury to the bladder, bowel, and other nearby structures.

Once the trocars are placed, the robot must be docked. Side docking is usually preferred as it allows for superior vaginal access and uterine manipulation during the course of surgery [20, 21]. In side docking, the robot is aligned at the outside of either the patient's left or right leg, depending on the specific operating room set-up and the surgeon's preference. Once the robotic arms are docked, it is important to confirm that the full range of motion of the arms will not cause inadvertent injury to the patient's extremities or face. There are usually two assistants required to allow for abdominal assistance and uterine manipulation.

18.7 Surgical Technique: Recognizing Endometriosis

Laparoscopic assessment of the abdominopelvic cavity with histologic examination of the surgical specimens remains the gold standard for the diagnosis of endometriosis. Surgeons must be knowledgeable in the most common locations and physical appearance of endometriosis in order to make an accurate diagnosis and provide complete treatment. Peritoneal implants are most commonly localized to the uterosacral ligaments, posterior cul-de-sac, ovarian fossa, and adjacent pelvic sidewalls. Less frequently, implants may also be found in the upper abdomen, ovaries, bladder, bowel and diaphragm. Careful inspection of the entire peritoneal cavity should be performed, including turning the camera to the upper abdomen prior to robot docking [22].

The magnification and three-dimensional camera of the robot may offer an improved ability to identify implants of endometriosis. Complete removal of endometriotic implants is difficult because of variability in appearance, visibility, and location on sensitive structures such as the ureter. Lesions are described using different terminology. "Powder burn" lesions are some of the most commonly described lesions that appear as a dark burn on the peritoneum or organ surface (Fig. 18.1). They represent foci of disease and usually contain endometrial glands and stroma. Hemosiderin deposits, which appear as brown pigmentations, are also commonly associated with endometriosis. Atypical and non-pigmented lesions are seen as clear vesicles, pink vascular patterns, white-scarred lesions, red lesions, yellow-brown patches, and peritoneal windows. The peritoneum must be examined from different angles and at different degrees of illumination to see vesicles or whitish lesions, and the peritoneal folds must be stretched and searched for small, atypical lesions. When surgery is performed on patients with chronic pelvic pain, a biopsy of the uterosacral ligaments is strongly recommended, even if they appear grossly normal. The uterosacral ligaments often contain microscopic disease and its excision may help the patient's pain [23].

An increased awareness of the variations in the appearance of endometriotic lesions has resulted in an increase in the diagnosis of endometriosis at laparoscopy [22]. It is essential that that gynecologic surgeons become adept at recognizing manifestations of endometriosis, in order to completely treat the disease at the time of surgery.

Endometriomas are one of the most common manifestations of endometriosis diagnosed by general gynecologists. An endometrioma is an ovarian cyst that contains endometrial glands and stoma and usually contains a thick fluid the color of chocolate. Nezhat and coworkers classified endometriomas according to their characteristics and histology [4, 24]. Type I endometriomas are primary endometriomas. They are small, usually less than 2 cm in size, and histologically contain only endometrial glands and stroma (Fig. 18.2). They develop from invagination of surface endometriotic implants and are difficult to excise surgically because they adhere to the surface of the ovary. The ovarian stroma may be compromised by surgically removing these cysts if improper surgical technique is used. They can be treated by either vaporization or excision; however, excision is the preferred method because it has a lower likelihood of recurrence. If the surgeon is unable to remove the cyst wall without compromising ovarian stroma, then the cyst wall should be left attached to the ovary and ablated. This technique is surgically simpler and less time-consuming than excising the cyst wall in its entirety [25]. Type II endometriomas are functional cysts that have been invaded by endometriosis. They are much easier to remove than type I endometriomas and can be further subdivided into three classes. Endometrioma type IIA has less than 50 % of the cyst wall invaded by endometrial glands and stroma. In type IIB, endometrial glands and stroma invade 50 % of the cyst wall, and in type IIC, endometrial glands and stroma invade more than 50 % of the cyst wall. As endometriomas progress from type IIA to type IIC, they become increasingly difficult to excise. Endometriomas almost always need to be surgically treated because they do not spontaneously resolve [24].

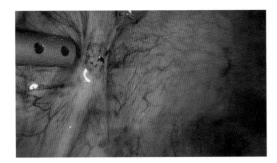

Fig. 18.1 Powder burn lesions [1]

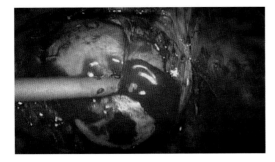

Fig. 18.2 Endometriomas immediately prior to resection [1]

18.8 Surgical Management: Conservative Surgery

In young patients who desire fertility, conservative surgery should be attempted. The goals of conservative operative procedures are to remove all implants, resect adhesions, reduce the risk of recurrence, and restore the involved organs to a normal anatomic and physiologic condition. When endometriosis is severe and obliterates the surgical planes, dissection can be very difficult, making the da Vinci robot helpful. In patients with severe disease and the desire for fertility, the posterior cul-de-sac (Fig. 18.3) and tubo-ovarian anatomy must be normalized to increase fertility [1]. Much debate has been raised over ablation versus resection of endometriosis. As long as the lesions are completely eradicated the method of removal is inconsequential.

Conservative surgery should not be considered definitive treatment for endometriosis. Although such procedures are seldom curative, they often improve the likelihood of pregnancy and offer temporary pain relief and improved quality of life [1, 4, 26]. Reoperation is not uncommon because of recurrence of endometriosis or progression of residual microscopic disease. The rate of repeat intervention is directly related to the extent of disease, the completeness of removal, the ability to conceive postoperatively, the use of postsurgical suppressive therapy, and the use of fertility-enhancing medications [27]. Because pregnancy is a progesterone-dominant state, many women will have symptomatic improvement during pregnancy. In conjunction, women who undergo infertility treatment are more likely to have a recurrence of the disease because of the high estrogen state.

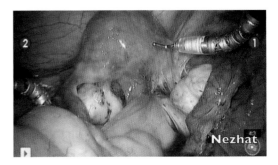

Fig. 18.3 Posterior cul-de-sac that has been obliterated by endometriosis, resulting in the loss of surgical planes and scarring of both ovaries

18.9   Surgical Management: Hysterectomy and Bilateral Salpingo-oophorectomy

Radical surgery is indicated for patients who no longer desire fertility and who have severe symptoms that are unresponsive to medical or conservative surgical treatment. Procedures include hysterectomy, salpingectomy, possible oophorectomy and the excision of deeply infiltrating endometriosis. This could involve partial resection of the bowel, bladder, or ureter in extreme cases [20]. Bilateral oophorectomy is done for the purpose of decreasing the estrogen that sustains and stimulates the ectopic endometrium, but there is a more recent trend towards ovarian preservation. In advanced disease, the ovaries may be encased and densely adherent to the pelvic sidewall. Ovarian dissection entails the risk of injury to the ureter, major blood vessels, and the bowel. A retroperitoneal approach can isolate the ureter throughout its course to ensure complete removal of ovarian tissue and prevent ovarian remnant syndrome. Some advocate the preservation of one ovary to avoid the long-term health risks associated with premature surgical menopause. However, such surgeries are not considered definitive and future surgery may be required to remove the remaining ovary for. In 2009, a large prospective study with 24 years of follow up reported that patients who underwent bilateral oophorectomy before the age of 65 had an increased risk of all-cause death. Since publication, many gynecologists have hesitated to perform oophorectomy. In general, it is better to begin with conservative surgery and then proceed to definitive surgery that may include oophorectomy. Oophorectomy should be considered only after the patient has had a trial of GnRH agonists to induce short-term cessation of ovarian function.

It must be noted that because of the obliteration of tissue planes from endometriosis, ovarian remnant are sometimes left behind during definitive surgery. That remnant can continue to cause proliferation of endometriosis. An ovarian remnant may be palpable on pelvic examination or may be visualized on pelvic ultrasound. Because of the scarring involved, it is often difficult to locate and excise these lesions. Ureteral stents can be helpful in patients with suspected ovarian remnant syndrome to help identify the ureters during surgery.

18.10   Postoperative Management

Although surgery can eradicate the visible endometriotic lesions, there is a role for post-operative medical suppression of the microscopic lesions. The goal of medical therapy is to avoid the estrogen surge that comes with ovulation and promote decidualization of the endometriotic lesions [28]. Patients who do not desire immediate fertility generally benefit from an oral contraceptive pill or a progesterone containing intra-uterine device. Gonadotropin-releasing hormone agonists, which decrease total estrogen, can be used short term post-operatively, but are slightly controversial in terms of pain improvement of decreased recurrence [29, 30]. Gonadotropin-releasing hormone agonists might be beneficial in women with severe disease who are undergoing a two-stage surgical procedure to suppress regrowth of endometriosis between the two surgeries.

In pre-menopausal women who have undergone total hysterectomy and bilateral salpingo-oophorectomy, treatment with a low dose of estrogen not only avoids the symptoms of menopause, but also maintains cardiovascular and bone health. A joint patient-physician decision must consider the suppression of endometriosis, patient comfort, and overall health.

For women with chronic pelvic pain, the role of a multi-disciplinary team for long-term pain management and treatment is indicated. This team could include a chronic pelvic pain specialist, pelvic floor physical therapist, psychologist, pain management anesthesiologist and acupuncturist.

18.11 Extragenital Endometriosis

Although endometriosis is classically found in pelvic organs, it can be found outside of the genital tract in up to 12 % of cases [3]. The most common sites for extragenital endometriosis are the urinary system and the bowel, but endometriosis can also be found in the lung, diaphragm, liver, and even brain.

Endometriosis may spread to the urinary system in 1–5 % of women with symptomatic endometriosis [3]. Urinary tract endometriosis most commonly affects the bladder, but can also be seen as involving the ureter and the kidney. Endometriosis of the urinary tract tends to be superficial, but may be invasive and cause significant symptoms. The signs and symptoms of bladder endometriosis include suprapubic pain, dysuria, hematuria, frequency, and dyspareunia. These symptoms may be cyclic in nature, but often are not associated with the menstrual cycle. Clinicians should consider endometriosis in cases of refractory and unexplained urinary complaints. If bladder endometriosis is suspected, a computed tomography (CT) scan with IV contrast and delayed images to evaluate the ureters should be completed. In cases of recurrent hematuria or a strong suspicion for endometriosis, a cystoscopic examination is indicated. If any lesions are noted on cystoscopy, a biopsy is recommended to confirm the diagnosis of bladder endometriosis. The majority of cases of bladder endometriosis are superficial lesions. For full-thickness lesions, segmental bladder resection may be indicated [3, 20].

Ureteral endometriosis is less common than that of the bladder, but can have more devastating consequences due to obstruction. The distal third of the ureter is the most common site of involvement, with the left ureter being involved more often than the right. Signs of ureteral endometriosis include hematuria, flank pain, back pain, abdominal pain, and dysuria. As with bladder endometriosis, symptoms may or may not be cyclical. Computed tomography with IV contrast or IV pyelogram may show hydroureter or hydronephrosis (Fig. 18.4). If the ureter is compressed by endometriosis, causing hydroureter or hydro-

nephrosis, surgical treatment via ureterolysis is mandatory (Fig. 18.5). Ureteral stent placement may be helpful in these cases. If the endometriosis invades through the ureter, segmental resection with either reimplantation or uretero-ureterostomy is indicated, depending on the level of the obstruction [20].

Endometriosis of the kidney is exceedingly rare and only merits a brief mention in this chapter. Signs and symptoms are similar to those of ureteral endometriosis. In addition, a renal mass may be noted on imaging. When this occurs, the mass is generally treated with partial or complete nephrectomy [3].

The gastrointestinal tract is involved in 3–37 % of women with endometriosis [31]. Endometriotic implants are most commonly found on the rectosigmoid colon, appendix, rectum, and cecum. Bowel endometriosis may be completely asymptomatic, but often will present with diarrhea, constipation, rectal bleeding, dyschezia, hematochezia or abdominal pain. The evaluation of a patient with suspected gastrointestinal endometriosis should include a fecal occult blood test, a colonoscopy, and possibly a CT scan or MRI prior to surgery. These tests rarely change in the treatment of the patient with endometriosis, but are helpful to rule out other causes of bowel dysfunction, especially malignancy [3, 32]. Operative laparoscopy, often facilitated by the robot, is performed to treat endometriotic implants on the intestinal wall, appendix, and rectovaginal space (Fig. 18.6) [33]. The surgery performed varies, depending on the patient, but can include appendectomy, disc excision, or bowel resection. Bowel resection should be reserved only for those patients who continue to have symptoms despite more conservative forms of treatment or present with obstructive symptoms.

Thoracic endometriosis, although less common than endometriosis of the genitourinary or gastrointestinal system, is another important site of extragenital endometriosis. The most common presenting symptoms are chest pain, catamenial pneumothorax, catamenial hemoptysis, catamenial hemothorax, or lung nodules [34, 35]. Women should be asked about pleuritic, shoulder, or upper abdominal pain occurring with menses because they often do not correlate the symptoms. The diagnosis requires a high clinical suspicion and a thorough history during the evaluation. The evaluation of the patient with suspected thoracic endometriosis may include chest radiograph, chest CT, chest MRI, bronchoscopy, and thoracentesis to evaluate for other etiologies of the symptoms. If it has been determined

preoperatively that the patient may have thoracic endometriosis, robotic or laparoscopic thoracic surgery should be performed by a cardiothoracic surgeon at the time of pelvic surgery [35]. During the video-assisted thoracoscopic surgery, any endometriotic implants should be ablated or resected and any scarring of the lung to the thoracic side wall should be treated surgically (Fig. 18.7 and 18.8).

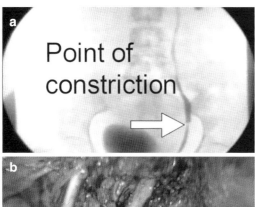

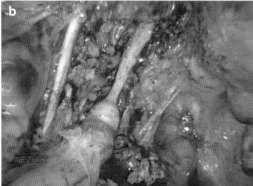

Fig. 18.4 (**a**) Intravenous pyelogram showing a ureteral stricture with hydroureter. (**b**) Confirmed pyelogram

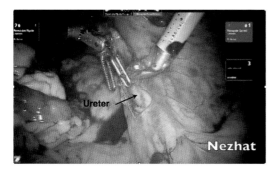

Fig. 18.5 Ureterolysis initiated by incision of the pelvic peritoneum at the pelvic brim

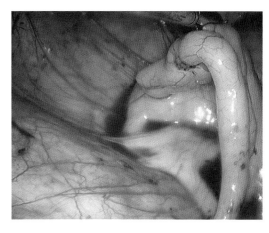

Fig. 18.6 Black and red endometriosis spots on appendix [1]

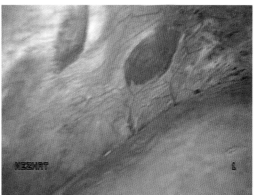

Fig. 18.7 Endometriosis as seen and ablated on the thoracic side wall, improving the patient's symptoms postoperatively [1]

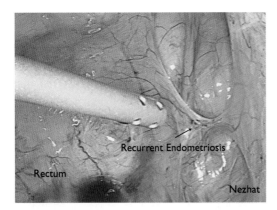

Fig. 18.8 Endometriosis recurrence at left pararectal site of previous excision [1]

18.12 The Future of Endometriosis and Robotic-Assisted Surgery

Despite the prevalence of endometriosis and decades of research and surgical experience, there are still many questions about this enigmatic disease. It is likely that each of the pathogenesis theories plays a role in endometriosis. There is currently promising research into the genetics and biochemical pathways of endometriosis, but much is still unknown. Until we have a better understanding of the basic etiology of the disease, and why some women are preferentially affected by their endometriosis, we will not be able to target individualized treatment.

Women with endometrioses are challenging because they often have multiple symptoms and multiple diagnoses involving the genitourinary and gastrointestinal tract. Endometriosis treatment often requires a multidisciplinary approach. This could include the gynecologist, a pelvic pain specialist, a physical therapist, a pain management team, a urogynecologist, and a gastroenterologist.

Until the day of individualized medicine arrives, practitioners will continue to manage symptomatic endometriosis with the tools currently available: generalized hormonal management and surgery. Computer-enhanced technology has revolutionized the surgical arena. The advent and popularization of laparoscopy was the initial technological advance to markedly improve patient care and outcomes by the introduction of abdominal minimally invasive surgery [1]. Robotic-assisted surgery has increased both physician and patient access to minimally invasive surgery by making laparoscopy technically easier. It also has the potential to increase minimally invasive surgery on a global scale via telesurgery and telementoring. Although there is debate over the future role of robotic-assisted surgery, if it increases the incidence of minimally invasive procedures and decreases the incidence of laparotomy, this is an undeniably positive outcome for patients. As more physicians become competent in minimally invasive techniques via laparoscopy or robotic surgery, we will see better patient outcomes and improved patient satisfaction.

Acknowledgment This chapter has been supported in part by an educational grant from the Zimmerman Foundation.

References

1. Nezhat C, Nezhat F. Endometriosis: ancient disease, ancient treatments. Fertil Steril. 2012;98(6S Suppl): S1–62.
2. Giudice LC, Kao LC. Endometriosis. Lancet. 2004;364:1789–99.
3. Veeraswamy A, Lewis M, Mann A, Kotikela S, Hajhosseini B, Nezhat C. Extragenital endometriosis. Clin Obstet Gynecol. 2010;53:449–66.
4. Nezhat C, Nezhat F, Nezhat CH. Nezhat's video-assisted and robotic-assisted laparoscopy and hysteroscopy. 4th ed. New York: Cambridge University Press; 2013. p. 1–17. 267–302.
5. Sampson JA. Peritoneal endometriosis due to menstrual dissemination of endometrial tissue into the peritoneal cavity. Am J Obstet Gynecol. 1927;14:422–69.
6. Halme J, Hammond MG, Hulka JF, et al. Retrograde menstruation in healthy women and in patients with endometriosis. Obstet Gynecol. 1984;64(2):151–4.
7. Rosenfeld DL, Lecher BD. Endometriosis is a patient with Rokitansky-Kuster-Hauser-syndrome. Am J Obstet Gynecol. 1981;139(1):105.
8. Schrodt GR, Alcorn MO, Ibanez J. Endometriosis of the male urinary system: a case report. J Urol. 1980; 124(5):722–3.
9. Javert CT. The spread of benign and malignant endometrium in the lymphatic system with a note on coexisting vascular involvement. Am J Obstet Gynecol. 1952;64(4):780–806.
10. Huang JQ, Lathi RB, Lemyre M, Rodriguez HE, Nezhat CH, Nezhat C. Coexistence of endometriosis in women with symptomatic leiomyomas. Fertil Steril. 2010;94:720–3.

11. Lee HJ, Lee JE, Ku SY, et al. Natural conception rate following laparoscopic surgery in infertile women with endometriosis. Clin Exp Reprod Med. 2013; 40(1):29–32.

12. Littman E, Giudice L, Lathi R, Berker B, Milki A, Nezhat C. Role of laparoscopic treatment of endometriosis in patients with failed in vitro fertilization cycles. Fertil Steril. 2005;84:1574–8.

13. Nezhat C, Crowgey SR, Garrison CP. Surgical treatment of endometriosis via laser laparoscopy. Fertil Steril. 1986;45:778–83.

14. Nezhat CR. When will video-assisted and robotic-assisted endoscopy replace almost all open surgeries? J Minim Invasive Gynecol. 2012;19:238–43.

15. Wright JD, et al. AAGL position statement: robotic-assisted laparoscopic surgery in benign gynecology. J Minim Invasive Gynecol. 2013;20:2–9.

16. Nezhat C, Lewis M, Kotikela S, Veeraswamy A, Saadat L, Hajhosseini B. Robotic versus standard laparoscopy for the treatment of endometriosis. Fertil Steril. 2010;94:2758–60.

17. Nezhat C, Lavie O, Lemyre M, et al. Robot-assisted laparoscopic surgery in gynecology: scientific dream or reality? Fertil Steril. 2009;91(6):2620–2.

18. Barbash GI, Glied SA. New technology and health care costs: the case of robot-assisted surgery. N Engl J Med. 2010;363:701–4.

19. Gainsburg DM, Wax D, Reich DL, Carlucci JR, Samadi DB. Intraoperative management of robotic-assisted versus open radical prostatectomy. JSLS. 2010;14(1):1–5.

20. Nezhat C, Hajhosseini B, King LP. Robotic-assisted laparoscopic treatment of bowel, bladder, and ureteral endometriosis. JSLS. 2011;15:387–92.

21. Einarsson JI, Hibner M, Advincula AP. Side docking: an alternative docking method for gynecologic robotic surgery. Rev Obstet Gynecol. 2011;4:123–5.

22. Schipper E, Nezhat C. Video-assisted laparoscopy for the detection and diagnosis of endometriosis: safety, reliability, and invasiveness. Int J Womens Health. 2012;4:383–93.

23. Nascu PC, Vilos GA, Ettler HC, Abu-Rafea B, Hollet-Caines J, Ahmad R. Histopathologic findings on uterosacral ligaments in women with chronic pelvic pain and visually normal pelvis at laparoscopy. J Minim Invasive Gynecol. 2006;13: 201–4.

24. Nezhat C, Nezhat F, Seidman DS. Classification of endometriosis. Improving the classification of endometriotic ovarian cysts. Hum Reprod. 1994;9:2212–3.

25. Donnez J, Squifflet J, Jadoul P, Lousse JC, Dolmans MM, Donnez O. Fertility preservation in women with ovarian endometriosis. Front Biosci (Elite Ed). 2012;4:1654–62.

26. Davis CJ, McMillan L. Pain in endometriosis: effectiveness of medical and surgical management. Curr Opin Obstet Gynecol. 2003;15:507–12.

27. Paka C, Miller J, Nezhat C. Predictive factors and treatment of recurrence of endometriosis. Minerva Ginecol. 2013;65(2):105–11.

28. Seracchioli R, Mabrouk M, Manuzzi L, et al. Post-operative use of oral contraceptive pills for prevention of anatomical relapse or symptom recurrence after conservative surgery for endometriosis. Hum Reprod. 2009;24:2729–35.

29. Vercellini P, Crosignani PG, Fadini R, et al. A gonadotrophin-releasing hormone agonist compared with expectant management after conservative surgery for symptomatic endometriosis. Br J Obstet Gynaecol. 1999;106:672–7.

30. Busacca M, Somigliana E, Bianchi S, et al. Post-operative GnRH analogue treatment after conservative surgery for symptomatic endometriosis stage III-IV: a randomized controlled trial. Hum Reprod. 2001;16(11):2399–402.

31. Ferrero S, Camerini G, Maggiore ULR, Venturini PL, Biscaldi E, Remorgida V. Bowel endometriosis: recent insights and unsolved problems. World J Gastrointest Surg. 2011;3(3):31–8.

32. Nezhat C, Hojhosseini B, King LP. Laparoscopic management of bowel endometriosis: predictors of severe disease and recurrence. JSLS. 2011;15:431–8.

33. Berker B, Lashay N, Davarpanah R, Marziali M, Nezhat CH, Nezhat C. Laparoscopic appendectomy in patients with endometriosis. J Minim Invasive Gynecol. 2005;12:206.

34. Joseph J, Sahn SA. Thoracic endometriosis syndrome: new observations from an analysis of 110 cases. Am J Med. 1996;100:164–70.

35. Nezhat C, Nicoll LM, Bhagan L, et al. Endometriosis of the diaphragm: four cases treated with a combination of laparoscopy and thoracoscopy. J Minim Invasive Gynecol. 2009;16:573–80.

Robotic Surgery in Gynecologic Oncology

19

Javier F. Magrina

The application of robotic technology for abdominal and pelvic surgery has had a strong impact in gynecologic oncological surgery. The most influential result is a decrease in the number of procedures performed by laparotomy. Many centers have evolved from a laparotomy to a robotic approach, and centers that were performing advanced laparoscopic procedures have discovered the advantages of robotic technology for gynecologic oncological operations. When analyzing perioperative outcomes for laparotomy, laparoscopy, and robotic surgery, three major benefits appear in almost all studies: reduced blood loss, shorter hospitalization, and shorter recovery to normal activities. Operating times are similar or longer, and postoperative complications are similar or reduced, for laparoscopy and robotic surgery patients. In our experience, when comparing laparoscopy and robotic perioperative outcomes, the advantages of the robotic procedures were shorter operating times for radical hysterectomy and a lower conversion rate for endometrial cancer. Otherwise, outcomes for blood loss, hospital days, and intraoperative and postoperative complications were similar.

J.F. Magrina, MD
Department of Gynecology, Division of Gynecologic Oncology, Mayo Clinic in Arizona,
5779 East Mayo Boulevard,
Phoenix, AZ 85054, USA
e-mail: jmagrina@mayo.edu

19.1 Endometrial Cancer

Endometrial adenocarcinoma is the most common malignancy of the female reproductive tract. In 2009, the Centers for Disease Control and Prevention reported 44,192 new cases in the United States [1]. The risk factors for this condition include obesity, hypertension, diabetes mellitus, chronic anovulation, and exogenous estrogen. As obesity has become an epidemic in the United States, the numbers of endometrial cancers has increased. For instance, there were 44,692 cases in 2009 whereas there will be 49,560 in 2013 [1].

The treatment for endometrial cancer is surgical. Historically, this included an exploratory laparotomy. However, a prospective randomized trial by the Gynecologic Oncology Group demonstrated that a minimally invasive approach is feasible, with minimal intraoperative complications [2] and recurrence and survival rates similar to those for laparotomy [3]. Robotic laparoscopic assistance overcomes some of the challenges of conventional laparoscopy, allowing a minimally invasive approach to more patients, while providing perioperative results similar to those of laparoscopy and better than laparotomy [4–7]. In our experience, we have observed a 3 % conversion rate with robotics and 10 % for laparoscopy patients [4].

P.F. Escobar, T. Falcone (eds.), *Atlas of Single-Port, Laparoscopic, and Robotic Surgery*,
DOI 10.1007/978-1-4614-6840-0_19, © Springer Science+Business Media New York 2014

19.2 Robotic Total Hysterectomy with Bilateral Pelvic and Para-aortic Lymphadenectomy

19.2.1 Patient Position and Preparation

During any robotic procedure, it is crucial to ensure that the patient is secured to the operating room table. We prefer inexpensive, disposable foam egg crate beneath the entire torso to prevent significant patient slippage during steep Trendelenburg (Fig. 19.1).

The patient is positioned in the dorsal lithotomy position, with the legs in either Allen stirrups or Yellofin stirrups. It is advised that the buttocks be positioned approximately 2 in. beyond the edge of the operating room table to allow the second assistant better access to the uterine manipulator and to prevent extreme patient positioning change. The patient's arms should always be tucked, with either arm extenders or padding to avoid nerve injury.

The patient is prepared and draped in the usual sterile fashion. An orogastric or nasogastric tube is placed to decompress the stomach, and a Foley catheter is placed to decompress the bladder and monitor urine output during the procedure.

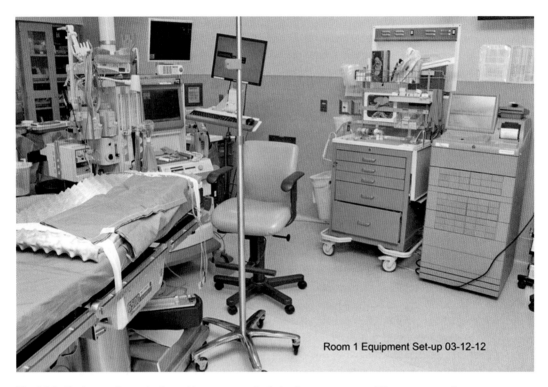

Room 1 Equipment Set-up 03-12-12

Fig. 19.1 Equipment for a robotic total hysterectomy includes foam egg crate padding to prevent slippage

19.2.2 Equipment and Robotic Column

Two monitors, being held by ceiling booms, are located at each side of the operating table at the level of the patient's knees. The robotic tower and the tower containing electrosurgical generators and active smoke evacuators are positioned to the right or left of the patient's feet, depending on the operating room organization.

19.2.3 Trocar Placement and Docking

We prefer the open Hasson transumbilical entry technique with a 12-mm trocar. A CO_2 pneumoperitoneum is created once intraperitoneal entrance is confirmed. The robotics laparoscope is used to perform a survey of the upper abdomen and pelvis. Two 8-mm robotic trocars are placed bilaterally, 10 cm distal to and at the level of the umbilicus. An accessory 10-mm trocar is placed 3 cm cranial and equidistant between the umbilical and left lateral ports. An additional 8-mm robotic trocar is placed in the right lower quadrant at the level of the cecum (Fig. 19.2). The patient is placed in enough Trendelenburg to shift the small bowel and sigmoid out of the pelvis.

The robotic column is side-docked to the patient's right in our operating room. An EndoWrist monopolar spatula or scissors (Intuitive Surgical Inc., Sunnyvale, CA), depending on the surgeon's preference, is inserted through the right lateral trocar and an EndoWrist PK bipolar grasper (Intuitive Surgical Inc., Sunnyvale, CA) is inserted through the left lateral trocar. EndoWrist ProGrasp forceps (Intuitive Surgical Inc., Sunnyvale, CA) is inserted through the right lower quadrant trocar as the fourth arm, and is used for retraction.

A Thermoflator (Karl Storz, El Segundo, CA) and a high-flow insufflator at 30 L/min are used. Reusable insufflation tubes are attached to the trocar valves for passive smoke evacuation and dropped by gravity into a bottle containing saline solution.

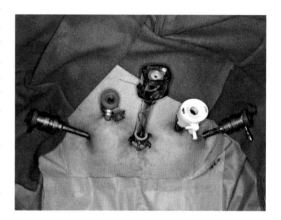

Fig. 19.2 Trocar placement for a robotic total hysterectomy

19.2.4 Hysterectomy Technique

This section follows our technique of robotic hysterectomy and bilateral salpingo-oophorectomy [8]. The pelvic peritoneum is incised at the level of the pelvic brim laterally and parallel to the ovarian vessels to identify the ureter (Fig. 19.3). A peritoneal window is created between the ovarian vessels and the left ureter, isolating the ovarian vessels and preventing ureteral injury (Fig. 19.4). The ovarian vessels are sealed and transected by the first assistant using a vessel-sealing device. The broad ligament is opened anteriorly and posteriorly and the cardinal ligament, left (Fig. 19.5) and right (Fig. 19.6), is sealed and divided by the assistant next to the cervix. The vesicovaginal space is dissected by pulling ventrally on the bladder anteriorly, assisted by placing a vaginal manipulator in the anterior vaginal fornix. With the vesicovaginal space fully dissected, the cervicovaginal junction is then identified without (Fig. 19.7a) and with the assistance of a vaginal manipulator (Apple probe) (Fig. 19.7b). This is an important aspect of any endoscopic hysterectomy.

A colpotomy is started anteriorly at the 12 o'clock location and completed in a circumferential fashion. The uterus and adnexa are removed through the vagina, and a sterile occluding balloon, inflated with 60 mL of water, is placed in the vagina to maintain the pneumoperitoneum until the cuff is closed. The cuff is left open until the nodal dissection is completed,

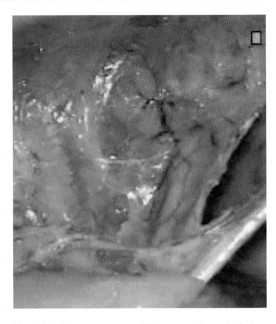

Fig. 19.4 To prevent ureteral injury, a peritoneal window is created between the infundibulopelvic (IP) ligament and the left ureter

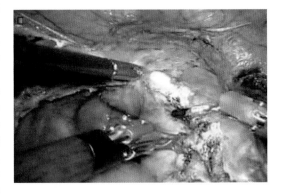

Fig. 19.5 The left cardinal ligament is sealed and divided

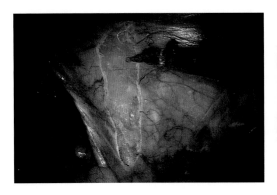

Fig. 19.3 The pelvic peritoneum is incised to identify the ureter

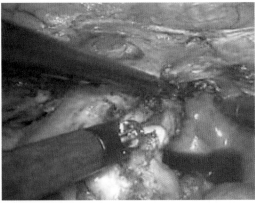

Fig. 19.6 The right cardinal ligament is sealed and divided

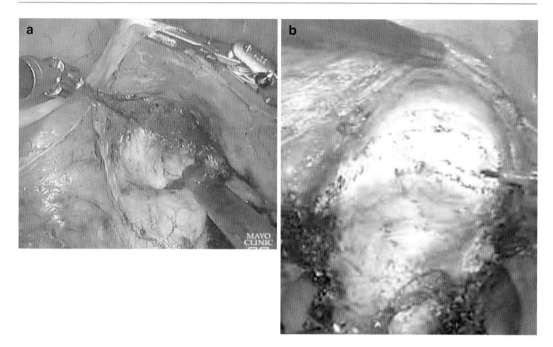

Fig. 19.7 The cervicovaginal junction is then identified without a vaginal manipulator (**a**) and with the assistance of a manipulator (Apple probe) (**b**)

allowing the removal of the nodes through the vagina. When this is completed, the cuff is closed with interrupted figure-of-eight sutures or a continuous suture using 2-0 polydioxanone (Fig. 19.8), incorporating uterosacral ligaments at each angle.

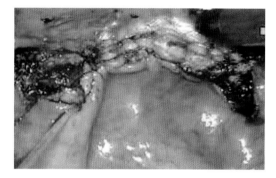

Fig. 19.8 After the colpotomy, the cuff is closed with interrupted figure-of-eight sutures or a continuous suture using 2-0 polydioxanone

19.2.5 Pelvic Lymphadenectomy Technique

A pelvic lymphadenectomy is performed by dissecting the paravesical space (Fig. 19.9) and occasionally the pararectal space (Fig. 19.10). The anatomic borders of the paravesical space are medially, the superior vesical artery; laterally, the external iliac artery; anteriorly, the pubic ramus; and posteriorly, the parametrium. The dissection is carried down to the levator ani, being careful to identify the obturator nerve. The margins of the pararectal space are medially, the ureter; laterally, the internal iliac artery; anteriorly, the parametrium; and inferiorly, the levator muscle. The superior margin of the pelvic lymphadenectomy is the bifurcation of the common iliac arteries (Fig. 19.11) and the distal margin is the inguinal ligament. The external iliac nodes overlying and lateral to the external iliac vessels are removed (Fig. 19.12), followed by the superficial lateral common iliacs (Fig. 19.11), and the internal iliac and obturator nodes (Fig. 19.13). The common iliac artery and vein, the external iliac and internal iliac arteries, the anterior bifurcation vessels of the internal iliac artery and the obturator nerve, should be clearly visible at the completion of the pelvic lymphadenectomy (Fig. 19.14). The nodes are sent for intraoperative frozen section. If the pelvic nodes are positive or tumor extends to the cervical stroma, the remaining nodal groups of the internal iliac artery and the deep lateral and medial common iliac nodes are removed.

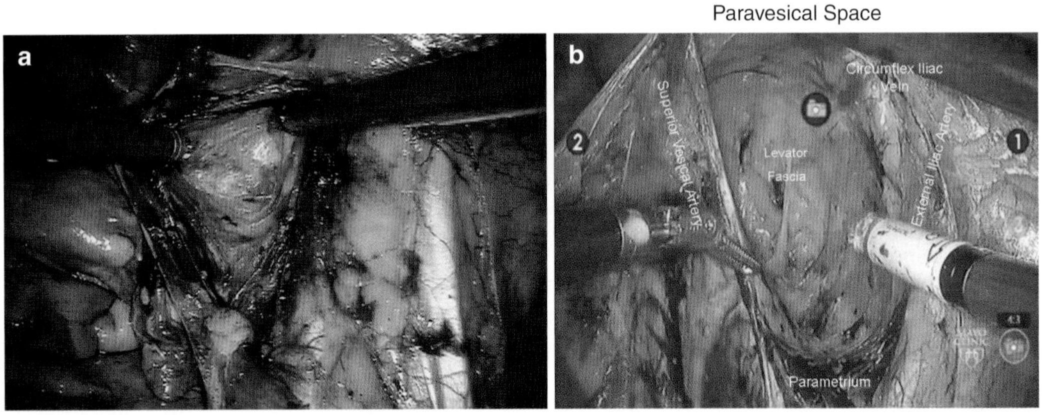

Fig. 19.9 (**a**, **b**) Pelvic lymphadenectomy is performed by dissecting the paravesical space

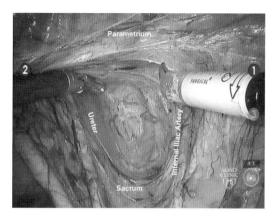

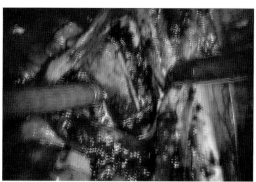

Fig. 19.13 Obturator nodes

Fig. 19.10 Pelvic lymphadenectomy occasionally involves dissecting the pararectal space

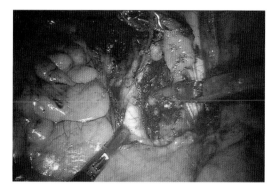

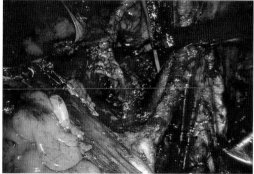

Fig. 19.11 Lateral common iliac arteries. The bifurcation of these arteries is the superior margin of the pelvic lymphadenectomy

Fig. 19.14 At the completion of the pelvic lymphadenectomy, the common iliac artery and vein, the external iliac and internal iliac arteries, the anterior bifurcation vessels of the internal iliac artery, and the obturator nerve should be clearly visible

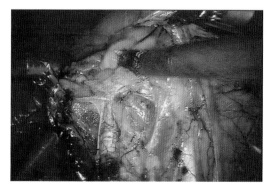

Fig. 19.12 The external iliac nodes overlying and lateral to the external iliac vessels are removed

19.2.6 Aortic Lymphadenectomy

Indications for aortic lymphadenectomy include myometrial invasion greater than 50 %, lymphovascular invasion, and positive pelvic nodes. In the presence of indications for aortic lymphadenectomy, the robotic column is undocked after completion of the pelvic operation, and three additional trocars are placed in the lower pelvis. A 12-mm trocar is inserted two or three fingerbreadths suprapubically and one or two fingerbreadths to the left of the midline. Two accessory trocars are placed 2 cm caudally and equidistant to the right and left of the 12-mm trocar (Fig. 19.15). The operating table is rotated 180°, so that the patient's head is now where her feet were located before and vice versa. (This rotation requires a longer intravenous line, longer endotracheal tubing, and cessation of assisted ventilation for about 30 s.)

The robotic column is then advanced to the patient's head or side-docked to the right shoulder. An EndoWrist monopolar spatula or scissors (Intuitive Surgical Inc., Sunnyvale, CA) is placed through the left robotic trocar and attached to the right robotic arm. An EndoWrist PK bipolar grasper (Intuitive Surgical Inc., Sunnyvale, CA) is placed through the right lower quadrant robotic trocar and attached to the left robotic arm. The assistant sits or stands between the patient's legs and uses a fan retractor with the left hand to retract the duodenum and pancreas ventrally while the right hand is used for a vessel-sealing device, suction-irrigation, and lateral retraction of the sigmoid mesentery.

A small incision is made on the peritoneum overlying the mid portion of the right common iliac artery and extended to the aortic bifurcation (Fig. 19.16). The left renal vein is identified and the duodenum and pancreas are retracted ventrally by the assistant, with a fan retractor (Fig. 19.17). The right aortic nodes over the vena cava and aorta are excised first, as well as the interaortic nodes if there is a separation between those two vessels (Fig. 19.18). The dissection is extended cranially until no nodal tissue is present, usually slightly above the right gonadal vein

entrance site into the vena cava. The inframesenteric left aortic lymph nodes are exposed by extending the peritoneal incision about 5 cm from the aortic bifurcation caudally and overlying the left common iliac artery (Fig. 19.18). The sigmoid mesentery is retracted laterally by the assistant. The left inframesenteric nodes are removed from the bifurcation of the aorta to the inferior mesenteric artery.

The infrarenal nodal area is exposed by dividing the inferior mesenteric artery with a vessel sealing device at its origin from the aorta and by lateral retraction of the left colon mesentery by the assistant (Fig. 19.19). The infrarenal nodes are removed from the stump of the inferior mesenteric artery to the left renal vein, and medial to the left ovarian vein (Fig. 19.20). A second lumbar vein is found passing through this nodal group in about one-third of patients, originating in the lumbar spine and draining directly to the left renal vein or, less frequently, to the left gonadal vein.

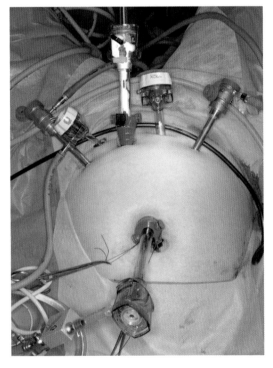

Fig. 19.15 Trocar placement for aortic lymphadenectomy

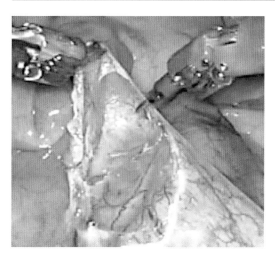

Fig. 19.16 A small incision is made on the peritoneum overlying the mid portion of the right common iliac artery and extended to the aortic bifurcation

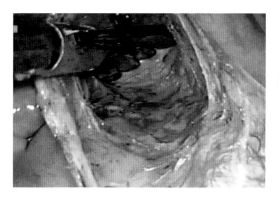

Fig. 19.17 The duodenum and pancreas are retracted ventrally by the assistant, with a fan retractor

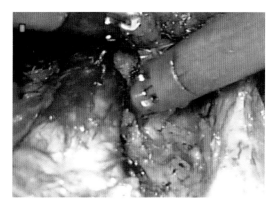

Fig. 19.18 The right aortic nodes, as well as the interaortic nodes if there is a separation between those two vessels, are excised first. The inframesenteric left aortic lymph nodes are exposed by extending the peritoneal incision about 5 cm from the aortic bifurcation caudally and overlying the left common iliac artery

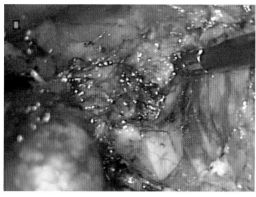

Fig. 19.19 Exposing the infrarenal nodal area

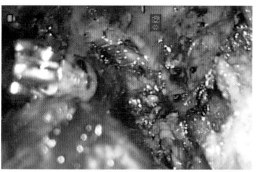

Fig. 19.20 Removal of the infrarenal nodes

19.3 Cervical Cancer

There are about 12,000 new cases of cervical cancer each year in the United States, but the number is decreasing [1]. Treatment for early invasive stage IA2 to IIA disease involves either a modified radical or radical hysterectomy with pelvic and para-aortic lymphadenectomy, if indicated. Traditionally, this procedure has been performed through an open approach. However, with advances in minimally invasive technology and particularly with the advent of robotics, studies have demonstrated the feasibility of these approaches in association with decreased blood loss and shorter hospital stay, compared with laparotomy [9, 10]. Operating times are similar or longer, and complication rates, recurrence, and survival outcomes are unchanged [9, 10].

19.3.1 Robotic Radical Hysterectomy

Patient position and preparation, equipment and robotic column, and trocar placement and docking are the same for robotic radical hysterectomy as described above for robotic total hysterectomy with bilateral pelvic and para-aortic lymphadenectomy.

19.3.2 Pelvic Lymphadenectomy Technique

In cervical cancer, a pelvic lymphadenectomy is performed first, as the procedure may be aborted depending on the size, number, and location of positive nodes. The paravesical space (Fig. 19.9) and pararectal space (Fig. 19.10) are dissected, similar to the technique described above for total hysterectomy (see Figs. 19.11, 19.12, 19.13, and 19.14). The nodes are sent for intraoperative frozen section. If the pelvic nodes are positive, the remaining nodal groups of the internal iliac artery and the deep lateral and medial common iliac nodes are removed.

19.3.3 Radical Hysterectomy Technique

The technique described here has been previously described [11] and corresponds to type C1 according to the recently reviewed classification of radical hysterectomy [12].

A peritoneal window is created between the ovarian vessels and the left ureter, isolating the ovarian vessels and preventing ureteral injury (Fig. 19.4). If adnexectomy is indicated, the ovarian vessels are sealed and transected by the first assistant, using a vessel-sealing device. The broad ligament is opened anteriorly and posteriorly.

The parametrium is transected at its origin from the internal iliac artery and vein, using a vessel-sealing device (Fig. 19.21), starting with the superior vesical and uterine arteries ventrally and dorsally to the deep uterine vein, joining the paravesical and pararectal spaces once the division is completed (Fig. 19.22).

The rectovaginal space (Fig. 19.23) is dissected to the lower vaginal half (Fig. 19.24) isolating both uterosacral ligaments. The uterosacral ligaments are transected at or distal to the anterior rectal wall, depending on tumor size and proximity to posterior vaginal wall, allowing further mobilization of the uterus (Fig. 19.25).

The vesicovaginal space (Fig. 19.26) is dissected to the mid portion of the anterior vaginal wall, by ventral retraction of the bladder and with the assistance of a vaginal manipulator (Apple probe).

The entrance of the ureter into the parametrial tunnel is identified by pulling on the transected uterine artery (Fig. 19.27). following figures have to be renumbered. The avascular space located at 12 o'clock over the ureter is dissected, isolating the ventral bladder pillar. which is divided with a vessel-sealing device or monopolar spatula (Fig. 19.28). The ureter is then gently mobilized laterally, isolating the dorsal bladder pillar (Fig. 19.29), which is divided with a vessel sealing device (Fig. 19.30). This allows ventral retraction of the ureter, exposing the underlying paravaginal tissue.

The paravaginal tissue is transected with a vessel-sealing device to the lateral aspect of the vaginal wall, incorporating the entire resected parametrium and uterosacral ligaments. A vaginal manipulator (Apple probe) is used to assist in performing the colpotomy and in indicating the cervicovaginal junction, which is used to determine the level of transection of the vagina to obtain adequate margins (Fig. 19.31). The colpotomy is performed in a circumferential fashion starting at the 12 o'clock position of the vagina. The uterus is removed through the vagina. The vaginal cuff is closed with a continuous suture or interrupted figure-of-eight sutures using 2-0 polydioxanone (Fig. 19.32).

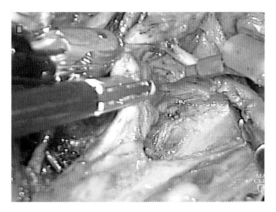

Fig. 19.21 The parametrium is transected at its origin from the internal iliac artery and vein

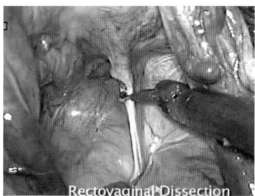

Fig. 19.23 Rectovaginal dissection

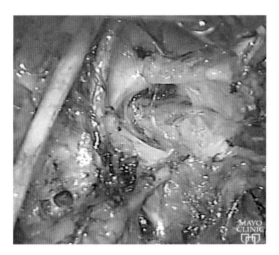

Fig. 19.22 Transection of the parametrium joins the paravesical and pararectal spaces (*left side shown*)

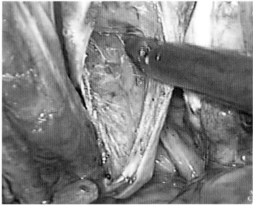

Fig. 19.24 The rectovaginal space is dissected to the lower vaginal half, isolating both uterosacral ligaments

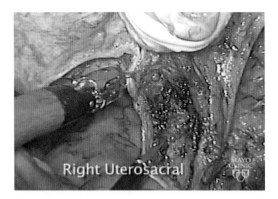

Fig. 19.25 Further mobilization of the uterus is achieved by transecting the uterosacral ligaments at or distal to the anterior rectal wall

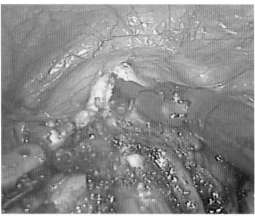

Fig. 19.27 Ventral bladder pillar

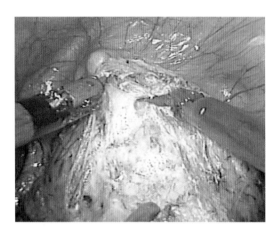

Fig. 19.26 The vesicovaginal space is dissected to the mid portion of the anterior vaginal wall, by ventral retraction of the bladder and with the assistance of a vaginal manipulator

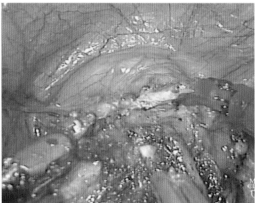

Fig. 19.28 Division of the ventral bladder pillar

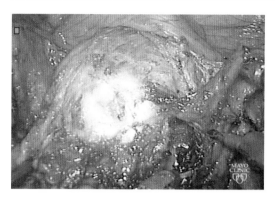

Fig. 19.29 The ureter is gently mobilized laterally, isolating the dorsal bladder pillar

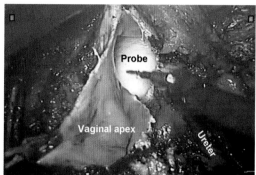

Fig. 19.31 A vaginal manipulator is used in determining the level of transection of the vagina

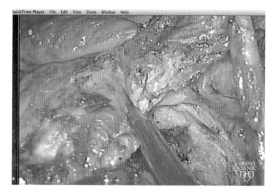

Fig. 19.30 Division of the dorsal bladder pillar

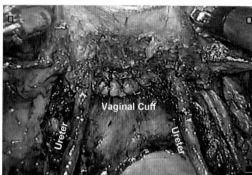

Fig. 19.32 Closure of the vaginal cuff

19.3.4 Aortic Lymphadenectomy

Indications for an aortic lymphadenectomy are positive pelvic nodes, cervical cancer more than 5 cm in diameter, and/or enlarged aortic nodes on pre-operative imaging. If an aortic lymphadenectomy is indicated, it must include the infrarenal nodes because nodal metastases can bypass the ipsilateral inframesenteric nodes [13]. A transperitoneal approach is used when aortic lymphadenectomy is performed concomitant to radical hysterectomy and pelvic lymphadenectomy [14]. An extra-peritoneal approach is preferable in patients with advanced cervical cancer who are undergoing pre-irradiation aortic lymphadenectomy [15].

The robotic column is undocked after completion of the pelvic operation, and three additional trocars are placed in the lower pelvis. A 12-mm trocar is inserted two or three fingerbreadths suprapubically and one or two fingerbreadths to the left of the midline. Two accessory trocars are placed 2 cm caudally and equidistant to the right and left of the 12-mm trocar (Fig. 19.15). The operating table is rotated 180°, so that the patient's head is now where her feet were located before and vice versa. (This rotation requires a longer intravenous line, longer endotracheal tubing, and cessation of assisted ventilation for about 30 s.)

The robotic approach and technique for infrarenal aortic lymphadenectomy are as described for endometrial cancer above and are not repeated here.

19.4 Ovarian Cancer

Some select patients with ovarian cancer are candidates for a robotic approach. Robotic procedures are preferable for patients with limited disease requiring one or two major procedures in addition to hysterectomy, adnexectomy, and omentectomy [16]. Laparotomy is preferable for patients with advanced disease who require three or more major procedures, because operating time is much shorter and the postoperative complications and hospital stay are similar to those with robotics [16].

The techniques of robotic hysterectomy and adnexectomy are similar to those described for endometrial cancer. The following section describes a robotic approach for diaphragmatic and hepatic metastases.

19.4.1 Resection of Diaphragmatic and Hepatic Metastases

Resection of any diaphragmatic or hepatic metastasis is indicated when the patient will be rendered disease-free (ie, complete cytoreduction). Resection of diaphragm or liver disease in the presence of other unresectable disease does not improve survival and may increase morbidity. A subhepatic approach is always preferable whenever possible; a suprahepatic approach is used for lesions not amenable to a subhepatic approach. Most hepatic metastases are superficially invasive and can be excised as described here. Metastases deep in the hepatic parenchyma that do not involve the surface may require partial or complete segmentectomy, bisegmentectomy, or partial hepatectomy. In our institution, these procedures are performed by a liver surgeon.

19.4.1.1 Patient Position
The patient is positioned supine, or in low Allen stirrups if pelvic lesions will also be resected. There is no need for Trendelenburg; on occasion, reverse Trendelenburg or lateral decubitus is necessary.

19.4.1.2 Trocar Placement, Robotic Column, and Instruments
The location and extent of the diaphragmatic lesions is important, as it will affect trocar placement. For lesions on the ventral portion of both diaphragms and of the left diaphragm, a subhepatic approach, using the same trocar position as for pelvic surgery, is preferable, as shown above. An additional right subcostal trocar for a fan retractor is necessary to retract the liver cranially, requiring a second assistant. For lesions of the dome of the liver and dorsal right diaphragm, all trocars, including the optical trocar, must be supraumbilical, and the left trocar and both right

trocars must be in a subcostal position. The right robotic trocar is close to the subcostal margin, and the left lateral robotic trocar is on the anterior axillary line. The assistant trocar is to the right or left of the optical trocar, depending on the location of the lesion. The right robotic trocar is inferior to the costal margin, and the left lateral robotic trocar is on the anterior axillary line. The assistant trocar is to the right or left of the optical trocar, depending on the location of the lesion. A 30-degree scope is used to improve visualization over the right hepatic lobe.

The robotic column is placed at the patient's head or side-docked at the right or left shoulder of the patient.

The robotic instruments are the same as used for pelvic surgery and are attached to the same robotic arms. The first assistant uses a fan retractor over the right hepatic lobe to provide diaphragm exposure.

19.4.1.3 Technique

The lesion to be removed is outlined with proper margins with the monopolar spatula, both in the liver and diaphragm (Fig. 19.33). It is excised from the diaphragm using a monopolar spatula, including transdiaphragmatic resection if invading the diaphragm muscle (Fig. 19.34). Positive pressure ventilation prevents lung collapse once the pleural cavity is entered. Lesions are resected from the liver using a monopolar spatula or scissors on a coagulating setting, a bipolar device, or a vessel-sealing device. Closure of the diaphragmatic defect is performed with one or more running, locking 2-0 polydioxanone sutures, each precut to 15 cm length and with a Lapra-Ty clip (Ethicon Endo-Surgery; Cincinnati, OH) at their distal end. Before closure is completed, remaining fluids and CO_2 in the pleural cavity are aspirated through a red Robinson catheter connected to

continuous suction. A Lapra-Ty clip is applied at the end of each 2-0 polydioxanone suture. Pleural leaks are checked with Valsalva under water, and a chest X-ray is obtained intraoperatively to check for residual pneumothorax.

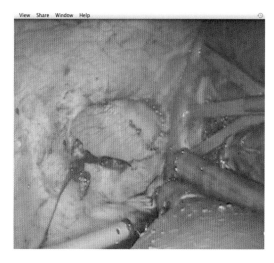

Fig. 19.33 The diaphragm lesion has been excised full-thickness and the defect is shown

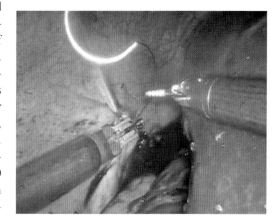

Fig. 19.34 The diaphragm defect has been closed with a continuous locking suture using 2–0 PDS. A lapraty is being applied at the end of the suture after the remaining CO_2 in the pleural cavity has been suctioned

References

1. American Cancer Society. Cancer facts & figures. 2013. http://www.cancer.org/research/cancerfacts-figures/cancerfactsfigures/cancer-facts-figures-2013. Accessed 16 Dec 2013.
2. Walker JL, Piedmonte MR, Spirtos NM, Eisenkop SM, Schlaerth JB, Mannel RS, et al. Laparoscopy compared with laparotomy for comprehensive surgical staging of uterine cancer: Gynecologic Oncology Group Study LAP2. J Clin Oncol. 2009;27:5331–6.
3. Walker JL, Piedmonte MR, Spirtos NM, Eisenkop SM, Schlaerth JB, Mannel RS, et al. Recurrence and survival after random assignment to laparoscopy versus laparotomy for comprehensive surgical staging of uterine cancer: Gynecologic Oncology Group LAP2 Study. J Clin Oncol. 2012;30:695–700.
4. Magrina JF, Zanagnolo V, Giles D, Noble BN, Kho RM, Magtibay PM. Robotic surgery for endometrial cancer: comparison of perioperative outcomes and recurrence with laparoscopy, vaginal/laparoscopy and laparotomy. Eur J Gynaecol Oncol. 2011;32:476–80.
5. Bandera C, Magrina JF. Robotic surgery in gynecologic oncology. Curr Opin Obstet Gynecol. 2009;21:25–30.
6. Boggess JF, Gehrig PA, Cantrell L, Shafer A, Ridgway M, Skinner EN, et al. A comparative study of 3 surgical methods for hysterectomy with staging for endometrial cancer: robotic assistance, laparoscopy, laparotomy. Am J Obstet Gynecol. 2008;199:360.e1–9.
7. Magrina JF. Minimally invasive surgery in gynecologic oncology. Gynecol Oncol. 2009;114(2 Suppl):S22–3.
8. Kho R, Hilger W, Hentz J, Magtibay P, Magrina JF. Robotic hysterectomy: technique and initial outcomes. Am J Obstet Gynecol. 2007;197:113.e1–4.
9. Magrina JF, Kho R, Weaver A, Magtibay P. Robotic radical hysterectomy: comparison with laparoscopy and laparotomy. Gynecol Oncol. 2008;109:86–91.
10. Magrina JF. Robotic surgery in gynecology. Eur J Gynaecol Oncol. 2007;28:77–82.
11. Magrina JF, Kho R, Magtibay PM. Robotic radical hysterectomy: technical aspects. Gynecol Oncol. 2009;113:28–31.
12. Querleu D, Morrow C. Classification of radical hysterectomy. Lancet Oncol. 2008;9:297–303.
13. Gil-Moreno A, Magrina JF, Perez-Benavente A, Diaz-Feijoo B, Sanchez-Iglesias JL, Garcia A, et al. Location of aortic node metastases in locally advanced cervical cancer. Gynecol Oncol. 2012;125:312–4.
14. Magrina JF, Long JB, Kho RM, Giles DL, Montero RP, Magtibay PM. Robotic transperitoneal infrarenal aortic lymphadenectomy: technique and results. Int J Gynecol Cancer. 2010;20:184–7.
15. Magrina JF, Kho R, Montero RP, Magtibay PM, Pawlina W. Robotic extraperitoneal aortic lymphadenectomy: development of a technique. Gynecol Oncol. 2008;113:32–5.
16. Magrina JF, Zanagnolo V, Noble BN, Kho RM, Magtibay PM. Robotic approach for ovarian cancer: preoperative and survival results and comparison with laparoscopy and laparotomy. Gynecol Oncol. 2011;121:100–5.

Techniques for Robotic Urogynecology and Pelvic Reconstructive Surgery

Megan E. Tarr and Marie Fidela Paraiso

Laparoscopic urethropexy was introduced in the early 1990s, and the first robot-assisted sacral colpopexy was reported in 2004 [1]. Over the past 10–15 years, laparoscopic and robot-assisted laparoscopic techniques have been applied to many prolapse and incontinence procedures. After the United States Food and Drug Administration approved its use in gynecologic surgery in 2005, the da Vinci Surgical System (Intuitive Surgical, Inc.; Sunnyvale, CA) gave gynecologic surgeons another minimally invasive option for surgeries that had been previously performed by laparotomy, vaginally, or by the traditional laparoscopic technique.

In the field of female pelvic reconstructive surgery, robotic-assisted laparoscopy is most widely used for sacrocolpopexy. Retrospective cohort studies show that robotic-assisted sacrocolpopexy is associated with less intraoperative blood loss, earlier hospital discharge, and better short-term anatomic outcomes when compared with open sacrocolpopexy [2, 3]. Additionally, robotic-assisted laparoscopy may enable surgeons who have not been extensively trained or are not appropriately skilled in traditional laparoscopic techniques to perform complex abdominal surgery by minimally invasive access, as there is some evidence that the learning curve may be shorter [4–6]. Finally, although this has not been widely studied in live surgery, robotic-assisted laparoscopy may offer ergonomic advantages over traditional laparoscopy [7–10].

There are many advantages of robotic sacrocolpopexy when compared with open sacrocolpopexy; however, there are several potential barriers to adopting robotic-assisted laparoscopic technology. Surgeons, surgical assistants, and operating room teams must be comprehensively trained, and patient-centered outcomes of surgical cases should be tracked. Surgeons must be wary of extending patient anesthesia time, especially during the early robotic learning curve. Finally, instrumentation cost and robotic maintenance fees must be considered in the adoption and maintenance of robotic technology at a particular institution.

Robotic technology has expanded the use of minimally invasive prolapse techniques, most especially in sacrocolpopexy. As robotic techniques for female pelvic floor disorders are taught and refined, we must continue to be cognizant of other minimally invasive surgery options, patient and societal costs, and most importantly, patient safety and satisfaction.

M.E. Tarr, MD, MS • M.F. Paraiso, MD (✉)
Department of Obstetrics and Gynecology,
Women's Health Institute, Cleveland Clinic,
9500 Euclid Avenue, A-81, Cleveland,
OH 44195, USA
e-mail: tarrm@ccf.org

P.F. Escobar, T. Falcone (eds.), *Atlas of Single-Port, Laparoscopic, and Robotic Surgery*,
DOI 10.1007/978-1-4614-6840-0_20, © Springer Science+Business Media New York 2014

20.1 Perioperative Considerations

Similar criteria are used to select patients for both laparoscopic and robotic-assisted laparoscopic pelvic reconstructive procedures. Patients should be able to tolerate pneumoperitoneum and the steep Trendelenburg position needed to facilitate cephalad bowel retraction for optimal visualization of pelvic anatomy. Consequently, patients with certain cardiopulmonary conditions may not be optimal candidates for robotic or laparoscopic pelvic floor procedures. In addition, unlike traditional laparoscopic procedures, use of the surgical robot prohibits use of operative table movement during cases. Consequently, patients are usually placed in the maximally required Trendelenburg position (often 30° from horizontal) and are maintained in this position for the duration of the robotic portion of the case. This position can cause difficulty in ventilating the patient and can contribute to intraoperative hemodynamic changes [11]. Prolonged Trendelenburg position increases chest wall resistance and dead space with a consequent decrease in the alveolar-arterial diffusion of oxygen. Pulmonary compliance and functional residual capacity are reduced; these effects are often more pronounced in obese patients [12–14].

The surgeon also needs to carefully consider the effects of intra-abdominal CO_2 insufflation and its hemodynamic and metabolic effects in patients with chronic obstructive pulmonary, cardiovascular, and chronic renal diseases [13–16]. Be aware of patients with contraindications to increases in intracranial pressure and patients who are potentially hypovolemic preoperatively; a laparoscopic or robotic procedure may be contraindicated in these patients. These concerns are particularly amplified in prolonged minimally invasive cases [17, 18]. Patients with such underlying cardiopulmonary conditions should be preoperatively counseled as to the need for a possible conversion to an open procedure if indicated by intraoperative physiologic parameters.

Robotic sacrocolpopexy and concomitant procedures frequently take over 3 h to perform; therefore, a patient may be exposed to prolonged general anesthesia and increased risks for thromboembolism, hypothermia, and nerve injury. Because prolongation of surgery is known to be associated with certain degrees of morbidity, a robotic surgeon should be mindful of surgical case progression. We often use time goals whereby a trainee is given a set amount of time to perform a portion of the surgery while at the surgeon console. If the time goal is met, they continue to sit at the console. If not, the attending surgeon assumes the role of the console surgeon. This technique is useful when teaching resident and fellow surgeons portions of a complex surgery.

20.2 Operating Room Set-up and Patient Positioning

We typically use either the da Vinci S or Si Surgical System (Intuitive Surgical, Inc.; Sunnyvale, CA). The Dual Console Si system is helpful when teaching a resident or fellow surgeon as long as an experienced bedside assistant is present. Our surgical team is typically composed of the robotic surgeon(s) at the surgeon console, a bedside assistant standing on the patient's right near the assistant port, a vaginal assistant who operates the vaginal and rectal sizers, a scrubbed surgical nurse or technician, and a circulating nurse.

Figure 20.1 demonstrates the robotic room set-up for sacrocolpopexy and reconstructive pelvic surgery. There is typically one table for laparoscopic and robotic abdominal instruments, one table for vaginal instruments and cystoscopy equipment, and a large Mayo stand upon which the robotic endoscopic camera sits (after it has been removed from the warmer) until it is placed into the peritoneal cavity. The Vision cart is usually on the left side of the operating table so that the bedside assistant on the patient's right can have an optimal viewing angle.

Patient positioning for robotic sacrocolpopexy is similar to that for laparoscopic sacrocolpopexy (*see* Chap. 7) in that the patient is placed on an antislip pad, foam egg crate pad, or bean bag. After induction of anesthesia and placement of an orogastric tube for stomach decompression, the patient is moved down the operating room table and placed in the dorsal lithotomy position with the buttocks slightly beyond the end of the table to facilitate movement of the vaginal and rectal sizers. The arms are tucked in by the patient's sides, and the hands and all bony prominences are padded for neural safety. We also typically place a padded chest strap at the nipple line to further secure the torso. After the patient is prepped and draped, a three-way Foley catheter is placed. We routinely recheck for optimal positioning of the patient during the case.

After intraperitoneal access has been gained, the bed is placed in the maximal Trendelenburg position, and the 8-mm robotic ports and laparoscopic assistant ports are placed (see section below). Once this has been safely accomplished, the bedside assistant temporarily stands on the patient's left and supervises the parallel docking of the robot on the patient's left side.

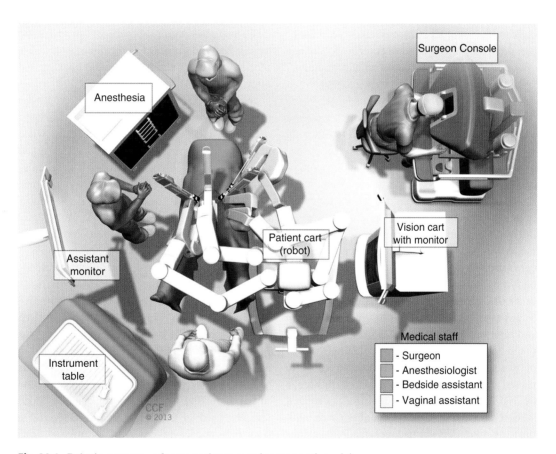

Fig. 20.1 Robotic room set up for sacrocolpopexy and reconstructive pelvic surgery

20.3   Prolapse Procedures

20.3.1 Sacrocolpopexy

Robotic sacrocolpopexy is performed using a technique similar to the laparoscopic sacrocolpopexy (*see* Chap. 7). The da Vinci Surgical System is currently the only widely used robotic surgical system in the United States, and the four-armed da Vinci S or da Vinci SI systems are currently the most commonly used. The robotic approach to sacrocolpopexy differs from the laparoscopic approach on a few parameters: trocar locations, docking the robotic patient cart, and use of intracorporeal knot tying, although this is also an option for the standard laparoscopic technique.

Figure 20.2b demonstrates robotic trocar placement compared with laparoscopic (Fig. 20.2a) trocar placement. Although there are a few ways in which the robotic and laparoscopic trocars can be positioned, we advocate using five trocars placed in a shallow "W" formation: two of the 8-mm robotic ports are placed bilaterally, 9 cm lateral and inferior from the umbilicus, and the third robotic trocar is placed in the left upper quadrant, 9 cm lateral to the more medial left-sided port. A 12-mm umbilical trocar is used for the robotic laparoscope, and a 10- or 8-mm assistant trocar is placed 9 cm lateral or medial to the right-sided robotic trocar. The 8-mm assistant trocar allows for the introduction and removal of suture with SH needles and does not require fascial closure, minimizing the risk of postoperative pain. The robotic trocars are placed approximately 9–10 cm apart to minimize the risk of robotic arm collision. If a patient has a short torso, a shallow "Z" configuration with the right robot port in the upper quadrant and the right lower quadrant accessory port three finger breaths cephalad and medial to the right anterosuperior iliac spine will decrease arm collision.

The robotic patient cart is then docked with the operating table in a 30-degree Trendelenburg position (Fig. 20.3). After the robotic trocars are safely placed and the patient is placed in the maximal Trendelenburg position (about 30°), the robotic patient cart is docked under the instruction of the bedside surgeon.

Although many methods of robotic patient cart docking have been described, we feel that parallel docking on the patient's left side allows easy access for vaginal manipulation during vaginal and rectal dissections in sacrocolpopexy and results in minimal issues with robotic arm collision (Fig. 20.4).

After first affixing the camera arm, the other robotic arms are connected to the robotic trocars with care taken to position them to minimize the risk of collisions (Fig. 20.5). A 30-degree angle between the instruments' arms and the camera is good, but a 45-degree angle is usually better. Positioning the fourth robotic arm (arm 3) at the most left lateral trocar is usually done last because of the need for its almost horizontal docking and often, its inferior angle to the patient.

We then place the appropriately calibrated robotic endoscope in the camera trocar. We typically use a 0-degree robotic endoscope when performing the vesicovaginal and rectovaginal dissection, but a 30-degree upward-facing endoscope can aid in the rectovaginal and perineal dissections and suture placement. A 30-degree downward-facing endoscope can be particularly helpful for the presacral dissection. We typically place the robotic monopolar scissors in arm 1, a bipolar instrument (either PK Dissecting Forceps [Gyrus Medical; Maple Grove, MN] or bipolar forceps) in arm 2, and a ProGrasp (Intuitive Surgical, Inc.; Sunnyvale, CA) in arm 3 for the initial dissection. If a hysterectomy is being performed, the Tenaculum forceps can be placed in arm 3 rather than the ProGrasp; however, this is rarely used in order to control costs. Once the initial dissection for the sacrocolpopexy is done (as discussed in Chap. 7), we typically use a SutureCut needle driver (Intuitive Surgical, Inc.; Sunnyvale, CA) in arm 1, a Needle Driver in arm 2, and a ProGrasp in arm 3 to suture robotically with 8-inch monofilament 2-0 or 0 polypropylene and polydioxanone. All knot tying in robotic sacrocolpopexy is performed using an intracorporeal technique. Suture and polypropylene graft placement do not differ between laparoscopic and robotic sacrocolpopexy (Fig. 20.6).

There are a few points of caution for robotic-assisted laparoscopic sacrocolpopexy. The lack of haptic feedback is important to acknowledge when distinguishing robotic from laparoscopic sacrocolpopexy. Consequently, the console surgeon has to pay close attention to visual cues when placing tension on tissues or sutures and judging the depth of suture placement. This is particularly important when determining where the sacral promontory is located for the presacral dissection. After identifying the right ureter, aortic bifurcation at the L4–L5 level, common iliac vessels, and retracting the sigmoid laterally, we typically have the bedside assistant palpate the promontory laparoscopically. Caution is also taken when placing sutures in the anterior longitudinal ligament at the level of S1; care must be taken not to penetrate the vertebral periosteum or intravertebral disk with deep suture placement. Finally, we also try to minimize robotic manipulation of the sigmoid and epiploica with the ProGrasp in arm 3 by initially retracting the bowel cephalad and laterally with a bowel grasper in the right upper quadrant assistant port. We then use the ProGrasp, with its closed or slightly open tips angled toward the sacrum,

to maintain gentle, lateral traction on the sigmoid. Alternatively, suture can also be passed through several sigmoid epiploica and brought through the left lower quadrant lateral to the left upper and lower quadrant port sites (arms 2 and 3, respectively) with a Carter Thomason suture carrier (Cooper Surgical; Trumbull, CT). Both suture ends are secured with minimal tension at the skin surface with a hemostat clamp, retracting the sigmoid laterally.

Other points of caution for robotic sacrocolpopexy include the following: (1) Once the robotic system is docked, the patient bed position cannot be changed without first removing instruments and undocking the robotic arms. (2) The tip of the robotic endoscopic camera becomes very hot and must be cleaned outside of the peritoneal cavity. (3) The abilities to clutch, exchange instruments, focus the camera, and to use monopolar and bipolar energy modalities differ between the different generations of da Vinci Robotic Surgical Systems. Consequently, a surgeon should be comfortable with the features of the particular robotic system prior to its use.

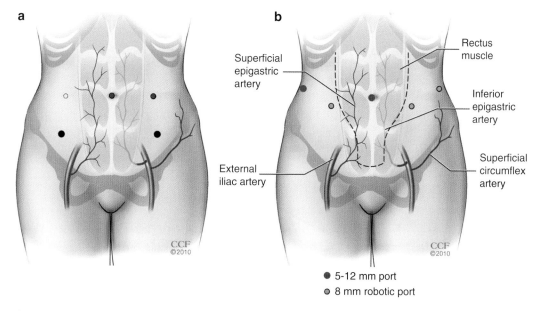

a

b

Superficial epigastric artery

Rectus muscle

Inferior epigastric artery

External iliac artery

Superficial circumflex artery

CCF ©2010

CCF ©2010

● 5-12 mm port
◉ 8 mm robotic port

Fig. 20.2 (**a**) Laparoscopic trocar placement compared with (**b**) robotic trocar placement

Fig. 20.3 Robotic patient cart docked with operating table in 30° Trendelenburg position

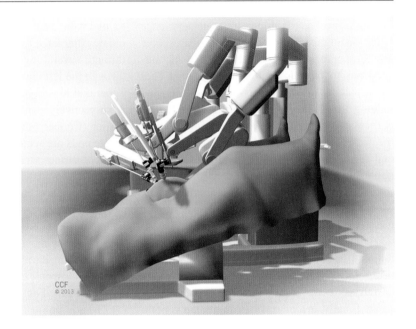

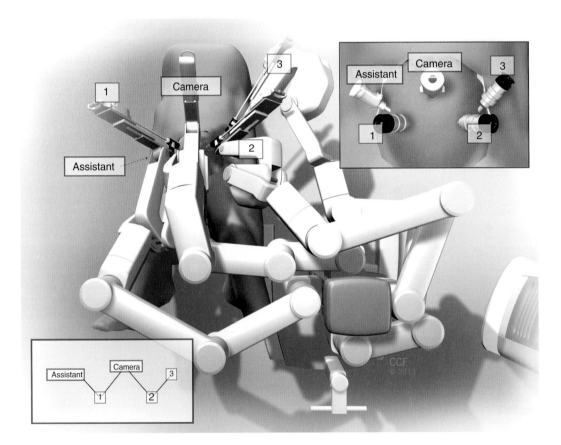

Fig. 20.4 Parallel docking of robotic patient cart

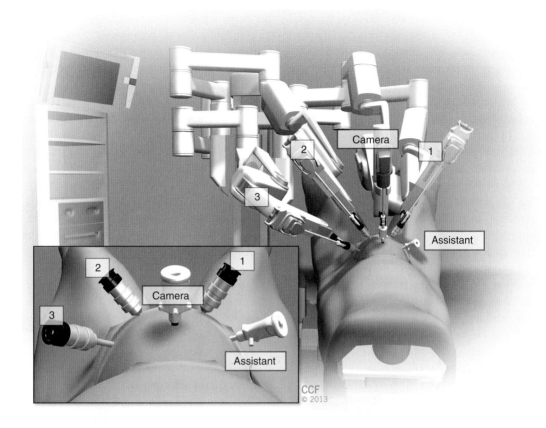

Fig. 20.5 Robotic arms connected to the robotic trocars

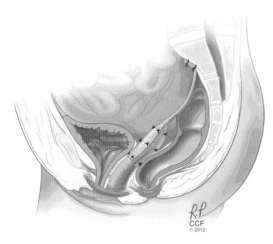

Fig. 20.6 Suture and polypropylene graft placement for sacrocolpopexy

20.3.1.1 Robotic Sacrocolpopexy Outcomes and Complications

In the recent update of the Cochrane review of surgical management of pelvic organ prolapse, Maher and coworkers [19] stated that abdominal sacrocolpopexy had lower rates of recurrent vaginal apex prolapse (3.5 % versus 15 %; RR 0.23, 95 % CI 0.07–0.77), a reduced grade of residual prolapse (5.7 % versus 20 %; RR, 95 % CI 0.09–0.97), and less dyspareunia (16 % versus 36 %; RR 0.39, 95 % CI 0.18–0.86) when compared with vaginal sacrospinous colpopexy. Abdominal sacrocolpopexy, however, was associated with a longer operative time (mean difference [MD] 21 min, 95 % CI 12–30), longer time to recovery (MD 8.3 days; 95 % CI 3.9–12.7), and was more expensive (weighted MD USD $1,334; 95 % CI $1,027–$1,641) than the non–mesh augmented vaginal approach. Well- designed randomized trials included in the meta-analysis by Paraiso and colleagues [20], Freeman and colleagues [21], and Maher and associates [22] compared laparoscopic sacrocolpopexy with either robotic [20], open [21], or total vaginal mesh [22].

Only a few well-designed comparative studies for robotic sacrocolpopexy exist, and many have varying objective and subjective outcomes. One single-center, blinded, randomized trial from our institution randomized women with posthysterectomy Stages 2–4 vaginal apex prolapse to either laparoscopic or robotic sacrocolpopexy groups [20]. The primary outcome was total operative time from incision to closure, but secondary outcomes included postoperative pain, functional activity, bowel and bladder symptoms, quality of life, anatomic vaginal support, and cost from a health care perspective. Total operative time was significantly longer in the robotic group (227 ± 47 vs 162 ± 47 min, p<.001), with docking only accounting for an average additional 14 min. In addition, sacrocolpopexy suture tying was longer for the robotic group (98 ± 22 versus 68 ± 16 min, p<.001). Although pain scores were not significantly different on postoperative day 1, the robotic group reported more pain at rest and with normal activities at several points during the 6-week postoperative period. We believe that increased pain in the robotic group was caused by muscular pain associated with manipulation and fascial closure of the right paracolic gutter accessory port. Hence, we have changed port size from 10 or 12 mm to 8 mm. At 6 and 12 months follow-up, anatomic and quality of life outcomes did not differ between the two groups. There were no significant differences in intraoperative and perioperative complications between robotic and laparoscopic sacral colpopexy [20]. The most frequent complication was in the area of urinary tract infections, of which there were three in the laparoscopic and five in the robotic groups (9 % versus 14 %, respectively, p=.71). There were two cystotomies recognized intraoperatively in both groups and one enterotomy in the robotic group. The robotic group had two patients with a

mesh erosion (6 % versus 0 %, p=.49), and three with abdominal wall pain necessitating trigger point injections (9 % versus 0 %, p=.24).

The majority of other studies comparing robotic and laparoscopic sacrocolpopexy with open sacrocolpopexy are retrospective cohorts from either one or two institutions, and the length of follow-up included in these studies ranged from 3 to 44 months. Overall, these studies show that both anatomic and subjective cure rates are comparable between robotic and laparoscopic sacrocolpopexy. Similar to the randomized trial by Paraiso and coworkers [20], Antosh's retrospective cohort trial comparing robotic and laparoscopic sacrocolpopexy did not show a significant difference in perioperative and postoperative complications [23]. There was no difference in the respective number of cystotomies (three versus one, p=1.0) or blood transfusions (one versus two, p=0.17) in either group. There were no conversions to laparotomy in either group. There were also no significant differences in urinary tract infection (nine versus six cases, p=.20), fever (one case in both groups, p=.46), wound infection/abscess (two versus one case, p=1.0) or mesh erosion (two versus 0 cases, p=1.0).

20.3.2 Sacrocolpoperineopexy

Although we perform traditional laparoscopic sacrocolpoperineopexy, we believe that the use of the robotic system may be particularly helpful for dissecting and suturing the most distal aspects of the vagina, perineum, and levator fascia and muscles, particularly when performing this procedure. A 30-degree upward-facing robotic endoscope is particularly helpful when performing this dissection. We typically place the robotic monopolar scissors in arm 1, a bipolar instrument (either PK Dissecting Forceps or bipolar forceps) in arm 2, and a Prograsp in arm 3 for the initial dissection.

The anatomic landmarks for laparoscopic or robotic rectocele repair, ventral rectopexy, and sacrocolpopexy/colpoperineopexy include the rectovaginal septum, made up of Denonvilliers fascia and its lateral attachment to the medial aspect of the levator ani muscles. The terms *rectovaginal fascia, rectovaginal septum,* and *Denonvilliers fascia* are synonymous. The posterior dissection for sacrocolpoperineopexy is started by opening the rectovaginal septum using an electrocautery or harmonic scalpel, facilitated using both vaginally and rectally placed end-to-end anastomosis (EEA) sizers. Blunt dissection, with the aid of hydrodissection or sharp dissection, may be used to open the rectovaginal space down to the perineal body and the levator ani. This should be relatively bloodless if performed correctly along anatomic planes. The rectovaginal septum is the posterior point of attachment of the sacrocolpopexy mesh. In contrast, a posterior T-shaped mesh is attached to the perineum and bilaterally to the levator ani fascia and muscles during sacral colpoperineopexy. Most surgeons prefer rectocele repair by the vaginal route for patients with distal stool trapping. We utilize the sacrocolpoperineopexy with attachment of a posterior mesh to the perineum and medial aspect of the pubococcygeus and iliococcygeus fascia and muscles for patients who have perineal descent with outlet dysfunction constipation or for patients who undergo concomitant ventral rectopexy (Fig. 20.7). We sometimes place absorbable plicating stitches into the rectovaginal muscularis in order to repair the rectovaginal defect causing the rectocele.

Some surgeons skilled in minimally invasive sacrocolpopexy, however, routinely perform sacrocolpoperineopexy for patients with a rectocele and perineal descent. The original approach for this surgery was a combined vaginal and open abdominal approach, described by Cundiff and coworkers in 1997 [24]. The posterior vaginal mesh was placed in the rectovaginal septum, anchored to the perineal body vaginally, passed through a colpotomy incision, and then affixed to the posterior vagina and anterior longitudinal ligament abdominally. This technique has been used laparoscopically [25]. A retrospective cohort study compared abdominal ($n=17$) versus vaginal ($n=51$) introduction of posterior polypropylene mesh overlaid with Pelvicol (Bard; Murray Hill, NJ) with attachment to the perineal body and rectovaginal septum for colpoperineopexy, followed by laparoscopic attachment of a second mesh to the anterior vagina with laparoscopic affixation of both meshes to the anterior longitudinal ligament [25]. At 6 months follow-up, there were no significant differences in perioperative outcomes and objective anatomic cure. Four patients in the abdominal group had symptoms of recurrent prolapse compared with one in the vaginal group ($p=.010$). Although there were no patients with mesh erosion in the abdominal group, the vaginal group had four ($p=0.6$), with one being apical and three noted at the posterior, distal vagina; all required surgical excision. Mesh erosion rates have been estimated to be approximately 6 % with sacrocolpoperineopexy [26, 27], and there are conflicting data regarding mesh erosion associated with sacrocolpoperineopexy and sacrocolpoperineopexy with concomitant hysterectomy [26, 28, 29].

There are limited data on minimally invasive sacrocolpoperineopexy with robotic assistance. We published a case series of ten patients who underwent robotic sacrocolpoperineopexy for combined rectal and vaginal prolapse that showed feasibility and minimal operative morbidity with the procedure [30]. Another retrospective cohort study of 84 women compared robot-assisted sacrocolpopexy and sacrocolpoperineopexy with a polypropylene mesh introduced transvaginally [31]. They showed comparable apical and posterior anatomic outcomes at a mean of 5 months' follow-up, but anterior recurrent prolapse was higher in the robotic sacrocolpoperineopexy group. In addition, there was significantly higher intraoperative blood loss in the sacrocolpoperineopexy group when compared with the sacrocolpopexy group (125 [50–1,000] versus 50 [50–400], $p=0.020$). Vaginal mesh exposure rate was 23 and 7 % in the sacrocolpopexy and sacrocolpoperineopexy groups, respectively. This high erosion rate was associated with incidental anterior vaginotomy, the surgeon's robotic experience, use of Ethibond suture (Ethicon; Somerville, NJ), and dissection with cautery. There are no larger studies with long-term follow-up for robot-assisted sacrocolpoperineopexy.

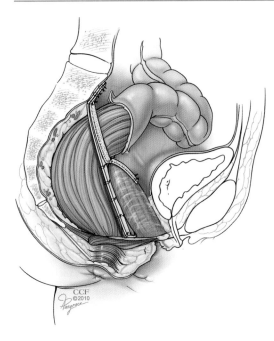

Fig. 20.7 Attachment of posterior mesh to pubococcygeus and iliococcygeus for ventral rectopexy performed in combination with sacrocolpopexy

20.3.3 Ventral Rectopexy

Rectal prolapse, full-thickness prolapse of the rectum through the anal muscles (Fig. 20.8), and rectal intussusception, full-thickness descent of the rectum through the anal muscles, can be addressed with a ventral rectopexy during a minimally invasive sacrocolpopexy [32, 33]. The colorectal surgeon can perform his or her dissection either prior to or after the vaginal and presacral dissections for the sacrocolpopexy. If performed laparoscopically, two 5-mm ports are utilized in the right and left lower quadrants with a 12-mm port placed suprapubically to the right of the midline for sigmoid retraction. When performed robotically, we utilize the "W" port configuration, as previously discussed in the sacrocolpopexy section. Other authors report using more of an arch configuration, with two robotic ports on the patient's right lower (arm 1) and right upper quadrants (arm 2). The third robotic port is in the left upper quadrant (arm 3). One 12-mm assistant port is in the left lower quadrant, and a 5-mm assistant port used for sigmoid retraction is located suprapubically [34].

A steep Trendelenburg position is utilized to retract the bowel cephalad, and the uterus is retracted anteriorly if needed. The presacral and rectovaginal dissections are performed in similar fashion to those for sacral colpopexy. If perineal descent is present, the dissection can be carried further caudad to the perineal body and pubococcygeus muscles. A polypropylene or biologic mesh measuring 8–9 × 15–20 cm is introduced through the 12-mm port, and 2-0 polydiaxone sutures are used to secure the mesh to the pelvic floor muscles laterally (Figs. 20.9 and 20.10). The width and length of the mesh depend on the dimensions of the pelvis and are chosen to ensure that the mesh is not placed on any tension. Six to eight sutures are then used to secure the mesh to the anterior seromuscular rectum, with caution used to avoid full-thickness rectal bites. The mesh is then secured to the anterior longitudinal ligament of the sacrum with sutures without any tension. At the conclusion of the prolapse repair, the peritoneum is closed over both the rectopexy and sacrocolpopexy meshes (Fig. 20.7).

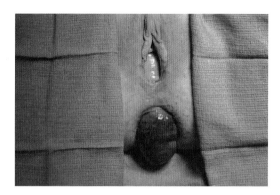

Fig. 20.8 Full-thickness rectal prolapse

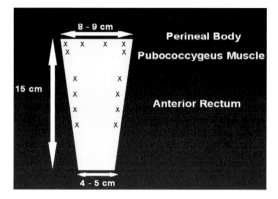

Fig. 20.9 Dimensions of ventral rectopexy mesh and points of attachment

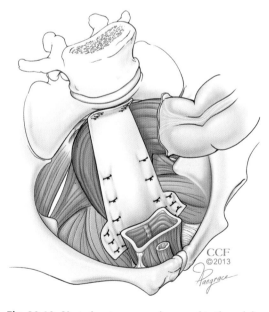

Fig. 20.10 Ventral rectopexy mesh secured to the pelvic floor muscles laterally and anterior seromuscular rectum

20.3.3.1 Ventral Rectopexy: Clinical Results and Complications

Several case series discuss the feasibility and safety of combined laparoscopic vaginal and rectal prolapse procedures [35, 36]. Slawik and colleagues reported a case series of 74 patients who underwent laparoscopic ventral rectopexy, posterior colporrhaphy, and sacrocolpopexy [35]. The median operative time was 125 min (range, 50–210 min), with only one conversion to an open procedure. Patients had only minor postoperative complications (three fecal impactions, one port-site infection, one urinary tract infection, one chest infection). These women were followed for a median time of 54 months (range, 20–96 months). Although no patient developed recurrent full- thickness rectal prolapse, four had symptoms of postoperative residual hypertrophied rectal mucosal prolapse. Wexner fecal incontinence scores improved in 91 % of patients, and obstructed defecation resolved in 80 %; three patients, however, reported new-onset minor issues with defecation. Although they did not report objective or subjective outcomes for vaginal prolapse or urinary incontinence, no mesh erosions were reported.

A recent systematic review of ventral rectopexy for rectal prolapse and rectal intussusception included 12 case series with a total of 728 patients [37]. Weighted mean percentage decrease in fecal incontinence was 45 % (95 % CI, 35.6 %–54.1 %), and weighted mean decrease in constipation was 24 % (95 % CI, 6.8 %–40.9 %). Recurrent rates of rectal prolapse ranged from 0 to 15.4 % over mean follow-up periods ranging from 3 to 106 months. The most common complications were urinary tract infections ($n = 11$) and port site or incisional hernias ($n = 16$). There were four reported mesh-related complications; there was one mesh erosion and two mesh detachments. One patient died from sepsis attributed to infection of a nylon mesh. Long-term outcome data on minimally invasive ventral rectopexy, however, are limited.

Other studies have compared operative, clinical, and cost results between ventral rectopexy performed laparoscopically and robotically [34, 38, 39]. Overall, small comparative studies report no difference in perioperative complications. One study found similar short-term outcomes for robotic and laparoscopic procedures. Another prospective cohort of 82 patients found recurrent rectal prolapse more frequent after laparoscopic and robotic procedures compared with open rectopexy (27, 20, and 2 %, respectively; p = .008). Robotic cases took longer than laparoscopic rectopexy (221 ± 39 versus 162 ± 60 min; p = .0001) and cost more to perform ($4,910 versus $4,165; p = .012) [34, 38]. Robot-assisted laparoscopy, however, may help with ease of suturing for those colorectal surgeons who are not accustomed to suturing laparoscopically.

20.3.4 Other Robotic Prolapse Procedures

Robotic uterosacral vault suspension, hysteropexy, sacrohysteropexy, and enterocele repair are all performed in a similar manner to their laparoscopic correlates, as described in detail in Chap. 7. All robotic suture tying, however, is performed with an intracorporeal technique. We utilize the same port placement as described for robotic sacrocolpopexy but move robotic ports into more of a sunburst or arch configuration for larger uteri. Posterior vaginal dissection, however, can be greatly hindered if the robotic ports are too far cephalad.

20.4 Incontinence Procedures

20.4.1 Burch Colposuspension and Paravaginal Defect Repair

Although robotic and single-port laparoscopic technology have been applied to laparoscopy for prolapse repair, it is not currently widely used for colposuspension; however, we have increased utilization of retropubic procedures in patients who do not prefer vaginally introduced synthetic mesh. When we perform a Burch colposuspension robotically, it is done with an intraperitoneal technique similar to that described for laparoscopic colposuspension in Chap. 7. Owing to the

lack of haptic feedback with the robot, careful dissection technique must be used when clearing off Cooper's ligament. Cadaveric studies have shown that the obturator canal is located approximately 5.4 cm (range, 4.5–6.1 cm) lateral to the pubic symphysis and 1.7 cm (range, 1.5–2.6 cm) inferior to the iliopectineal line [40]. Additionally, the external iliac vessels are located approximately 1 cm lateral to the obturator canal and 7.3 cm (range, 6.3–8.5 cm) lateral to the pubic symphysis (Fig. 20.11) [41].

After the space of Retzius is exposed as described in Chap. 7, the vaginal or bedside assistant places two fingers or an end-to-end anastomosis (EEA) sizer in the vagina and identifies the urethrovesical junction with gentle traction on the Foley catheter. With elevation of the periurethral and paravaginal tissues, the vaginal wall lateral to the bladder neck is exposed by using a laparoscopic blunt-tipped dissector held by the bedside assistant. A No. 0 monofilament permanent suture on a CT-2 or SH needle can be placed first through the Cooper ligament, then through the periurethral endopelvic fascia in a figure-of-eight fashion, again through Cooper's ligament, and finally tied superior to the ligament in an intracorporeal fashion. The surgeon must take care to place stitches in the vaginal wall, excluding the vaginal epithelium at the level of, or just proximal to, the midurethra and bladder neck (Fig. 20.12). We typically place the midurethral sutures first and tie sutures immediately after placement to avoid tangling. A suture bridge of 1.5–2 cm between the paravaginal tissue and Cooper's ligament is common. When a paravaginal defect repair

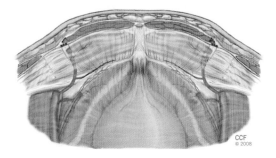

Fig. 20.11 Vascular anatomy of the retropubic space

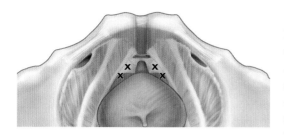

Fig. 20.12 Location of Burch colposuspension sutures

is performed at the same time as Burch colposuspension, the paravaginal sutures are placed prior to the Burch sutures in the same manner as described laparoscopically in order to optimize exposure in the surgical field (Figs. 7.7 and 7.8)

20.4.1.1 Burch Colposuspension: Clinical Results and Complications

Apart from a small case series that utilized an extracorporeal robotic technique, there is scant literature on robotic-assisted laparoscopic colposuspension [42]. A recent Cochrane review compared laparoscopic Burch colposuspension with open Burch colposuspension [43]. Twelve randomized trials were included, with a total of 1,260 women studied. Comparison of short-term success was limited by the combined estimates for subjective stress incontinence showing a wide confidence interval, favoring either approach (RR 0.97; 95 % CI 0.79–1.18). Only one trial with 64 participants was included in long-term analysis [44]. Although statistical significance was not reached, this seemed to favor laparoscopic Burch (RR 1.89; 95 % CI 0.99–3.59). In this trial, however, there was greater than 50 % incontinence rate following open Burch, which was much greater than that reported in other trials. Objective clinical data regarding stress incontinence outcomes, both in the short (six trials) and middle (seven trials) term did not show differences between laparoscopic and open Burch (RR 0.88; 95 % CI 0.64–1.21) and (RR 0.92; 95 % CI 0.71–1.19), respectively.

There were slight differences in some of the surgical parameters and perioperative complications between laparoscopic and open Burch [43]. The operative time for open Burch was significantly shorter (range, 15–41 min) than for laparoscopic surgery in three of the four trials comparing procedural time [45–48]. Five [46–50] of the seven trials reported a longer hospital stay for open Burch, with two trials showing no difference in length of stay [51, 52]. Four trials showed a higher rate of bladder perforation for the laparoscopic Burch (0.6 % versus 3 %; RR 0.22; 95 % CI 0.06–0.87) [47, 49, 50, 52]. Six trials showed no significant difference in de novo detrusor overactivity (8 % versus 11 %; RR 0.82; 95 % CI 0.48–1.38) or voiding difficulties (10 % versus 9 %; RR 1.12; 95 % CI 0.70–1.79) between laparoscopic and open Burch [44, 46, 48, 51–53]. Two trials reported a total of 39 new or recurrent prolapse events, rate 11 % versus 9 %, with no significant difference between laparoscopic and open Burch (RR 0.76; 95 % CI 0.39–1.52) [51, 52].

Conclusions

Robotic-assisted laparoscopy is a means of less invasive surgical access but should not be considered a unique surgical procedure. We believe that the minimally invasive and open prolapse and incontinence procedures should be identical in operative techniques. The benefits of improved visualization of anatomic structures and the small incisions associated with minimally invasive approaches are desirable, particularly in obese patients. The advantages of less postoperative pain, shorter hospitalization, shorter recovery period, and earlier return to work are very popular with patients, but these advantages are partially offset by increased operating time and, in many cases, increased costs.

Although the quality of surgical trials for minimally invasive prolapse and incontinence procedures has increased over the past 5 years, the field of pelvic reconstructive surgery still needs long-term outcomes from multicenter, prospective, randomized trials. Surgical recovery and health-related quality of life indices must be included in further work. These patient-centered outcomes, along with surgical efficiency and cost containment, must be emphasized when training the next generation of minimally invasive pelvic reconstructive surgeons.

References

1. Di Marco DS, Chow GK, Gettman MT, Elliott DS. Robotic-assisted laparoscopic sacrocolpopexy for treatment of vaginal vault prolapse. Urology. 2004;63:373–6.
2. Geller EJ, Siddiqui NY, Wu JM, Visco AG. Short-term outcomes of robotic sacrocolpopexy compared with abdominal sacrocolpopexy. Obstet Gynecol. 2008;112:120–6.
3. Nosti PA, Umoh U, Kane S, et al. Outcomes of minimally invasive and abdominal sacrocolpopexy: a Fellows' Pelvic Research Network Study (abstract). Female Pelvic Med Reconstr Surg. 2012;18:S18.
4. Akl MN, Long JB, Giles DL, Cornella JL, Pettit PD, Chen AH, Magtibay PM. Robotic-assisted sacrocolpopexy: technique and learning curve. Surg Endosc. 2009;23:2390–4.
5. Lim PC, Kang E, Park DH. Learning curve and surgical outcome for robotic-assisted hysterectomy with lymphadenectomy: case-matched controlled comparison with laparoscopy and laparotomy for treatment of endometrial cancer. J Minim Invasive Gynecol. 2010;17:739–48.
6. Kho R. Comparison of robotic-assisted laparoscopy versus conventional laparoscopy on skill acquisition and performance. Clin Obstet Gynecol. 2011;54:376–81.
7. Lawson EH, Curet MJ, Sanchez BR, Schuster R, Berguer R. Postural ergonomics during robotic and laparoscopic gastric bypass surgery: a pilot project. J Robot Surg. 2007;1:61–7.
8. Lee EC, Rafiq A, Merrell R, Ackerman R, Dennerlein JT. Ergonomics and human factors in endoscopic surgery: a comparison of manual vs telerobotic simulation systems. Surg Endosc. 2005;19:1064–70.
9. Berguer R, Smith W. An ergonomic comparison of robotic and laparoscopic technique: the influence of surgeon experience and task complexity. J Surg Res. 2006;134:87–92.
10. van der Schatte Olivier RH, Van't Hullenaar CD, Ruurda JP, Broeders IA. Ergonomics, user comfort, and performance in standard and robot-assisted laparoscopic surgery. Surg Endosc. 2009;23:1365–71.
11. Falabella A, Moore-Jeffries E, Sullivan MJ, Nelson R, Lew M. Cardiac function during steep Trendelenburg position and CO_2 pneumoperitoneum for robotic-assisted prostatectomy: a trans-oesophageal Doppler probe study. Int J Med Robot. 2007;3:312–15.
12. Ogunnaike BO, Jones SB, Jones DB, Provost D, Whitten CW. Anesthetic considerations for bariatric surgery. Anesth Analg. 2002;95:1793–5.
13. Danic MJ, Chow M, Alexander G, et al. Anesthesia considerations for robotic-assisted prostatectomy: a review of 1,500 cases. J Robot Surg. 2007;1:119–23.
14. Baltayian S. A brief review: anesthesia for robotic prostatectomy. J Robot Surg. 2008;2:59–66.
15. London ET, Ho HS, Neuhaus AM, Wolfe BM, Rudich SM, Perez RV. Effect of intravascular volume expansion and renal function during prolonged CO_2 pneumoperitoneum. Ann Surg. 2000;231:195–201.
16. Tekelioglu UY, Erdem A, Demirhan A, Akkaya A, Ozturk S, Bilgi M, et al. The prolonged effect of pneumoperitoneum on cardiac autonomic functions during laparoscopic surgery: are we aware? Eur Rev Med Pharmacol Sci. 2013;17:895–902.
17. Murdock CM, Wolff AJ, Van Geem T. Risk factors for hypercarbia, subcutaneous emphysema, pneumothorax, and pneumomediastinum during laparoscopy. Obstet Gynecol. 2000;95:704–9.
18. Routh JC, Bacon DR, Leibovich BC, Zincke H, Blute ML, Frank I. How long is too long? The effect of the duration of anesthesia on the incidence of nonurological complications after surgery. BJU Int. 2008;102:301–4.
19. Maher C, Feiner B, Baessler K, Schmid C. Surgical management of pelvic organ prolapse in women. Cochrane Database Syst Rev. 2013;(4):CD004014. doi: 10.1002/14651858.CD004014.pub5.
20. Paraiso MF, Jelovsek JE, Frick A, Chen CC, Barber MD. Laparoscopic compared with robotic sacrocolpopexy for vaginal prolapse. Obstet Gynecol. 2011;118:1005–13.
21. Freeman RM, Pantazis K, Thomson A, Frapell J, Bombieri L, Moran P, et al. A randomised controlled trial of abdominal versus laparoscopic sacrocolpopexy for the treatment of post-hysterectomy vaginal vault prolapse: LAS study. Int Urogynecol J. 2013;24:377–84.
22. Maher CF, Feiner B, DeCuyper EM, Nichlos CJ, Hickey KV, O'Rourke P. Laparoscopic sacral colpopexy versus total vaginal mesh for vaginal vault prolapse: a randomized trial. Am J Obstet Gynecol. 2011;204:360.e1–7.
23. Antosh DD, Grotzke SA, McDonald MA, Shveiky D, Park AJ, Gutman RE, Sokol A. Short-term outcomes of robotic versus conventional laparoscopic sacral colpopexy. Female Pelvic Med Reconstr Surg. 2012;18:158–61.
24. Cundiff GW, Harris RL, Coates K, Low VH, Bump RC, Addison WA. Abdominal sacral colpoperineopexy: a new approach for correction of posterior compartment defects and perineal descent associated with vaginal vault prolapse. Am J Obstet Gynecol. 1997;177:1345–53.
25. McDermott CD, Park J, Terry CL, Woodman PJ, Hale DS. Laparoscopic sacral colpoperineopexy: abdominal versus abdominal-vaginal posterior graft attachment. Int Urogynecol J. 2011;22:469–75.
26. Nosti PA, Lowman JK, Zollinger TW, Hale DS, Woodman PJ. Risk of mesh erosion after abdominal sacral colpoperineopexy with concurrent hysterectomy. Am J Obstet Gynecol. 2009;201:541.e1–4.
27. Su KC, Mutone MF, Terry CL, Hale DS. Abdominovaginal sacral colpoperineopexy: patient

perceptions, anatomical outcomes and graft erosions. Int Urogynecol J Pelvic Floor Dysfunct. 2007;18: 503–11.

28. Cundiff GW, Varner E, Visco AG, Zyczynski HM, Nager CW, Norton PA, et al. Risk factors for mesh/suture erosion following sacral colpopexy. Am J Obstet Gynecol. 2008;199:688.e1–5.

29. Visco AG, Weidner AC, Barber MD, Myers ER, Cundiff GW, Bump RC, Addison WA, et al. Vaginal mesh erosion after abdominal sacral colpopexy. Am J Obstet Gynecol. 2001;184:297–302.

30. Reddy J, Ridgeway B, Gurland B, et al. Robotic sacrocolpoperineopexy with ventral rectopexy for the combined treatment of rectal and pelvic organ prolapse: initial report and technique. J Robot Surg. 2011;5:167–73.

31. Wehbe SA, El-Khawand D, Arunachalam D, et al. Comparative outcomes of robotic assisted sacrocolpopexy and sacrocolpoperineopexy. A cohort study (abstract). Neurourol Urodyn. 2012;31:261–2.

32. Cullen J, Rosselli JM, Gurland BH. Ventral rectopexy for rectal prolapse and obstructed defecation. Clin Colon Rectal Surg. 2012;25:34–5.

33. D'Hoore A, Cadoni R, Penninckx F. Long-term outcome of laparoscopic ventral rectopexy for total rectal prolapse. Br J Surg. 2004;91:1500–05.

34. Wong MT, Meurette G, Rigaud J, Regenet N, Lehur PA. Robotic versus laparoscopic rectopexy for complex rectocele: a prospective comparison of short-term outcomes. Dis Colon Rectum. 2011;54:342–6.

35. Slawik S, Soulsby R, Carter H, Payne H, Dixon AR. Laparoscopic ventral rectopexy, posterior colporrhaphy and vaginal sacrocolpopexy for the treatment of recto-genital prolapse and mechanical outlet obstruction. Colorectal Dis. 2007;10:138–43.

36. Sagar PM, Thekkinkattil DK, Heath RM, Woodfield J, Gonsalves S, Landon CR. Feasibility and functional outcome of laparoscopic sacrocolpopexy for combined vaginal and rectal prolapse. Dis Colon Rectum. 2008;51:1414–20.

37. Samaranayake CB, Luo C, Plank AW, Merrie AE, Plank LD, Bissett IP. Systematic review on ventral rectopexy for rectal prolapse and intussusception. Colorectal Dis. 2009;12:504–14.

38. Heemskerk J, de Hoog DENM, van Gemert WG, Baeten CG, Greve JW, Bouvy ND. Robot-assisted vs conventional laparoscopic rectopexy for rectal prolapse: a comparative study on costs and time. Dis Colon Rectum. 2001;50:1825–30.

39. de Hoog DE, Heemskerk J, Nieman FH, van Gemert WG, Baeten CG, Bouvy ND. Recurrence and functional results after open versus conventional laparoscopic versus robot-assisted laparoscopic rectopexy for rectal prolapse: a case–control study. Int J Colorectal Dis. 2009;24:1201–6.

40. Drewes PG, Marinis SI, Schaffer JI, Boreham MK, Corton MM. Vascular anatomy over the superior pubic rami in female cadavers. Am J Obstet Gynecol. 2005;193:2165–8.

41. Pathi SD, Castellanos ME, Corton MM. Variability of the retropubic space anatomy in female cadavers. Am J Obstet Gynecol. 2009;201:524.e1–5.

42. Khan MS, Challacombe B, Rose K, Dasgupta P. Robotic colposuspension: two case reports. J Endourol. 2007;21:1077–9.

43. Lapitan MCM, Cody JD. Open retropubic colposuspension for urinary incontinence in women. Cochrane Database Syst Rev. 2012;(6):CD002912. doi: 10.1002/14651858.CD002912.pub5.

44. Morris AR, Reilly ET, Hassan A, et al. 5–7 year follow up of a randomized trial comparing laparoscopic colposuspension and open colposuspension in the treatment of genuine stress incontinence (abstract). Int Urogynecol J. 2001;12 Suppl 3:S6.

45. Ankardal M, Ekerydh A, Crafoord K, Milsom I, Stjerndahl JH, Engh ME. A randomized trial comparing open Burch colposuspension using sutures with laparoscopic colposuspension using mesh and staples in women with stress urinary incontinence. BJOG. 2004;111:974–81.

46. Fatthy H, El Hao M, Samaha I, Abdallah K. Modified Burch colposuspension: laparoscopic versus laparotomy. J Am Assoc Gynecol Laparosc. 2001;8:99–106.

47. Stangel-Wojcikiewicz K. Laparoscopic Burch colposuspension compared to laparotomy for treatment of urinary stress incontinence. Neurourol Urodyn. 2007;27:714 (Abstract).

48. Su TH, Wang KG, Hsu CY, Wei HJ, Hong BK. Prospective comparison of laparoscopic and traditional colposuspension in the treatment of genuine stress incontinence. Acta Obstet Gynecol Scand. 1997;76:576–82.

49. Kitchener HC, Dunn G, Lawton V, Reid F, Nelson L, Smith AR, COLPO Study Group. Laparoscopic versus open colposuspension—results of a prospective randomized controlled trial. BJOG. 2006;113:1007–13.

50. Tuygun C, Bakirtas H, Eroglu M, Alisir I, Zengin K, Imamoglu A. Comparison of two different surgical approaches in the treatment of stress urinary incontinence: open and laparoscopic Burch colpopsuspension. Turk Uroloji Dergisi. 2006;32:248–53.

51. Cheon WC, Mak JH, Liu JY. Prospective randomized controlled trial comparing laparoscopic open colposuspension. Hong Kong Med J. 2003;9:10–4.

52. Carey MP, Goh JT, Rosamilia A, Cornish A, Gordon I, Hawthorne G, et al. Laparoscopic versus open Burch colposuspension: a randomized controlled trial. BJOG. 2006;113:999–1006.

53. Ustun Y, Engin-Ustun Y, Gungor M, Tezcan S. Randomized comparison of Burch urethropexy procedures concomitant with gynecologic operations. Gynecol Obstet Invest. 2005;59:19–23.

Techniques for Robotic Tubal Surgery

21

Rebecca Flyckt

Robotic tubal reanastomosis allows less experienced laparoscopic surgeons to offer a minimally invasive approach to sterilization reversal. Robotic techniques present several advantages for the surgeon: easier dissection of the tubal ends, better visualization of the tubal lumina for reapproximation, more delicate tissue handling, and more precise placement of fine sutures. Data on pregnancy outcomes after robotic tubal reversal appear comparable with those obtained after classic laparotomy with microsurgery. For women desiring childbearing after tubal ligation, robotic tubal reanastomosis should be considered a viable alternative to in vitro fertilization, especially in younger patients.

21.1 Introduction

Tubal ligation remains the most common form of contraception in the United States among married women and women over the age of 30 [1]. Although it is a safe and efficacious method, tubal sterilization is associated with a high risk of desire for reversal, and approximately 1–2 % of patients seek tubal reversal for further fertility [2]. Young age at the time of sterilization is the most common factor related to feelings of regret

[3]. Couples desiring children after tubal ligation can chose between in vitro fertilization (IVF) or surgical tubal reanastomosis.

Traditionally, tubal reanastomosis was performed through a Pfannenstiel laparotomy incision using microsurgical techniques. Success rates for this technique have been quoted to be as high as 85 % [4]. However, this technique has the standard limitations of a laparotomy, including longer recovery time, increased postoperative pain, and increased risk of adhesion formation. Typically, patients remain in the hospital overnight and cannot return to work and normal activities for at least 2 weeks. Laparoscopic tubal reversals became more common in the 1990s with the rise of minimally invasive surgery [5]. Unfortunately, this method requires advanced training in complex laparoscopy and experience with laparoscopic suturing using very fine suture material. In addition, two experienced surgeons are often needed to complete a laparoscopic tubal reanastomosis, and the procedure can take from 2 to 4 h.

As IVF success rates climbed over the past several decades and comfort with complex laparoscopic suturing has diminished, some centers have dismissed the surgical approach to treating infertility after tubal ligation. However, robotic tubal reanastomosis is attainable for less experienced laparoscopic surgeons and offers the advantages of improved visualization of the tubal lumina, simpler knot tying, and finer dissection and manipulation of the fallopian tubes. Patients can be discharged home the same day. For patients seeking restoration of fertility, robotic tubal reanastomosis represents

R. Flyckt, MD
Department of Obstetrics and Gynecology,
Cleveland Clinic, 9500 Euclid Avenue,
Cleveland, OH 44195, USA
e-mail: flycktr@ccf.org

a one-time, minimally invasive method of tubal reversal with a high chance of subsequent successful spontaneous conception. In comparison with IVF, tubal reversal surgery dramatically reduces the risk of twins and higher order multiples, along with their attendant concerns of increased cost and medical risks. An additional benefit of tubal reversal is that one procedure can result in more than one subsequent pregnancy.

21.2 Set-up and Positioning

A preoperative semen analysis should be performed for all couples electing this procedure. Patients of advanced maternal age may also be assessed for ovarian reserve. Standard preconception counseling can be undertaken at the time of the preoperative visit.

The patient is placed in the lithotomy position. Choosing a uterine manipulator with the capability for chromopertubation is essential. Because the appropriateness of the patient's tubes for surgery cannot be assessed preoperatively, a 5-mm trocar is placed at the umbilicus for the introduction of the 5-mm laparoscope, and pelvic survey is performed before extending the umbilical incision to accommodate a 12-mm trocar for the robotic laparoscope. The tubes must be of adequate length (at least 4 cm) and free of significant adhesions for the procedure to be successfully performed [6]. The 8-mm robotic trocars are then placed at a 10- to 15-degree angle approximately 8–10 cm from the umbilicus on either side. Five-mm robotic trocars and instruments are also now available and can be used for this procedure.

An important aspect of the approach for tubal reanastomosis is the placement of an accessory port low in the abdomen. We place either a 5- or 10-mm accessory port in the right or left lower quadrant to allow the assistant to easily introduce needles under direct visualization into the operator field. The needles for tubal reanastomosis are small and difficult to handle and can be easily lost if not transferred slowly and carefully. Once lost, the chances of finding and retrieving the needle are small.

21.3 Docking of the Robot

The column of the robot is located at the patient's side, which allows easy access to the manipulator by an assistant. The camera is placed into the umbilical port, and the two robotic arms are attached to the two lateral robotic trocars. A recent adaptation is the use of the first and third robotic arms for tubal reanastomosis to allow a wider angle of approach. The final arm can be docked with the placement of an additional 8-mm trocar if needed, but this scenario is rare.

21.4 Robotic Instrumentation

After the robot has been docked, the robotic instruments are introduced into the pelvis under operator visualization. The instruments needed for the procedure are the EndoWrist monopolar cautery hook or shears (Intuitive Surgical Inc., Sunnyvale, CA) and the EndoWrist PK grasper (Intuitive Surgical Inc., Sunnyvale, CA) with bipolar energy attached. For right-handed surgeons, the EndoWrist PK grasper is loaded into the left port and the monopolar energy source is in the right port. If the final remaining arm is utilized, the EndoWrist Prograsper (Intuitive Surgical Inc., Sunnyvale, CA) can be introduced here. For suturing, we prefer an EndoWrist Black Diamond Micro Forceps (Intuitive Surgical Inc., Sunnyvale, CA) in either hand as the needle drivers.

21.5 Surgical Procedure

The goal of robotic tubal reanastomosis is to duplicate the steps of the open procedure using robotic instruments and techniques.

21.5.1 Preparation of Proximal and Distal Segments

The serosa is incised, and the stump is exposed. Initially, lysis of tubal adhesions is performed, and any tubal clips or rings are removed. Dilute vaso-pressin (20 U in 100–200 mL of normal saline) is then injected into the mesosalpinx for hemostasis and to assist with identifying tissue planes. Transcervical injection of indigo carmine dye can then be performed to ensure proximal tubal patency and identify the end of the proximal tube for dissection. The serosa covering the occluded end is then incised using the monopolar cautery, and the serosa is peeled back to expose the proximal stump.

Scissors are used without energy to reveal tubal lumina. The robotic scissors are then used to move across the exposed area, excising the scar and revealing the tubal lumina. Energy is not applied during this step, and minimal cautery is used to coagulate bleeders to minimize subsequent scarring or reocclusion. A similar procedure is performed to expose the distal tubal lumina, and the fimbriated end of the tube can be cannulated to confirm patency by injection of indigo carmine dye.

This step is particularly amenable to a robotic approach. Visualization of the tubal lumina is enhanced by robotic magnification, and tremor reduction allows a more careful dissection of the tubal ends.

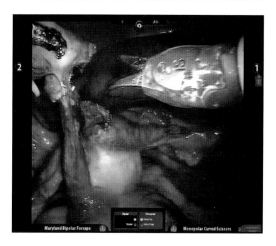

Fig. 21.2 Scissors are used without energy to reveal the tubal lumen

21.5.2 Reapproximation of Mesosalpinx

Often, the mesosalpinx separates widely after preparation of the tubal ends. To align the tubes and relieve tension on the anastomosis site, one or more 6-0 Vicryl (Ethicon, EndoSurgery Inc., Somerville, NJ) stitches are placed into the mesosalpinx to bring its edges closer together. Also at this time, a catheter is placed into the proximal and distal tubal ends to facilitate suturing of the lumina.

For a tubal stent we use the inner plastic cannula from the Novy Cornual Cannulation set (Cook Medical Inc., Bloomington, IN), cut to a 6- to 9- cm length. Other luminal stents and adaptations have been described, including simply using a piece of 0-Vicryl suture for this purpose.

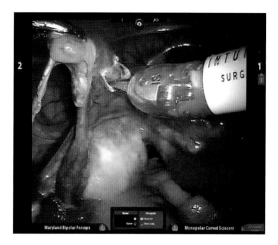

Fig. 21.1 The serosa is incised, and the stump is exposed

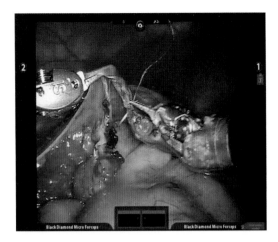

Fig. 21.3 Reapproximated mesosalpinx

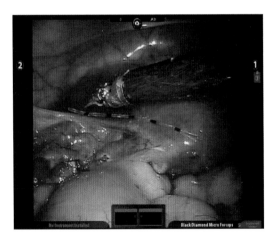

Fig. 21.4 Plastic cannula as tubal stent

21.5.3 Tubal Reanastomosis

The tubal reanastomosis is performed using interrupted sutures of 8-0 Vicryl through the tubal muscularis and mucosal layers. In order, we place sutures at the 6, 3, 9, and 12 o'clock locations and tie them with intracorporeal knot-tying techniques. The suturing should position the knot outside of the tubal lumen. Precise placement of these sutures is another distinct advantage when using the surgical robot. We do not tie down the 3 and 9 o'clock knots until the 12 o'clock stitch is placed; otherwise, it may be difficult to identify

the lumina and place the 12 o'clock stitch correctly. Great care must be taken to handle the tissue delicately while suturing and not to avulse the needle.

As with all robotic surgery, visual rather than tactile feedback can be used to provide the appropriate tissue tension. Transcervical injection of indigo carmine dye is again used to confirm tubal patency at the conclusion of this portion of the procedure. Revisions can occur if patency has not been established. Usually an additional suture placed at an area of dye leakage at the anastomosis site is all that is needed.

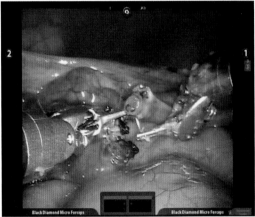

Fig. 21.5 Chromopertubation

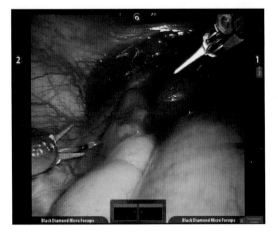

Fig. 21.6 Serosal stitches

21.5.4 Serosal Repair

In a similar fashion to the above, the serosa is repaired with circumferential interrupted stitches of 8-0 Vicryl. Chromopertubation is again performed to ensure that the reanastomosis site has not been kinked or occluded by the placement of serosal sutures.

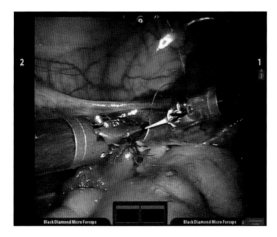

Fig. 21.7 Repair of serosa with circumferential stitches

21.6 Postoperative Care

In most cases, patients undergoing robotic tubal reanastomosis can be discharged home the same day with oral pain medications. A follow-up visit should be scheduled within 6 weeks. Patients can initiate attempts to conceive after two menstrual cycles. We recommend a hysterosalpingogram if the patient has not conceived within six cycles.

21.7 Discussion

In comparison to standard microsurgical tubal reanastomosis via laparotomy, robotic tubal reversal offers a same day approach with the benefits of a minimally invasive recovery. Given that few surgeons possess the skills needed for laparoscopic tubal reanastomosis, robotic reversal should be considered as a first-line alternative to IVF in carefully selected women.

Cumulative pregnancy rates after robotic tubal reanastomosis are largely dependent on the woman's age and range from 60 to 90 % [5, 7]. Chances for conception are highest in the first year after surgery. In a recent large series of robotic tubal reanastomosis, even women between 40 and 42 years old had high pregnancy and birth rates of 50 and 44 %, respectively [7]. Ectopic risk after tubal reanastomosis appears to be consistently 2–3 % [2, 4, 8, 9].

Two publications with small sample sizes have compared outcomes of women undergoing robotic tubal reanastomosis with reanastomosis by laparotomy or outpatient minilaparotomy [5, 10]. Pregnancy and ectopic rates were similar, although the robotic approach took longer and was more costly. As expected, hospitalization times and return to normal activities were shorter after robotic surgery than laparotomy. When weighing robotic surgery versus IVF, one must take into consideration the individual success rates of the IVF program versus the surgeon's comfort and ability with the procedure and the patient's prognosis for success. Higher cumulative pregnancy rates and lower cost per delivery have been described for tubal reanastomosis versus IVF in women less than 37 years old [11].

In conclusion, robotic tubal reanastomosis offers an alternative to open surgery or IVF for women seeking sterilization reversal. This type of surgery appears uniquely suited to robotics owing to the need for delicate tissue handling, increased magnification for identification and preparation of the tubal ends, and fine intracorporeal suturing. The limited data available support the efficacy and safety of this approach.

References

1. Zite N, Borrero S. Female sterilisation in the United States. Eur J Contracept Reprod Health Care. 2011;16:336–40.
2. Yoon TK, Sung HR, Kang HG, Cha SH, Lee CN, Cha KY. Laparoscopic tubal anastomosis: fertility outcome in 202 cases. Fertil Steril. 1999;72:1121–6.
3. Hillis SD, Marchbanks PA, Tylor LR, Peterson HB. Poststerilization regret: findings from the United States Collaborative Review of Sterilization. Obstet Gynecol. 1999;93:889–95.
4. Dubuisson JB, Chapron C, Nos C, Morice P, Aubriot FX, Garnier P. Sterilization reversal: fertility results. Hum Reprod. 1995;10(10):1145–51.
5. Dharia Patel SP, Steinkampf MP, Whitten SJ, Malizia BA. Robotic tubal anastomosis: surgical technique and cost effectiveness. Fertil Steril. 2008;90:1175–9.
6. Rock JA, Guzick DS, Katz E, Zacur HA, King TM. Tubal anastomosis: pregnancy success following reversal of Falope ring or monopolar cautery sterilization. Fertil Steril. 1987;48:13–7.
7. Caillet M, Vandromme J, Rozenberg S, Paesmans M, Germay O, Degueldre M. Robotically assisted laparoscopic microsurgical tubal reanastomosis: a retrospective study. Fertil Steril. 2010;94:1844–7.
8. Kim JD, Kim KS, Doo JK, Rhyeu CH. A report on 387 cases of microsurgical tubal reversals. Fertil Steril. 1997;68:875–80.
9. Gordts S, Campo R, Puttemans P, Gordts S. Clinical factors determining pregnancy outcome after microsurgical tubal reanastomosis. Fertil Steril. 2009;92:1198–202.
10. Rodgers AK, Goldberg JM, Hammel JP, Falcone T. Tubal anastomosis by robotic compared with outpatient minilaparotomy. Obstet Gynecol. 2007;109:1375–80.
11. Boeckxstaens A, Devroey P, Collins J, Tournaye H. Getting pregnant after tubal sterilization: surgical reversal or IVF? Hum Reprod. 2007;22:2660–4.

Management of Laparoscopy-Related Complications

22

Jill H. Tseng, Amanda Nickles Fader, and Stacey A. Scheib

22.1 Introduction

The benefits of laparoscopy have been well established and are numerous. However, laparoscopy is not without complications. The overall complication rate ranges from 0.2 to 10.3 % [1, 2]. The rate of complications is clearly correlated with the complexity of the surgery and the skill set and experience of the surgeon. More than half of laparoscopic injuries occur during abdominal entry [1, 2]. Additionally, 20–25 % of complications are not recognized intraoperatively. The complication rate for surgeons who have performed less than 100 laparoscopies is more than four times greater than a surgeon with more experience [4].

Prevention is the key to avoiding complications and their sequelae. Experience in avoidance and management of adverse events related to minimally invasive surgery leads to improved patient outcomes.

J.H. Tseng, MD (✉) • A.N. Fader, MD
S.A. Scheib, MD
Department of Gynecology and Obstetrics,
Johns Hopkins Hospital,
600 N. Wolfe Street, Phipps 264,
Baltimore, MD 21287, USA
e-mail: jtseng3@jhmi.edu; afader1@jhmi.edu,
amandanfader@gmail.com; sscheib1@jhmi.edu

22.2 Complications Related to Entry

A number of laparoscopic insertion techniques are available, and laparoscopic entry injuries may occur with any technique. Although the complications of operative laparoscopy are low, they can be severe and life-threatening. A search of the Manufacturer and User Facility Device Experience Database (MAUDE) from the Medical Device section of the Food and Drug Administration's web site lists 25 serious iatrogenic injuries involving Veress needle entry between March 1992 and May 2000 [1]. Seventeen (68 %) vascular injuries and 4 (16 %) bowel perforations occurred, all requiring emergent laparotomy. One death, as a result of an aortic laceration, was reported. Insertion of the Veress needle and primary trocar for initial entry remains perhaps one of the most hazardous parts of laparoscopy, accounting for 40 % of all laparoscopic complications and the majority of fatalities. It is critical that patients are positioned in the supine position and NOT in Trendelenburg position during initial trocar insertion.

Entry injuries may occur with the insertion of a Veress needle or primary trocar. Vascular, visceral, and urinary tract injuries as well as gas embolism have all been described in the literature as complications related to laparoscopic abdominal entry [2]. An abdominal entry may be closed or open. There are two closed entry techniques.

P.F. Escobar, T. Falcone (eds.), *Atlas of Single-Port, Laparoscopic, and Robotic Surgery*,
DOI 10.1007/978-1-4614-6840-0_22, © Springer Science+Business Media New York 2014

The first utilizes the Veress needle, which is inserted blindly into the peritoneal cavity, followed by insufflation of the peritoneal cavity and then the trocar is inserted with or without the use of a laparoscope. The second technique involves insertion of the trocar with or without the use of a laparoscope prior to insufflation of the peritoneal cavity. The open or Hasson technique involves identification and cutting down of the fascia and peritoneum, followed by the insertion of a blunt trocar under direct visualization (Fig. 22.1). Open entry and direct entry have a lower rate of failed entry compared with the use of the Veress needle for extraperitoneal insufflation and omental injury [3].

A recent update to the Cochrane Database Review regarding laparoscopic entry techniques demonstrated that no single entry technique is superior in terms of decreasing the risk of vascular or visceral injury [4]. The review included 28 randomized controlled trials with 4,860 individuals undergoing laparoscopy and evaluated 14 comparisons. Overall, there was no evidence of advantage of using any single technique in terms of preventing major vascular or visceral complications. Using an open-entry technique compared to a Veress needle demonstrated a reduction in the incidence of failed entry; however, the odds ratio was 0.12 (95 % CI 0.02–0.92). There were three advantages with direct-trocar entry when compared with Veress needle entry in terms of lower rates of failed entry (OR 0.21, 95 % Cl 0.14–0.31), extraperitoneal insufflation (OR 0.18, 95 % Cl 0.13–0.26), and omental injury (OR 0.28, 95 % CI 0.14–0.55). There was also an advantage with the radially expanding access system (STEP) trocar entry when compared with standard trocar entry in terms of trocar site bleeding (OR 0.31, 95 % Cl 0.15–0.62). Finally, there was an advantage of not lifting the abdominal wall before Veress needle insertion when compared to lifting in terms of failed entry, without an increase in the complication rate (OR 4.44, 95 % CI 2.16–9.13). However, studies were limited to small numbers, excluding many patients with previous abdominal surgery and women with a raised body mass index who may have higher complication rates.

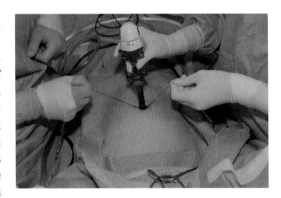

Fig. 22.1 Hasson or open entry technique

22.3   Vascular Complications

Vascular injuries are one of the most serious and potentially catastrophic complications of minimally invasive gynecologic surgery. Fortunately, the incidence of major vascular injuries is uncommon, occurring in 0.01–1 % of cases [1, 2, 4–6]. However, mortality can be as high as 9–23 % [2, 6].

22.3.1 Major Vascular Injuries

Major vessel injuries are almost five times as common during Veress needle insertion or placement of the primary trocar than during the laparoscopic operation itself [2]. The majority of major vascular injuries are arterial, with aortic and right common iliac artery injuries being the most frequent (Table 22.1). The most commonly injured venous structure is the vena cava [6, 7]. When gaining access to the peritoneal cavity using closed entry via the umbilicus, one must keep in mind the anatomic relationship of the umbilicus to the underlying retroperitoneal vessels. In non-obese patients (BMI <30 mg/m^2), the aortic bifurcation lies at or slightly caudal to the level of the umbilicus. At a 45-degree angle, the average abdominal wall thickness measures 2–3 cm, and at a 90-degree angle, the vessels are usually 6–10 cm from the skin but may be as close as 2 cm to the skin. Thus, inserting instruments through the base of the umbilicus at a 45-degree angle minimizes the risk of injury while still maintaining a high probability of successful entry. In obese women (BMI ≥30 kg/m^2), the aortic bifurcation is almost always cephalad to the level of the umbilicus. At a 45-degree angle, the average abdominal wall thickness in these patients is 11 cm, and at a 90-degree angle, the distance between the skin and the retroperitoneal vessels is greater than 13 cm. In obese patients, it is recommended that instruments be inserted through the base of the umbilicus at a 90-degree angle in order to maximize successful entry; injury to the aorta and vena cava are less likely to occur because they are further away. The angle of the surgical table must also be taken into account, since patients are often in the Trendelenburg position during laparoscopy. If the patient's feet are elevated 30° prior to instrument insertion, placing a trocar or Veress needle at a 45-degree angle to the horizontal will result in inserting the instrument at a 75-degree angle, which could result in serious consequences [7].

Many surgeons prefer open laparoscopy for placement of the primary port. Although a recent systematic review of randomized controlled trials looking at laparoscopic entry techniques reported that these studies were underpowered to detect differences in the incidence of vascular injury between various modalities [5], past literature reviews have reported vascular injuries to be a very rare complication of open entry [1, 2, 7]. All trocar types have been reported as associated with major vascular injuries; therefore technique seems to be a factor.

Major injury to the retroperitoneal vessels can also occur during secondary port placement. Lateral trocars are routinely placed 8 cm lateral to the midline and 5 cm superior to the mid-pubic symphysis to avoid injury to the vessels of the anterior abdominal wall. However, the external iliac vessels often lie directly deep to this specific location. Lateral trocars should thus be placed under direct visualization in a slow, controlled manner, along an axis perpendicular to the anterior abdominal wall. Using excessive force should be avoided, as an unexpected loss of resistance may drive the trocar directly into viscera or a major vessel.

Vascular injuries tend to be relatively easy to diagnose intraoperatively, and because of the potentially high risk of mortality, rapid recognition is imperative. Injuries involving the Veress needle or trocar can be recognized by the return of frank blood through the needle or trocar sheath. Lacerations to major retroperitoneal vessels will almost always result in brisk bleeding or an expanding hematoma. Major vascular injury should be considered if the patient becomes hemodynamically unstable during surgery. Sometimes vascular injuries can be hidden temporarily behind the omentum or retroperitoneally.

When a major vessel injury is discovered, the site should be immediately tamponaded with a blunt laparoscopic instrument. If the injury occurred as a result of a Veress needle or trocar puncture and it is still directly in the vessel, it should not be removed. Communication is key to patient outcome and survival. Anesthesia must be promptly notified, as well as vascular surgery, if available. Blood products and appropriate instruments should be called for. If the injury was from a secondary trocar or occurred during the procedure and the bleeding is controlled with pressure, the intraperitoneal cavity may remain insufflated while emergency resources are being established. Some vascular injuries can be repaired laparoscopically in the hands of experienced vascular or gynecologic oncology surgeons, but in most cases, a laparotomy will be required.

Uncontrolled bleeding warrants emergency laparotomy via midline vertical incision (from the xyphoid to the suprapubic region). Upon entry into the abdominal cavity, aortic compression should be performed immediately. Proximal and distal control of the bleeding vessel can be obtained once the site of injury is identified. Small arterial lacerations may be successfully sutured, while large arterial injuries and injuries to the great veins often require graft repair. With continued uncontrolled hemorrhage, the abdomen can be packed with laparotomy sponges while the situation is reassessed.

Small vascular injuries may not always be apparent during surgery. If a patient's blood count is inexplicably low, serial laboratory results should be obtained. Continued decrease in hematocrit level or signs of hemodynamic instability should be considered as secondary to ongoing hemorrhage until proven otherwise.

Table 22.1 Site and number of vascular injuries

Site	Number of vascular injuries
Right iliac artery	14
Right iliac vein	12
Left iliac artery	3
Left iliac vein	9
Aorta	4
Vena cava	2
Mesenteric	2
Interior epigastric[a]	2
Other	1
Total injuries	**49**

From Baggish [17]

[a]At origin from external iliac

22.3.2 Vascular Injuries to the Anterior Abdominal Wall

Major vascular injury to the anterior abdominal wall usually occurs during lateral trocar placement. The incidence of abdominal wall bleeding is 0.5 %, and in one study is less frequent with the use of blunt versus sharp-cutting trocars [2]. The inferior epigastric artery is the most commonly injured vessel. It branches off of the external iliac artery laterally, pierces the transversalis fascia, and courses medially and then superiorly in the rectus abdominis muscle, where it eventually anastomoses with the superior epigastric artery. Secondary trocars should be placed lateral to the rectus sheath.

The peritoneum covering the inferior epigastric vessels, also known as the lateral umbilical ligaments, can usually be identified as smooth ridges along the inner surface of the anterior abdominal wall, traveling superiorly and medially from the left lower quadrant and right lower quadrant toward the umbilicus. Thus, inserting the trocars under direct visualization after proper identification of these peritoneal folds can help reduce the risk of injury.

An injury to the inferior epigastric vessel can be diagnosed by bleeding from the trocar site into the abdomen or local hematoma formation. Although there is a potential for significant bleeding, these injuries can be managed in several ways. If the trocar is removed and the vessel has not retracted into the abdominal wall, bipolar coagulation may be used to achieve hemostasis. A Foley catheter can also be inserted through the trocar site and the balloon inflated to tamponade the bleeding vessel. Alternatively, if the surgeon desires to continue the surgery, the trocar can be left in place and the vessels ligated with suture cephalad and caudad to the injury. This can be performed with a large curved needle or, if the patient is obese, laparoscopically using a Keith needle that is passed through the entire thickness of the anterior abdominal wall.

In some instances, an injury to an anterior abdominal wall vessel may not be identified immediately. Severe pain around the trocar site, ecchymosis, and a palpable mass are signs of a rectus sheath hematoma. If the hematoma stays stable in size, expectant management is appropriate. However, if it continues to expand, or if there is a significant drop in the patient's hematocrit, exploration of the wound and ligation of the bleeding vessel are necessary [5].

22.4 Urinary Tract Injuries

Urinary tract injuries complicate 0.03–1.7 % of laparoscopic gynecologic surgeries [1, 2, 8]. Bladder injuries, which are more common than ureteral injuries, are up to 15 times more likely to be diagnosed intraoperatively compared with ureteral lesions [1, 8, 9]. Given the potential for significantly increased morbidity with delayed diagnosis, such as peritonitis, compromised renal function, or fistula formation, it is important for the gynecologic surgeon to be familiar with the risks of urinary tract injuries, strategies for prevention, diagnostic methods, and principles of treatment.

22.4.1 Urinary Bladder Injuries

The most common type of bladder injury is perforation [1, 2, 8, 9]. Laparoscopic assisted vaginal hysterectomies have the highest incidence of bladder injuries [8, 9]. Bladder injuries may occur in several ways. Puncture from a Veress needle generally causes a small perforation, whereas trocar injuries may result in larger lacerations. Placement of a midline suprapubic trocar can cause significant damage, especially when the bladder has not been decompressed. In addition, thermal injuries may occur when using electrocautery to dissect the bladder off of the lower uterine segment during a hysterectomy. Thus, it is important to insert a Foley catheter prior to making an abdominal incision. Secondary trocar placement should be performed under direct visualization, and consideration should be given to lateral trocar placement if a suprapubic port is not absolutely necessary. If tissue planes are unclear when dissecting the bladder from the lower uterine segment, especially in cases of endometriosis or severe adhesive disease, it is important to use sharp dissection. Blunt dissection can cause indiscriminate tearing at the site of least resistance, which may result in injury [9]. Retrograde filling of the bladder with saline or water can also help delineate its boundaries when anatomy is significantly distorted.

Signs of bladder compromise can be obvious, such as seeing or palpating the bulb of the Foley catheter in the surgical field or witnessing frank extravasation of urine. Pneumaturia or air in the Foley bag is also indicative of a bladder injury. While transient hematuria may result from manipulation or irritation of the bladder mucosa, persistent bloody urine should prompt a thorough investigation. If an injury is suspected but not apparent, it is helpful to backfill the bladder with dilute indigo carmine or methylene blue and watch for leakage of dye. This can also help identify areas that may have been weakened from dissection, where only the mucosa is left intact. Thermal injuries are often difficult to detect and may not be apparent until several days later. Signs or symptoms of concern for delayed diagnosis of bladder injury include abdominal pain, distention, ileus, ascites, and peritonitis, with or without leukocytosis.

Injuries diagnosed intraoperatively should be repaired prior to the completion of surgery. Expectant management is appropriate for minimal defects in the bladder dome, such as those created by a Veress needle. Defects less than 1 cm in diameter may be closed surgically or managed by prolonged decompression with a Foley catheter. Cystotomies 1 cm or larger are usually repaired with a simple two-layer closure using delayed absorbable suture, bringing together the mucosa and muscularis first and then the serosa for reinforcement (Fig. 22.2). The suture line should be tested for a watertight seal by instilling 300 mL of dye into the bladder and looking for leakage. A Foley catheter should be left in place for 4–14 days, depending on the size and location of the defect. Larger injuries and those located at the trigone may require more time to heal. Prior to removal of the catheter, a cystogram is should be obtained to ensure that appropriate epithelialization has occurred.

If a bladder injury is suspected after surgery, a cystogram can be performed for focused evaluation. Symptoms can be varied and can include nausea, vomiting, malaise, abdominal pain and/or distention, ileus, oliguria, or anuria. Blood tests may show an increase in creatinine levels. The diagnosis is confirmed with a cystogram. Similar to injuries that are diagnosed intraoperatively, small defects can be managed with bladder decompression using a Foley catheter, while larger defects may require surgical repair. In these cases, an urologist should be consulted for further guidance.

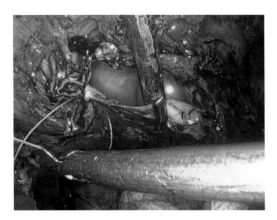

Fig. 22.2 Repair of cystotomy

22.4.2 Ureteral Injuries

The most common locations of ureteral injury in gynecologic surgery are at the cardinal ligament and at the level of the infundibulopelvic ligament [2, 9, 10]. In the cardinal ligament, the ureter passes beneath the uterine artery. It is usually less than 1 cm away from the uterine artery and 1.5 cm lateral to the cervix, although radiologic studies have shown that in cases involving cervical pathology, the ureter may be as close as 5 mm to the cervix [10]. At the level of the infundibulopelvic ligament, the ureter crosses over the pelvic brim and common iliac vessels and courses into the pelvis along the medial leaf of the broad ligament. Other sites where the ureter is particularly vulnerable to injury include the lateral border of the uterosacral ligament, the ovarian fossa, and the ureteric canal [2, 10].

Ureteral injuries can result from transection, crush, devascularization, or electrothermal damage. Because of the potential morbidity of these injuries, immediate recognition is important, although these are not commonly identified intraoperatively.

There are several measures that can be taken to avoid or reduce the risk of ureteral injury. Meticulous surgical technique and a thorough understanding of female pelvic anatomy are essential. Prior surgery, severe adhesive disease, endometriosis, enlarged uterus, fibroids, adnexal masses, and congenital anomalies all lead to distorted anatomy and tissue planes. Ideally, the ureter should be visualized before clamping any tissue pedicles. This can be done by retroperitoneal dissection, in which the round ligament is taken laterally and the peritoneum is dissected parallel to the infundibulopelvic ligament. After developing the pararectal and paravesical spaces, blunt dissection can be used to locate the ureter, which sits along or on the medial leaf of the broad ligament. Observation of vermiculation can help confirm that the correct structure has been identified.

In addition, when performing a hysterectomy, skeletonizing the uterine arteries, mobilizing the bladder down past the cervix, and deviating the uterus cranially with the use of a uterine manipulator will lateralize the ureters so that ligation of the uterine vessels and colpotomy can be performed safely [10]. Use of a cautery near the ureters should be minimized and, if necessary, hemostasis can be controlled with surgical clips. The degree of ureterolysis depends on the amount of visualization and mobilization necessary. In cases of extremely distorted pelvic anatomy, preoperative imaging or placement of ureteral stents may help to better delineate the course of the urinary tract.

If a ureteral injury is suspected, intravenous indigo carmine is administered. If there is no peritoneal extravasation, a cystoscopy is performed. The cystoscopy is used to assess for brisk efflux of dye from the bilateral ureteral orifices; sluggish efflux may be indicative of injury. Stents can also be fed through the ureters to evaluate for obstruction. If cystoscopy is not possible, stents can be fed through the ureters via cystotomy by making a small defect in the dome of the bladder. Retrograde filling of the bladder with dye and looking for leaks in the field may be useful in a limited number of cases; however, most injuries fail to demonstrate intra-operative intraperitoneal leaks [2]. Thermal injuries and partial transections are especially difficult to recognize, as they may not be identifiable by any of the above methods.

If a ureteral injury is discovered, an urologist should be consulted for intraoperative evaluation. The type of repair depends on the mechanism of injury, the severity, and the location. Laparotomy is usually necessary, although laparoscopic repair is possible with a trained surgeon. Complete ligation, crush injuries, and thermal injuries usually require complete resection of the involved segment [5, 10]. Stenting may be adequate for small burns and partial lacerations [5]. Ureteroureterostomy is usually performed for injuries of the upper third of the ureter, ureteroureterostomy with tension-free anastomosis for the middle third, and ureteroneocystostomy with a psoas hitch for the pelvic ureter.

Unfortunately, the majority of ureteral injury diagnoses are delayed. Symptoms often manifest 2–7 days postoperatively but can be as late as up to 33 days after surgery [9]. Thermal injuries sometimes appear after 10–14 days if there is delayed necrosis with partial obstruction of the ureteral wall [11]. Patients can exhibit a wide range of symptoms, including nausea, vomiting, malaise, flank pain, hematuria, vaginal drainage, leakage of fluid from trochar sites, abdominal pain and/or distention, ileus, and peritonitis. They may have leukocytosis and rising serum creatinine levels. A renal ultrasound is useful in identifying urinary leaks or hydronephrosis suggestive of obstruction. Computed tomography urograms (with intravenous contrast material if the patient has normal renal function) and retrograde pyelograms are also recommended imaging modalities. With delayed diagnosis of ureteral injuries, it is important to ensure adequate urinary drainage. This can be accomplished using percutaneous nephrostomy tubes and/or ureteral stents. Patients with successful antegrade or retrograde stent placement have a higher likelihood of recovering without open surgery [5]. Immediate treatment is supportive, including the drainage of ascites or urinomas. If surgical repair is necessary and there is tissue edema or inflammation present, or if the patient is in general poor health, a waiting period of 6 weeks or longer should be observed before proceeding [11].

22.4.3 Urinary Tract Fistulas

Fistulas are delayed postoperative complications (Fig. 22.3). Patients typically present with urine from the vagina or report incontinence. Inspection of the vagina may or may not reveal a fistula tract. In the office a tampon test can be performed in which the patient is given Pyridium orally, diluted indigo carmine is instilled into the bladder and a tampon is placed in the vagina. When the tampon is removed an hour later, orange on the tampon may point to a ureterovaginal fistula and blue may be consistent with a vesicovaginal fistula. With a fistula diagnosis, patient should be referred to a urogynecologist or urologist. Repair is typically delayed for 2–6 months.

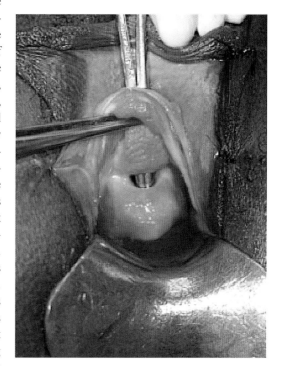

Fig. 22.3 Vesicovaginal fistula

22.4.4 Routine Cystoscopy

The use of routine cystoscopy after major gynecologic surgery has remained controversial because of the lack of high quality data demonstrating a clear benefit. In a recent prospective study of 839 patients undergoing hysterectomy, 97.4 % of the urinary tract injuries were diagnosed intraoperatively using routine cystoscopy [11]. The American Association for Gynecologic Laparoscopists cites a sensitivity of 80–90 % when using intraoperative cystoscopy for the detection of ureteral trauma and recommends that cystoscopy be available to all gynecologic surgeons performing laparoscopic hysterectomies (Fig. 22.4). However, they state that the level of evidence and limited data available preclude a recommendation for making cystoscopy an integral component of laparoscopic hysterectomy (Level B) [12]. The American College of Obstetricians and Gynecologists has recommended that cystoscopy be performed on all prolapse and incontinence procedures, since the ureters and bladder are at increased risk of injury (Level C) [13].

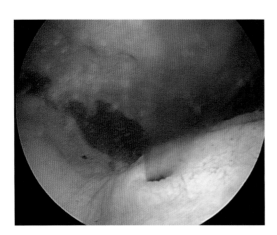

Fig. 22.4 Cystoscopy with intravenous indigo carmine

22.5 Visceral Injuries

The incidence of bowel injuries in gynecologic laparoscopic surgery ranges between 0.05 and 0.65 % [2, 3, 9]. The occurrence of small and large bowel injuries (Figs. 22.5 and 22.6) are approximately the same, collectively accounting for 82–91 % of cases, while the stomach is less frequently involved [2, 3]. Because most injuries are not diagnosed immediately, the risks of peritonitis and death are high. Bowel injuries have been reported as the most common or second most common cause of postoperative death related to laparoscopy [2, 3], with a mortality rate of 2.5–5 % [2, 9]. Mortality can be as high as 28 % with delayed diagnosis of a bowel injury [3]. Thus vigilance and early recognition are of utmost importance.

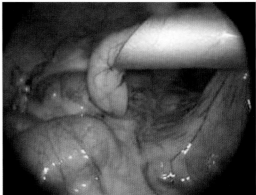

Fig. 22.5 Trocar-related bowel injury

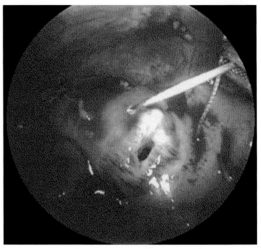

Fig. 22.6 Trocar-related colon injury

22.5.1 Injury and Prevention

Mechanisms of bowel injury during laparoscopy include puncture or laceration from a Veress needle or trocar placement, during tissue dissection or lysis of adhesions, or electrosurgical injury [9]. About a third to a half of injuries occur with abdominal entry [2, 3]. Of women who have had intraoperative bowel injuries, 87 % had adhesive disease at the time of surgery, mostly from endometriosis (Fig. 22.7) [3]. The three main risk factors for bowel complications are complexity of the surgery, the presence of intra-abdominal adhesions, and the experience of the surgeon [2].

In patients with prior abdominal surgery who are suspected to have adhesive disease, which eliminates safe entry using the Veress needle, using an open technique (Hassan method) or gaining primary access through Palmer point in the left upper quadrant should be considered. Visceral injuries from secondary trocar placement should almost never occur since after initial entry, additional trocars should be placed under direct visualization.

Injury to the stomach occurs most frequently during Veress or trocar placement, especially if Palmer point is being used for entry or if the stomach is distended. Care should be taken to reduce gastric insufflation, which can happen during mask induction with inhaled anesthetic agents or in the case of esophageal intubation [5]. A nasogastric or orogastric tube should be inserted for gastric decompression prior to Veress needle or trocar placement.

There are a number of strategies to prevent an electrosurgical injury. The insulation on instruments should be evaluated for breaks, since breaks increase the risk for electricity leaks. Avoid contact of the instrument with the bowel, including the shaft when electricity is in use. When using electricity, avoid prolonged activation of the electrode, since this increases the risks of capacitive coupling or an insulation breakdown. Activate the electrode only when it is in the view of the laparoscope and in contact with the target tissue, using the lowest possible setting. Consider cold cutting with scissors for bowel adhesions. Keep the entire tips of the

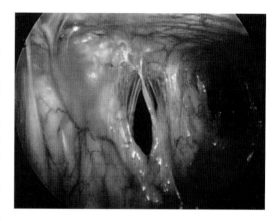

Fig. 22.7 Small bowel adhesions

instruments used in the visual field and isolate areas to be cauterized from the nearby bowel to prevent inadvertent direct burns, direct coupling, or capacitive coupling of injuries.

Postoperatively, it is not advised to prescribe antiemetics because they can mask signs of a visceral injury.

22.5.2 Diagnosis

Prognosis is dependent on prompt recognition of injuries, as mortality increases if diagnosis is delayed for longer than 72 h after surgery. Signs of direct visceral perforation during Veress needle placement and insufflation include aspiration of succus entericus or feces, asymmetric abdominal distention, and high initial insufflation pressure (although this can also be a sign of insufflating the preperitoneal space). Once a secondary trocar has been placed, the camera should be directed at the initial trocar site to evaluate for injury. A general abdominal and pelvic survey should also be performed looking for evidence of bleeding or bowel content leakage.

If an intraoperative small bowel injury is suspected or discovered, the entire small bowel should be run with bowel graspers and visually inspected to ensure that all sites of damage are accounted for. If a rectosigmoid injury is suspected, a bowel integrity test or "flat tire" test needs to be performed. This test is done by filling the pelvis with sterile water or saline and then injecting air into the rectum through a 60-mL bulb syringe. Laparoscopically, the sigmoid is compressed proximally with a blunt probe, which keeps the air distal. If there is a rectosigmoid perforation, bubbles can be seen in the fluid-filled pelvis. An alternative to the bowel integrity test is to fill the rectum with indigo carmine stained sterile water or saline. If one sees blue dye spillage or the dye can be seen through the bowel wall, the bowel needs to be repaired at that site immediately.

Visceral injuries often go unrecognized intraoperatively, especially thermal injuries, which may not be recognizable at the time of surgery. Patients with penetrating trauma usually present within 24–48 h, while unrecognized thermal injuries may not manifest until 4–10 days later. Initial signs and symptoms may be nonspecific, including abdominal pain, nausea, vomiting, distention, anorexia, or ileus; a low-grade fever and leukocytosis are also usually present. Later on, patients may develop generalized peritonitis or present with septic shock. Free air on a plain abdominal radiograph is usually not helpful because pneumoperitoneum can be seen up to 2 weeks after laparoscopy [5], although increasing free air on serial imaging is certainly important for visceral injury. A computed tomography scan of the abdomen and pelvis with oral contrast may demonstrate leakage of contrast into the peritoneal cavity or even a localized peritoneal abscess. If the imaging is inconclusive but suspicion is high, it is reasonable to proceed with a diagnostic laparoscopy along with a general surgery consultation.

22.5.3 Treatment

If injuries are recognized intraoperatively, they should be repaired immediately, the peritoneal cavity copiously irrigated, and the patient administered antibiotics. A puncture from a Veress needle can generally be managed expectantly as long as there is no associated bleeding. An experienced gynecologic surgeon may repair small defects laparoscopically, although the overall rate of conversion to laparotomy has been reported to be between 52.4 and 90 % [2].

Larger and more complicated injuries should be evaluated and repaired in consultation with a general surgeon.

Injuries of the stomach, other than those resulting from a Veress needle, require repair. The abdominal cavity should be copiously irrigated to reduce the risk of injury from gastric juices. Defects are closed in two layers using delayed absorbable suture, usually done by a general surgeon. Postoperatively, a nasogastric tube should be maintained until normal bowel function returns [9].

Small intestinal injuries are repaired in two layers, usually perpendicular to the long axis of the bowel to avoid stricture formation. The injured bowel segment can often be exteriorized through a laparoscopic incision (that is increased to 2 cm) and repaired extracorporeally with either a primary closure or a bowel resection and side-to-side, end-to-end anastomosis. One technique of primary bowel repair involves closing the mucosa and muscularis using a delayed absorbable suture in an interrupted fashion, followed by closure of the serosal layer using interrupted silk sutures. It is recommended that segmental resection be performed if the laceration is greater than one half of the diameter of the small bowel [9]. Smaller lacerations of the colon can be repaired in a similar manner to those of the small bowel, while larger injuries may require segmental resection or a colostomy.

Thermal bowel injuries usually require wider resection beyond the visible damage because underlying coagulation necrosis and absence of capillary ingrowth may be occurring in an otherwise normal-appearing bowel. Removal of 1–2 cm of viable tissue around the site of injury should ensure removal of all potentially damaged tissue [5, 9].

The presence of gross fecal contamination should not affect the treatment intraoperatively. The colorectal and general surgery literature has established that gross fecal contamination does not increase the risk of infection or leak [14].

Injuries with delayed identification should be evaluated by a general surgeon. Most likely these patients will need a segmental resection with reanastomosis or a diversion.

22.6 Injuries Related to Positioning

22.6.1 Nerve Injuries

Neurologic injuries are associated with incorrect positioning of the anesthetized patient or patient shifting during surgery. Risk factors for positional injuries include surgeries longer than 4 h, obesity, frequent adjustment of the legs, and a steep Trendelenburg position [2].

In the upper extremity the brachial plexus and ulnar nerves can be injured. Brachial plexus injuries occur in 0.16 % of laparoscopies [1]. The mechanism of injury can be from abduction of the arms and shoulder braces. Brachial plexus injuries are related to torsion, pinching, stretching, or ischemia of the cervical branches of the brachial plexus as it passes under the coracoid process and between the clavicle and the first rib [1]. Brachial plexus injuries are characterized by pain, paresthesias, and weakness of the entire upper extremity. The ulnar nerve injuries are caused by lateral elbow compression against the arm board. Ulnar nerve injuries manifest with pain, weakness, and paresthesias of the wrist and the fourth and fifth fingers.

Femoral, sciatic, and peroneal nerves may be involved with lower extremity nerve injury. The femoral nerve can be injured by compression against the inguinal ligament with hyperflexion of the leg or can be stretched if the leg is externally rotated and/or abducted at the hip. With a femoral injury, patients will show weakness of the quadriceps muscle. Therefore, they may have problems walking, climbing stairs, or a decreased patellar reflex. Usually, there is no pain with femoral nerve injuries. Sciatic nerve injuries occur because of stretch with high lithotomy when the knee is straightened in the stirrups or from direct compression in the morbidly obese patients during prolonged procedures. Symptoms from a sci-

atic nerve injury include posterior leg pain and weakness. Peroneal nerve injury is a result of compression of the lateral knee against the stirrup where the nerve crosses the head of the fibula. Patients have foot drop and weakness and or numbness of the dorsal foot.

The patient's position should be reevaluated periodically during the surgery. Upper extremity injury can be prevented by tucking the arms in the military position with careful attention to padding the elbow, wrist, and hands. If shoulder braces are necessary, they should be placed over the acromioclavicular joints while the arms are in the tucked position. When patients are in dorsal lithotomy position, care is needed to keep the leg in a neutral position with the ankle aligned with the knee and far shoulder. The hip angle should not be more than 170°. The knee should be flexed from 90 to 120°. The angle between the legs should be less than 90°. The lateral knee should be padded in the stirrup.

Treatment is supportive. Nerves take 3–4 months to regenerate. Neuropathic pain modulators can be used to treat the pain related to nerve injuries. Physical therapy is the mainstay of treatment, and the purpose is to maintain joint range of motion and muscle strength. If there is no improvement, refer to a neurologist.

22.6.2 Pressure Alopecia

Pressure alopecia is characterized by hair loss in the vertex of the scalp within 28 days of surgery. It is caused by constant pressure on the scalp and can be exacerbated by hypotension and hypoxemia. Trendelenburg positioning for 3 h or more increases the risk of permanent alopecia. Some patients experience tenderness, swelling, or ulceration of the scalp prior to the occurrence of alopecia. Alopecia can be prevented by regular head turning or by periodic scalp massage during surgery.

22.7   Complications Related to Pneumoperitoneum

22.7.1 Gas Embolism

Gas embolism is when carbon dioxide has direct entry into the vascular system and gets trapped in the right ventricle and in the pulmonary artery. There are two mechanisms by which this can occur. The first is when the Veress needle is inserted into a vein or parenchymal organ. The second instance is if there is a tear in an abdominal wall or peritoneal vessel that permits CO_2 to be forced into the bloodstream with pneumoperitoneum. When a gas embolism occurs, this leads to increased pulmonary artery pressure, increased resistance to right ventricular outflow and diminished pulmonary return with consequent decreased left ventricular preload, diminished cardiac output, asystole, and systemic cardiovascular collapse. It is characterized by hypotension, cyanosis, raised jugular venous pressure, high arterial pCO_2, a drop in end tidal carbon dioxide concentration, and "millwheel" murmur. Gas embolism is rare (0.0014 %) but very serious with a mortality rate of 28.5 % [2].

The first sign of gas embolism is usually a drop in end tidal carbon dioxide concentration. The first thing to do is to stop the insufflation, disconnect the tubing, and remove the Veress needle. Investigate to exclude this diagnosis. Anesthesia should stop all medications that cause myocardial depression, administer 100 % oxygen, and hyperventilate the patient to facilitate dissolution of the embolism. Keep the patient in the Trendelenburg position to maximize blood flow to the brain and to allow for central line placement. A central venous pressure catheter in the internal jugular or subclavian vein can be used to aspirate the gas from the right ventricle. Intracardiac gas aspiration is another option. Chest compressions have been shown to be effective in the setting of cardiovascular collapse. Above all, call a vascular surgeon immediately and prepare for a possible laparotomy. Once the patient is hemodynamically stable, the peritoneal cavity needs to be evaluated. Laparoscopy can be considered with a direct or open technique unless there are signs of intra-abdominal hemorrhage, such as abdominal distention, in which case an immediate laparotomy is indicated.

This patient should be admitted overnight with continuous cardiac monitoring because of the risk of a delayed development of a gas embolism several hours after surgery [6]. Hyperbaric oxygen treatment has been used for patients who have not regained full neurologic function to improve neurologic function [6].

To aid in injury prevention at the time of abdominal entry, the Veress needle should be placed with the tap open and without insufflation tubing connected. This allows the surgeon to see blood coming out of the open tap if there is a vascular injury. Abdominal entry should be avoided in the Trendelenburg position.

22.7.2 Subcutaneous and Preperitoneal Emphysema

Subcutaneous emphysema is when CO_2 is in the subcutaneous tissues and is noted in 0.3–2 % of laparoscopies [2]. This can occur from inserting the Veress needle at too shallow an angle and insufflation, when trochars or gas inflow slips retroperitoneally into the thickness of the abdominal wall, if trochar sites are stretched from the torque sufficiently to allow for gas influx above the peritoneal layer, or during the operation in the presence of peritoneal incisions (i.e., retroperitoneal dissections). It is diagnosed by crepitus under the skin and usually resolves by itself. If noted in the operating room, massage the affected area on the abdominal wall towards the closest trochar site to express the gas. The risk can be decreased with a direct entry with the trochar or open entry technique.

22.7.3 Pneumomediastinum and Pneumothorax

Pneumomediastinum and pneumothorax can occur in the setting of congenital defect of the diaphragm or, less commonly, from a perforation of the diaphragm during an upper abdominal procedure. Pneumomediastinum can also happen from ascending preperitoneal gas. One should be concerned about these complications if emphysema is noted in the neck, face, or chest. If noted in the neck, there can be concern for airway compromise and patients should remain intubated postoperatively until the swelling reduces.

A pneumothorax can rapidly evolve into a tension pneumothorax. A tension pneumothorax is characterized by cyanosis, engorged neck veins, and increased airway pressure. As soon as a pneumothorax is recognized, patient should be given 100 % oxygen, pneumoperitoneum desufflated, and a thoracostomy tube placed.

22.7.4 Cardiac Arrhythmias

There can be a reflex vagal response to distention of the peritoneum, which can occur in up to 27 % of laparoscopies [2]. In extreme cases, cardiac arrest has been reported in 0.002–0.003 % of cases [2]. This is usually managed successfully by deflating the abdomen and administering an anticholinergic agent. Once the arrhythmia has resolved, then the peritoneum can be reinsufflated slowly. Occasionally, the arrhythmia persists and the laparoscopy needs to be aborted.

22.7.5 Shoulder Pain

Shoulder pain is common, and the incidence is about 35–80 % and ranges from mild to severe [15]. The exact etiology is unclear, but it is thought to be caused by carbon dioxide– induced phrenic nerve irritation that refers pain to C4 projected to the shoulder. At the end of the procedure with the patient still in the Trendelenburg position, anesthesia administers five positive pressure breaths to help expel carbon dioxide from the peritoneal cavity [15].

22.8 Wound-Related Complications

22.8.1 Hematoma

Trocar sites associated with delayed bleeding can be associated with drops in the hemoglobin, and large abdominal or flank ecchymoses. The patient may report pain, swelling, ecchymoses, and even bleeding from the trochar site. In most cases, this can be managed conservatively. The hematoma may spontaneously drain and be self-limiting. In large hematomas, correction of the anemia may need to occur. If the hematoma is expanding or becomes infected, it should be evacuated.

22.8.2 Infection

Infections are rare after laparoscopic surgery. Most infections can be prevented with sterile surgical technique, the use of prophylactic antibiotics when indicated, and good hemostasis. If they do occur, they are treated easily with wound care, antibiotics, and drainage, if necessary.

22.8.3 Disruptions and Hernias

Trocar site hernias are usually caused by lack of closure or improper closure (Fig. 22.8). Disruptions in the skin should be probed because of a suspicion of a hernia. Most hernias (61.7–100 %) are at extraumbilical sites. The incidence is about 1 %, but studies have shown rates of 0.06–5 % [2]. Most are Richter type hernias, which involve the peritoneum alone, or the peritoneum and the fascia. Bowel incarceration is a risk with trochar site hernias, which in turn can result in ischemia and necrosis, peritonitis, and obstruction [2].

Patients can present with symptoms of nausea, vomiting, fever, pain, abdominal distention, and even acute abdomen. Ultrasound or CT scan can be diagnostic, especially if there is no evidence of a physical examination. All trocar sites greater than or equal to 10 mm should have their fascia closed (although approximately 18 % of hernias occur despite fascial closure) [2]. At sites where single-incision trochars are used, a delayed absorbable suture should be used to close the fascia [16]. Trochars should be removed under direct visualization to ensure that there is no herniation of peritoneal contents at the time of surgery. Hernia repair can be performed both laparoscopically and by laparotomy. If there was incarcerated bowel, the entire bowel should be run to assess for bowel injury and the need for resection.

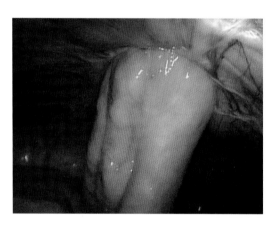

Fig. 22.8 Trocar incisions hernia

22.8.4 Port Site Metastasis

Port site metastasis is when cancer grows at the trochar site after a laparoscopic oncology procedure. It occurs in 1–2 % of laparoscopic cases, which is comparable to the rate with laparotomies. Risk factors include advanced disease and ascites.

22.9 Vulvar Edema

The mechanism is unclear. The edema is self-limited. Conservative management can include analgesia, ice packs and, in extreme cases, bladder catheterization. Swelling in the vulvar area can be related to vascular bleeding and requires intervention.

22.10 Conversion Requiring Laparotomy

The overall conversion rate to laparotomy is 2.1 %, with 1.2 % for minor laparoscopic procedures and 2 % for major laparoscopic procedures [2]. The most common reasons for conversion are vascular and visceral injuries. The need for laparotomy is influenced by the severity and location of the injury and the experience of the laparoscopist.

22.11 Mortality Related to Laparoscopy

The mortality rate associated with laparoscopy is 4.4 per 100,000 laparoscopies [1]. The biggest risk factor is the acuity of the procedure being performed. The main causes are related to the complications of the surgery and the anesthesia. Intestinal and vascular complications are the most common complications of surgery associated with mortality.

Conclusion

Complications related to laparoscopy in gynecologic patients are rare but may occur with increasing frequency given the rising obesity epidemic and number of gynecologic surgery patients with a history of previous abdominal or pelvic surgery. Over 50 % of complications related to gynecologic laparoscopy occur at entry, and 20–25 % percent are not recognized until the postoperative period. With proper preoperative planning and a thoughtful surgical approach, the vast majority of injuries may be avoided. Sound techniques performed by high volume surgeons contribute to improved outcomes for women who require laparoscopic surgery.

References

1. Manufacturer and User Facility Device Experience Database (MAUDE) [database online]. US Food and Drug Administration, Rockville. Available at http://www.fda.gov.
2. Magrina J. Complications of laparoscopic surgery. Clin Obstet Gynecol. 2002;45:469–80.
3. Makai G, Isaacson K. Complications of gynecologic laparoscopy. Clin Obstet Gynecol. 2009;52:401–11.
4. Ahmad G, O'Flynn H, Duffy JMN, Phillips K, Watson A. Laparoscopic entry techniques. Cochrane Database Syst Rev. 2012;(2):CD006583.
5. Capelouto CC, Kavoussi LR, Blebea J, Altose MD, Hurd WW. Complications of laparoscopic surgery. Urology. 1993;42:2–12.
6. Sandadi S, Johannigman JA, Wong VL, Blebea J, Altose MD, Hurd WW. Recognition and management of major vessel injury during laparoscopy. J Minim Invasive Gynecol. 2010;17:692–702.
7. Pickett SD, Rodewald KJ, Billow MR, Giannios NM, Hurd WW. Avoiding major vessel injury during laparoscopic instrument insertion. Obstet Gynecol Clin North Am. 2010;37:387–97.
8. Saidi MH, Sadler RK, Vancaillie TG, Akright BD, Farhart SA, White AJ. Diagnosis and management of serious urinary complications after major operative laparoscopy. Obstet Gynecol. 1996;87:272–6.
9. Sharp HT, Swenson C. Hollow viscus injury during surgery. Obstet Gynecol Clin North Am. 2010;37:461–7.
10. Elmira M, Cohen SL, Sandberg EM, Kibel AS, Einarsson J. Ureteral injury in laparoscopic gynecologic surgery. Rev Obstet Gynecol. 2012;5:106–11.
11. Ibeanu OA, Chesson RR, Echols KT, Nieves M, Busangu F, Nolan TE. Urinary tract injury during hysterectomy based on universal cystoscopy. Obstet Gynecol. 2009;113:6–10.
12. AAGL. AAGL Practice Report: Practice guidelines for intraoperative cystoscopy in laparoscopic hysterectomy. J Minim Invasive Gynecol. 2012;9:407–11.
13. Smilen HT, Weber AM, ACOG Committee on Practice Bulletins – Gynecology. ACOG Practice Bulletin No. 85: Pelvic organ prolapse. Obstet Gynecol. 2007;110:717–29.
14. Güenaga KF, Matos D, Wille-Jørgensen P. Mechanical bowel preparation for elective colorectal surgery. Cochrane Database Syst Rev. 2011;(9):CD001544.
15. Phelps P, Cakmakkaya OS, Apfel CC, Radke OC. A simple clinical maneuver to reduce laparoscopy-induced shoulder pain: a randomized controlled trial. Obstet Gynecol. 2008;111:1155–60.
16. Gunderson CC, Knight J, Ritter C, Escobar PF, Ibeanu O, Fader AN. The risk of umbilical hernia and other complications with laparoendoscopic single-site surgery. J Minim Invasive Gynecol. 2012;19:40–5.
17. Baggish MS. Analysis of 31 cases of major vessel injury associated with gynecologic laparoscopy operations. J Gynecol Surg. 2003;19:63–73.

Single-Site Robotics

23

Jason A. Knight, Jesus Manuel Salgueiro Bravo, and Pedro F. Escobar

Minimally invasive surgery has changed the landscape of gynecologic disorders and treatment over the last 30 years, most substantially via robotic-assisted surgical platforms. The only currently available system is the da Vinci robotic system (Intuitive Surgical Inc.; Sunnyvale, CA), providing the surgeon with an ergonomic three-dimensional platform with instrumentation that mimics the movements performed by the surgeon in an open procedure. The robotic system decreases incision burden, thereby lowering wound infection, improving cosmesis, and reducing postoperative pain. However, there is a learning curve associated with single-site surgery.

J.A. Knight, MD (✉)
Women's Health Institute, Section of Gynecologic Oncology, Cleveland Clinic, 9500 Euclid Avenue, Cleveland, OH 44195, USA
e-mail: knightj3@ccf.org

J.M.S. Bravo
Attending Physician, HIMA San Pablo Oncologico, Caguas, PR, USA

P.F. Escobar, MD
Director of Gynecologic Oncology,
Instituto Gyneco-Oncológico,
Hospital HIMA-Oncologico,
100 Luis Muñoz Marín Avenue,
Caguas, PR 00725, USA

Clinical Associate Professor of Surgery,
Cleveland Clinic Lerner College of Medicine,
Cleveland, OH USA
e-mail: escobarp@me.com

P.F. Escobar, T. Falcone (eds.), *Atlas of Single-Port, Laparoscopic, and Robotic Surgery*,
DOI 10.1007/978-1-4614-6840-0_23, © Springer Science+Business Media New York 2014

23.1   Introduction

Minimally invasive surgery has revolutionized the management of gynecologic disorders over the last 30 years. It is one of the most exciting areas of development and research in surgery. The most substantial development has come with the advent of robotic-assisted surgical platforms. These robotic platforms were initially funded and developed by the Stanford Research Institute, the United States Defense Department, and the National Aeronautics and Space Administration (NASA) in the hope of offering telesurgery to wounded soldiers in the battlefield. However, limitations in telecommunication and funding prevented its deployment in the battlefield despite the technological capability of the robotic platform. Instead, the robotic platform was adapted for civilian use and commercialized by Intuitive Surgical Inc. (Sunnyvale, CA) to create the da Vinci robotic system [1].

This is currently the only commercially available robotic surgical platform on the market. The da Vinci robotic platform provides the surgeon with an ergonomic three-dimensional vision system, EndoWrist robotic instrumentation (Intuitive Surgical Inc.; Sunnyvale, CA) with natural hand and wrist motions that mimic the movements performed in open surgery with the added benefit of reducing tremor. Similarly, Titan Medical Inc. (Toronto, Canada), a Canadian public company, has a robotic surgical platform under development. The platform consists of a surgeon-controlled robotic system and a workstation that provides the surgeon with an interface to the robotic platform for controlling instruments and providing a three-dimensional endoscopic view. Criticisms of the technology as it exists today are the lack of tactile feedback and the size or "bulk" of the current available systems. Surgical robots are likely to be further streamlined and incorporate advanced surgical instrumentation. The aim of this chapter is to discuss the newest technology, instrumentation, and novel platforms in robotic surgery.

23.2   Single-Site Robotics in Context

Decreased total incision length affords laparoscopy lower wound infection, improved cosmesis, and less postoperative pain compared with laparotomy. Single-site laparoscopy attempts to further reduce total incision length, promising further advances in these end points. Compared with multiport laparoscopy, improvement in hernia incidence has not been realized with single-site laparoscopy, probably because the length of the single incision is typically longer than any individual laparoscopy incisions [2].

Despite the promise of improved pain, less infection, and better cosmetic outcomes compared with multiport laparoscopy, the learning curve associated with single-site laparoscopy has limited its broad adoption in gynecology. Single-site robotic surgery promises to overcome the limitations of single-site laparoscopy by eliminating instrument clashing and reproducing conventional triangulation in a single incision environment. These advances are achieved using instruments with flexible shafts delivered through curved cannulae. The arc of the instruments allows them to enter the surgical field from opposing lateral aspects, thereby recreating triangulation intracorporeally while maximizing arm separation extracorporeally (Fig. 23.1).

The first iteration of single-site robotics in gynecology was reported by Escobar and colleagues using standard EndoWrist instruments directed through a GelPort (Applied Medical; Rancho Santa Margarita, CA) at the umbilicus. Limitations included arm clashing (crowding), reduced triangulation, and compromised pneumoperitoneum [3]. Since then, instrumentation designed specifically for single-site robotics has addressed these limitations. A specialized port maintains pneumoperitoneum in the presence or absence of cannulae (Fig. 23.2). Flexible instruments delivered through curved cannulae allow instruments to enter the surgical field from opposing lateral aspects, recreating triangulation intracorporeally while maximizing arm separation extracorporeally (Fig. 23.3). These flexible instruments are not wristed, thus creating an intracorporeal environment akin to "straight-stick" laparoscopy.

Fig. 23.1 From *left* to *right*:
two long curved laparoscope
cannulae, 300 mm; long
flexible obturator; two short
curved cannulae, 250 mm;
short flexible obturator;
assistant cannula, 5 mm;
assistant cannula, 10 mm

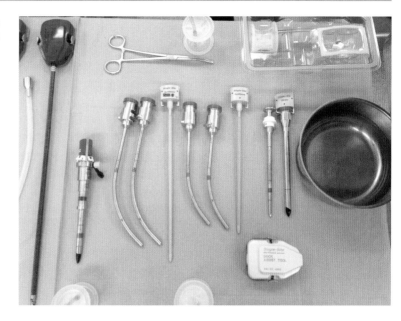

Fig. 23.2 Single-site port

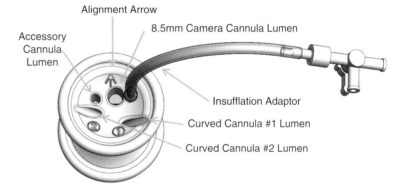

Fig. 23.3 Extracorporeal environment with robotic side
cart docked

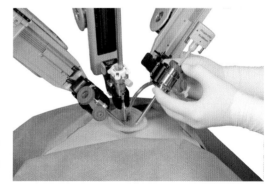

23.3 Technique

23.3.1 Extracorporeal Environment

A 2.5-cm skin incision at the umbilicus is required using the Hasson technique for intraperitoneal access. Port placement is similar to the SILS port (Covidien; Mansfield, MA) with the exception that the material is much more delicate and will fracture easily. Therefore, the port should be "fed" incrementally into the incision using a curved clamp with care to slide rather than drag the port into place.

Insufflation can begin after port placement and gas egress is minimal even in the absence of trocars. The camera trocar is placed, and the robot center docked. Under direct visualization the short curved cannulae are placed, arm two before arm one, with the trocar concavity facing the midline. Within the port, the cannula channels cross (Fig. 23.4). Therefore, when placing a cannula, the tip will come into view on the contralateral side. While handedness is maintained at the console (i.e., the surgeon's right hand controls the instrument tip field right), notice that arm two (patient left) holds the instrument in field right and arm one (patient right) holds the instrument in field left. Side docking is feasible; however, doing so limits the range of motion on the contralateral side. For most purposes, center docking is preferred (Fig. 23.5).

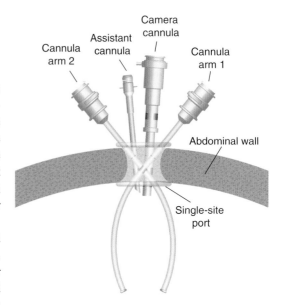

Fig. 23.4 Curved cannulas establish triangulation intracorporeally while achieving wide instrument separation extracorporeally

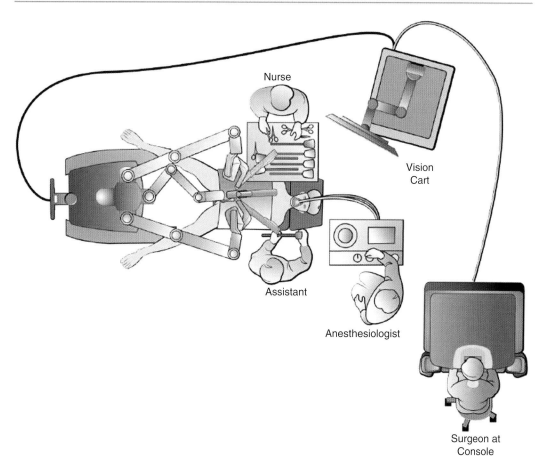

Fig. 23.5 Configuration of the robot for center docking. The second joint of arms 1 and 2 is kept at a straight angle. The second joint of the camera arm is kept at about a 45-degree angle to the right or left to keep the arm in the first or last third of the "sweet spot"

23.4   Intracorporeal Environment

The surgical environment is similar to straight-stick laparoscopy, since the current iteration of the single-site robotic platform does not include EndoWrist instruments.

All instruments, including the assistant's instrument, enter through a single trocar, forming a cluster that moves as a unit when the camera is moved. Therefore, all instruments should be maintained in the field of view to prevent unintended collisions with structures during gross camera movements. Furthermore, moving the camera while grasping tissue will cause traction and should be avoided. If static retraction is required, this can be achieved using a +1 configuration with either an accessory assistant port or the robot's third arm with a conventional robotic instrument docked laterally.

The flexible instrument shafts, necessary for instrument delivery through curved cannulas, limit the tolerated instrument load. Excessive load causes the shaft to bend. Upon releasing grasped tissue, the instrument recoils and may cause unintended effects. Therefore, load-bearing maneuvers such as manipulation of the uterus by grasping the cornua should be avoided.

23.5   Surgical Technique

Total robot-assisted hysterectomy and oophorectomy are feasible FDA approved applications of single-site robotics. Pelvic lymphadenctomy is a feasible off-label application of the platform. Typical instrument configuration includes the monopolar hook or shears in the dominant hand and a bipolar grasper in the nondominant hand. However, the optimal configuration is dependent on the comfort and experience of each surgeon.

Successful single-site robotic hysterectomy recapitulates the technique of the open and laparoscopic approach. The round ligament is divided and the retroperitoneal spaces are developed as needed to skeletonize the gonadal vessels and visualize the ureter. The vesicouterine peritoneum

is opened, and the bladder is reflected away from the lower uterine segment and cervix. The uterine arteries are skeletonized, coagulated, and divided. Posteriorly, the peritoneal incision is continued, dividing the uterosacral ligaments, taking care to avoid the ureters laterally and the rectum posteriorly. The colpotomy is performed and cuff closure can be achieved vaginally or robotically.

Pelvic lymphadenectomy requires development of the pararectal and paravesicle spaces with identification of the ureters, external and internal iliac vessels, genita femoral nerve, superior vesicle artery, and circumflex iliac vein. Lymphatic tissue is dissected from the ventral surface of the external iliac artery followed by development of the obturator space, identification of the obturator nerve, and then removal of obturator nodes. Nodal tissue can be removed vaginally, through the umbilical incision, or through a lateral accessory port.

Single-site robotic cuff closure without EndoWrist instruments is similar to laparoscopic suturing. The lack of instrument shaft rigidity adds another challenge and in many cases a quicker and more robust closure can be achieved vaginally. Exchanging the short curved cannulas with the long cannulas decreases the length of exposed flexible shaft, thereby decreasing the tendency to bend while driving the needle. Using curved forceps improves needle angulation.

References

1. Weinberg L, Rao S, Escobar PF. Robotic surgery in gynecology: an updated systematic review. Obstet Gynecol Int. 2011;2011:852061. doi:10.1155/2011/852061. Epub 2011 Nov 28.
2. Gunderson CC, Knight J, Ybanez-Morano J, Ritter C, Escobar PF, Ibeanu O, et al. The risk of umbilical hernia and other complications with laparoendoscopic single-site surgery. J Minim Invasive Gynecol. 2012; 19:40–5.
3. Escobar PF, Fader AN, Paraiso MF, Kaouk JH, Falcone T. Robotic-assisted laparoendoscopic single-site surgery in gynecology: initial report and technique. J Minim Invasive Gynecol. 2009;16:589–91.

Index

Printed in the United States of America